Peripheral Artery Disease: Pathogenesis, Endovascular Treatment and Angiography

Peripheral Artery Disease: Pathogenesis, Endovascular Treatment and Angiography

Editor: Ruth Washington

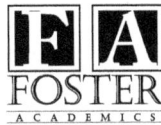

FOSTER
ACADEMICS

www.fosteracademics.com

www.fosteracademics.com

FA
FOSTER
ACADEMICS

Cataloging-in-Publication Data

Peripheral artery disease : pathogenesis, endovascular treatment and angiography / edited by Ruth Washington.
p. cm.
Includes bibliographical references and index.
ISBN 978-1-63242-918-6
1. Peripheral vascular diseases. 2. Arteries--Diseases. 3. Peripheral vascular diseases--Endoscopic surgery.
4. Angiography. I. Washington, Ruth.
RC694 .P47 2020
616.131--dc23

© Foster Academics, 2020

Foster Academics,
118-35 Queens Blvd., Suite 400,
Forest Hills, NY 11375, USA

ISBN 978-1-63242-918-6 (Hardback)

Contents

Preface

This book aims to highlight the current researches and provides a platform to further the scope of innovations in this area. This book is a product of the combined efforts of many researchers and scientists, after going through thorough studies and analysis from different parts of the world. The objective of this book is to provide the readers with the latest information of the field.

Peripheral artery disease (PAD) is the condition characterized by an abnormal narrowing of arteries that supply blood to all parts of the body other than the heart or brain. The underlying mechanisms of peripheral artery disease are atherosclerosis, blood clots, artery spasm, fibromuscular dysplasia, trauma and vasculitis. Depending on the severity of the disease, PAD can be managed through revascularization, medication and lifestyle changes. Revascularization can be done through an angioplasty, vascular bypass grafting, atherectomy, thrombolysis and thrombectomy. Endovascular treatment offers an alternative to open surgery in patients with PAD. The need for revascularization is determined on the basis of the clinical presentation of critical limb ischemia, claudication and acute limb ischemia. Angiography, in particular magnetic resonance angiography and high-resolution computed tomography angiography provides assessment of vascular anatomy, disease location and lesion character. Such imaging helps to localize the lesions that are targeted for revascularization. This book is a compilation of chapters that discuss the most vital concepts and emerging trends in the pathogenesis, diagnosis and treatment of peripheral artery disease. The topics included in this book on endovascular treatment and angiography are of utmost significance and bound to provide incredible insights to readers. It will help new researchers by foregrounding their knowledge in peripheral artery disease.

I would like to express my sincere thanks to the authors for their dedicated efforts in the completion of this book. I acknowledge the efforts of the publisher for providing constant support. Lastly, I would like to thank my family for their support in all academic endeavors.

Editor

Risk Factors in the Patients with Extracranial Carotid Atherosclerosis

Mei-Ling Sharon Tai, Julia Sien Yuin Liew,
Sheun Yu Mo and Mohamed Abdusalam Elwaifa

Abstract

There are vascular risk factors known to be associated with stroke. These risk factors have been shown to either directly or indirectly lead to stroke. The risk factors include hypertension (HT), diabetes mellitus (DM), smoking, hyperlipidaemia, ischemic heart disease (IHD) and atrial fibrillation (AF). Studies have shown that carotid atherosclerosis is a cause of stroke. Extracranial carotid atherosclerosis accounts for up to 40% of the ischemic strokes in the Western countries. The latest stroke guidelines recommend the routine use of Ultrasound Carotid Doppler to assess for extracranial carotid artery atherosclerotic diseases (carotid intima media thickness, plaques, carotid stenosis) in these patients. A previous study emphasized the value of carotid ultrasonography in the detection of early extracranial carotid atherosclerosis.

Keywords: extracranial, carotid, atherosclerosis, risk, factors

1. Introduction

Stroke is one of the most common diseases in the world and results in up to 10% of mortality globally [1]. Stroke is the third leading cause of mortality and long-term disability in the United States of America [2].

There are vascular risk factors known to be associated with ischemic strokes [3]. These risk factors have been shown to either directly or indirectly lead to stroke [3]. The risk factors include hypertension (HT), diabetes mellitus (DM), smoking, hyperlipidaemia, ischemic heart disease (IHD) and atrial fibrillation (AF) [3].

Studies have shown that carotid atherosclerosis is a cause of stroke [4]. Annually, about 20–30% of new strokes are due to atherosclerotic carotid artery disease [5]. The latest stroke guidelines recommend the routine use of ultrasound carotid Doppler to assess for extracranial carotid artery atherosclerotic diseases (carotid intima media thickness, plaques, carotid stenosis) in these patients [6].

Ultrasound carotid Doppler is a non-invasive and cost-effective test [7]. Carotid intima media thickness (CIMT) measurements and plaque location are evaluated on gray scale imaging (B-mode) [7]. Flow disturbance and stenosis is assessed on color Doppler [7]. The blood flow velocities are examined on spectral Doppler [7].

A previous study emphasized the value of ultrasound carotid Doppler in the detection of early extracranial carotid atherosclerosis [4]. In the world, an increased CIMT is found in 9.4% of the men and 11.7% of the women [4]. Assessment of CIMT increases with ultrasound carotid Doppler in the subjects without carotid atherosclerosis and free of previous vascular events predicts the occurrence of carotid plaque [8].

The prevalence of carotid plaque is 13.3% in the men and 13.4% in the women in the world [8]. The prevalence of extracranial carotid stenosis is 2.7% in the men and 1.5% in the women globally [8]. Stroke is associated with the plaques containing softer tissue, especially with thin fibrous cap [2].

Hyperlipidaemia is a common risk factor for extracranial atherosclerosis [9]. The risk factor of hyperlipidaemia was one of the two most common risk factors for stroke in Singapore (76.5–86.4%) [3]. Hyperlipidaemia results in an atheroma or a fibrofatty plaque leading to gradual occlusion of the arteries. As the plaques increase in size, they progressively occlude the lumen and compromise the blood flow causing stroke [10]. In the South Korean studies, extracranial atherosclerosis was associated with higher LDL levels [9, 11].

Furthermore, low levels of HDL cholesterol are associated with an increased risk of having echolucent, rupture-prone atherosclerotic plaques [12]. In addition, an increased risk of having an echolucent plaque is independently associated with increasing degree of stenosis [12]. The subjects with echolucent plaques have increased risk of ischemic cerebrovascular events and stroke independent of the degree of stenosis and cardiovascular risk factors [13].

A community-based study in Taiwan showed that hypertension strongly influenced extracranial carotid atherosclerosis and hypertension was the predictor of carotid stenosis ≥50% [14, 15]. The frequencies of hypertension among the stroke patients in the other Asian countries were: 59% in Pakistan [16], 38.3% in Japan [17], and 19–28% in China, Korea and Taiwan [17].

There are several mechanisms of stroke due to hypertension. High blood pressure results in endothelial damage, which leads to thrombi formation [18]. Hypertension is also known to accelerate the atherosclerotic process [18]. Moreover, in the general population, hypertension is a predictor of the occurrence of plaques [8]. Systolic blood pressure is significantly associated with severe extracranial carotid atherosclerosis (plaque, stenosis) [4].

The percentages of ischemic stroke patients with DM were 37% in Pakistan [16] and 30% in South Korea [11]. DM is an important risk factor for extracranial carotid atherosclerosis [14, 19]. DM affects the vascular endothelium and reduces the bioavailability of nitric oxide (NO), which is a major anti-atherosclerotic agent [20–22]. Hyperglycemia inhibits the production of NO by restraining the activation of endothelial NO synthase [23]. In addition, the prevalence of extracranial carotid atherosclerosis is significantly higher in the ketosis-onset DM patients than in the control subjects [24]. The frequency of extracranial carotid atherosclerosis in the ketosis-onset DM patients is similar to the non-ketotic type 2 DM patients [24].

Smoking is also known to be associated with atherosclerosis of the extracranial carotid vessels [14]. The percentage of the patients with smoking history was 25% in Wasay et al.'s study [16]. Smoking leads to damage of cells that line the arteries. In addition, smoking increases the build-up of plaque constituents in the arteries. Moreover, smoking results in thickening and narrowing of the arteries [25].

Smoking history is a determinant of the occurrence of a new carotid plaque in the subjects with no previous carotid atherosclerosis and also free of previous vascular events [8]. In addition, there is a significant association between severe extracranial carotid atherosclerosis and smoking [4]. Furthermore, smoking was found to be associated with carotid plaque and extracranial carotid stenosis in several studies [9, 26, 27]. Cessation of smoking will be helpful in the management of these stroke patients.

IHD and ischemic stroke are vascular diseases [28]. IHD was present in 11.8–20% of the Singapore stroke patients [3]. Moreover, IHD was associated with carotid stenosis in a study [27]. In another study conducted in Japan on consecutive patients who had coronary angiography, 6% of them had extracranial carotid stenosis [29].

AF is known cardiovascular risk factor of stroke [30]. AF can predispose to embolism and stroke [31]. AF is commonly associated with stroke in South Asia, Western Europe, North America and Australia [32]. Increased CIMT and presence of carotid plaque are associated with increased risk of ischemic stroke in the patients with AF [33]. Higher CIMT and the presence of carotid plaque are associated with higher incidence of AF incidence [34].

Age is an important risk factor for extracranial carotid atherosclerosis, especially in the Chinese and South Koreans [9, 11, 14, 19, 35]. These patients tend to be older in age [9, 11, 19, 35]. Age is a significant predictor of the occurrence of a new carotid plaque in the general population [8]. The incremental probability of the occurrence of plaque is higher in the subject's midlife [8]. In the subjects aged ≥40 years old, the severity of carotid atherosclerosis (plaques, stenosis) was significantly associated with age [4]. Moreover, the frequency of extracranial carotid atherosclerosis significantly increases with age in the DM patients (ketosis-onset and non-ketotic DM) [24].

Male gender is also risk factor for extracranial atherosclerosis [9, 19]. 14.8% of the patients with extracranial atherosclerosis, had family history of stroke [9]. In a Chinese study, 48.4% of the healthy population with extracranial carotid atherosclerosis had obesity [19].

Elevated CIMT is associated with an increased risk of stroke [20]. Plaque rupture with subsequent embolism can lead to stroke [20]. The presence of plaque is associated with an increased risk morbidity and mortality secondary to stroke [28].

One population study showed the relationship between extracranial carotid atherosclerotic lesions with the classic risk factors such hypertension, hyperlipidaemia and smoking [28].

An European Rotterdam Elderly Study showed that hypertension, smoking and reduced serum HDL were associated with carotid artery stenosis [36]. In that study, factor VIIc and factor VIIIc (hemostatic factor) activity was higher in the patients with extracranial carotid disease [36].

Altogether, the number of classic risk factors among the patients with extracranial athero-sclerosis was 1.67 in a South Korean study [11]. The number of traditional risk factors in the patients with severe extracranial atherosclerosis was almost similar (1.68) [11].

CIMT is a marker of subclinical atherosclerosis and hypertension has been known to be risk factor of atherosclerosis [28]. Therefore, proper monitoring of CIMT and treatment can poten-tially be helpful to these patients to prevent further progression to plaques and stenosis. In a previous study, 18.2% of the patients with extracranial atherosclerosis had history of previous stroke [11]. Among the patients with severe extracranial atherosclerosis, 21.6% of them had history of previous stroke [11].

Furthermore, a study by Amarenco et al. showed that there was a higher prevalence of coro-nary plaques, with concomitant carotid plaques, in patients with non-fatal ischemic stroke with no known IHD [37]. In a study done among Chinese patients, 7.8% of the patients with paroxysmal AF had a combination of extracranial carotid stenosis and IHD [30].

The miR-146a rs2910164 polymorphism may be associated with carotid vulnerable plaque risk in the Chinese patients with type 2 DM, particularly in older patients and women [38]. This polymorphism may be associated with carotid vulnerable plaque risk in the patients with DM duration of >10 years and the patients with hypertension [38].

In addition, the metabolically abnormal but normal weight subjects have increased CIMT compared to the metabolically healthy but obese subjects and metabolically healthy normal weight subjects [39]. The patients with extracranial carotid atherosclerosis are more likely to have contralateral extracranial carotid atherosclerosis [26].

In terms of ethnic variation, the South Asians have the higher prevalence of extracranial carotid atherosclerosis compared to the Europeans and Chinese [20]. The South Asians have an increased frequency of impaired glucose tolerance, hypercholesterolemia (higher total and LDL cholesterol), hypertriglyceridemia and lower HDL cholesterol [20]. In addition, the South Asians have higher concentrations of fibrinogen, homocysteine, lipoprotein (a), and plasminogen activator inhibitor-1 [20].

The Chinese have lower rates of cardiovascular disease than the Europeans [40]. Furthermore, the Chinese have a more favorable risk factor profile except for impaired glucose tolerance [40]. The Europeans are more likely to be current or former smokers [20]. The Caucasians with severe extracranial carotid stenosis are more obese than those without such stenosis, unlike the Japanese [41].

In conclusion, proper identification and optimization of the risk factors in the patients with extracranial carotid atherosclerosis in important. This will help to prevent or slow down the progression of the extracranial carotid atherosclerosis. By preventing the devel-opment of carotid stenosis, the occurrence of ischemic stroke can be minimized (**Figure 1** and **Table 1**).

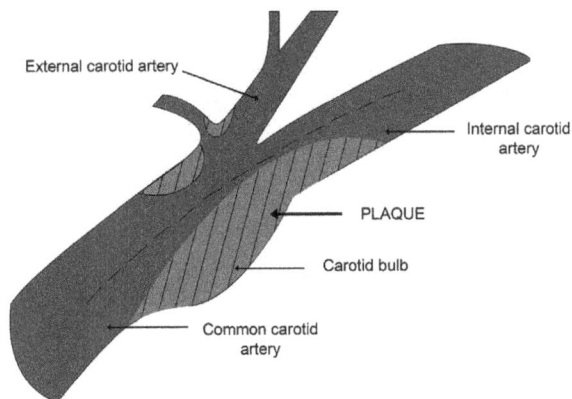

Figure 1. Diagram showing plaques at the carotid bulb extending to the internal carotid artery [2].

1. Hypertension

2. Diabetes mellitus

3. Hyperlipidaemia

4. Smoking

5. Ischemic heart disease

6. Atrial fibrillation

7. Advancing age

8. Male gender

9. miR-146a rs2910164 polymorphism

10. Metabolically abnormal but normal weight

Table 1. Risk factors of extracranial carotid atherosclerosis [9, 14, 18, 19, 28, 30, 38, 39].

Author details

Mei-Ling Sharon Tai*, Julia Sien Yuin Liew, Sheun Yu Mo and
Mohamed Abdusalam Elwaifa

*Address all correspondence to: sharont1990@gmail.com

Division of Neurology, Department of Medicine, Faculty of Medicine, University of Malaya, Malaysia

References

[1] Santulli G. Epidemiology of cardiovascular disease in the 21st century: Updated numbers and updated facts. Journal of Cardiovascular Disease. 2013;**1**:1-2

[2]   Allen JD, Ham KL, Dumont DM, Sileshi B, Trahey GE, Dahl JJ. The development and potential of acoustic radiation force impulse (ARFI) imaging for carotid artery plaque characterization. Vascular Medicine. 2011 Aug;**16**(4):302-311

[3]   Sharma VK, Tsivgoulis G, Teoh HL, Ong BK, Chan BP. Stroke risk factors and outcomes among various Asian ethnic groups in Singapore. Journal of Stroke and Cerebrovascular Diseases. 2012 May;**21**(4):299-304

[4]   Prati P, Vanuzzo D, Casaroli M, Di Chiara A, De Biasi F, Feruglio GA, Touboul PJ. Prevalence and determinants of carotid atherosclerosis in a general population. Stroke. 1992 Dec;**23**(12):1705-1711

[5]   Timsit S, Sacco R, Mohr J, Foulkes M, Tatemichi T, Wolf P, Price T, Hier D. Early clinical differentiation of cerebral infarction from severe atherosclerotic stenosis and cardioembolism. Stroke. 2007;**23**:486-491

[6]   Brott TG, Halperin JL, Abbara S, Bacharach JM, Barr JD, Bush RL, Cates CU, Creager MA, Fowler SB, Friday G, Hertzberg VS, McIff EB, Moore WS, Panagos PD, Riles TS, Rosenwasser RH, Taylor AJ. 2011 ASA/ACCF/AHA/AANN/AANS/ACR/ASNR/CNS/SAIP/SC'AI/SIR/SNIS/SVM/SVS guideline on the management of patients with extracranial carotid and vertebral artery disease: Executive summary: A report of the American College of Cardiology Foundation/American Heart Association task force on practice guidelines, and the American Stroke Association, American Association of Neuroscience Nurses, American Association of Neurological Surgeons, American College of Radiology, American Society of Neuroradiology, Congress of Neurological Surgeons, Society of Atherosclerosis Imaging and Prevention, Society for Cardiovascular Angiography and Interventions, Society of Interventional Radiology, society of NeuroInterventional surgery, Society for Vascular Medicine, and society for vascular surgery. Stroke. 2011;**42**:e420-e463

[7]   Gaitini D, Soudack M. Diagnosing carotid stenosis by Doppler sonography: State of the art. Journal of Ultrasound in Medicine. 2005 Aug;**24**(8):1127-1136

[8]   Prati P, Vanuzzo D, Casaroli M, Bader G, Mos L, Pilotto L, Canciani L, Ruscio M, Touboul PJ. Determinants of carotid plaque occurrence. A long-term prospective population study: The san Daniele project. Cerebrovascular Diseases. 2006;**22**(5-6):416-422

[9]   Kim JS, Nah HW, Park SM, Kim SK, Cho KH, Lee J, Lee YS, Kim J, Ha SW, Kim EG, Kim DE, Kang DW, Kwon SU, Yu KH, Lee BC. Risk factors and stroke mechanisms in atherosclerotic stroke: Intracranial compared with extracranial and anterior compared with posterior circulation disease. Stroke. 2012 Dec;**43**(12):3313-3318

[10] Khan MRK. Hyperlipidemia as a Risk Factor for Ischaemic Stroke. www.orion-group.net/journals/Journals/vol19_Sept2004/199.htm

[11] Kim YD, Choi HY, Jung YH, Nam CM, Yang JH, Cho HJ, Nam HS, Lee KY, Heo JH. Classic risk factors for atherosclerosis are not major determinants for location of extracranial or intracranial cerebral atherosclerosis. Neuroepidemiology. 2009;**32**(3):201-207

[12] Mathiesen EB, Bønaa KH, Joakimsen O. Low levels of high-density lipoprotein choles-terol are associated with echolucent carotid artery plaques: The tromsø study. Stroke. 2001 Sep;**32**(9):1960-1965

[13] Mathiesen EB, Bønaa KH, Joakimsen O. Echolucent plaques are associated with high risk of ischemic cerebrovascular events in carotid stenosis: The tromsø study. Circulation. 2001 May 1;**103**(17):2171-2175

[14] Liu CY, Chen CQ. Intra- and extracranial atherosclerotic stenosis in China: Epidemiology, diagnosis, treatment and risk factors. European Review for Medical and Pharmacological Sciences. 2014 Nov;**18**(22):3368-3379

[15] Su TC, Jeng JS, Chien KL, Sung FC, Hsu HC, Lee YT. Hypertension status is the major determinant of carotid atherosclerosis: A community-based study in Taiwan. Stroke. 2001;**32**:2265-2271

[16] Wasay M, Azeemuddin M, Masroor I, Sajjad Z, Ahmed R, Khealani BA, Malik MA, Afridi MB, Kamal A. Frequency and outcome of carotid atheromatous disease in patients with stroke in Pakistan. Stroke. 2009 Mar;**40**(3):708-712

[17] Kim YD, Jung YH, Saposnik G. Traditional risk factors for stroke in East Asia. Journal of Stroke. 2016 Sep;**18**(3):273-285

[18] Johansson BB. Hypertension mechanisms causing stroke. Clinical and Experimental Pharmacology & Physiology. 1999 Jul;**26**(7):563-565

[19] Pan XF, Lai YX, Gu JQ, Wang HY, Liu AH, Shan ZY. Factors significantly associated with the increased prevalence of carotid atherosclerosis in a northeast Chinese mid-dle-aged and elderly population: A cross-sectional study. Medicine (Baltimore). 2016 Apr;**95**(14):e3253

[20] Anand SS, Yusuf S, Vuksan V, Devanesen S, Teo KK, Montague PA, Kelemen L, Yi C, Lonn E, Gerstein H, Hegele RA, McQueen M. Differences in risk factors, atherosclero-sis, and cardiovascular disease between ethnic groups in Canada: The study of health assessment and risk in ethnic groups (SHARE). Lancet. 2000 Jul 22;**356**(9226):279-284

[21] Beckman JA, Creager MA, Libby P. Diabetes and atherosclerosis: Epidemiology, pathophysiology, and management. Journal of the American Medical Association. 2002;**287**:2570-2581

[22] Lloyd-Jones DM, Bloch KD. The vascular biology of nitric oxide and its role in athero-genesis. Annual Review of Medicine. 1996;**47**:365-375

[23] De Vriese AS, Verbeuren TJ, Van de Voorde J, Lameire NH, Vanhoutte PM. Endothelial dysfunction in diabetes. British Journal of Pharmacology 2000;**130**:963-974

[24] Li LX, Zhao CC, Ren Y, Tu YF, Lu JX, Wu X, Zhang WX, Zhu JA, Li MF, Yu LB, Bao YQ, Jia WP. Prevalence and clinical characteristics of carotid atherosclerosis in newly diagnosed patients with ketosis-onset diabetes: A cross-sectional study. Cardiovascular Diabetology. 2013 Jan 16;**12**:18

[25] Centre for Disease Control and Prevention (CDC)-Health Effects-Heart Disease-Smoking &TobaccoUse. http://www.cdc.gov/tobacco/basic_information/health_effects/heart_disease/

[26] Chen H, Hong H, Xing S, Liu G, Zhang A, Tan S, Zhang J, Zeng J. Intracranial versus Extracranial symptomatic carotid atherosclerosis in Chinese patients: Risk factors, stroke mechanisms, and long-term prognosis. Journal of Stroke and Cerebrovascular Diseases. 2015 Nov;**24**(11):2632-2639

[27] Leung SY, Ng TH, Yuen ST, Lauder IJ, Ho FC. Pattern of cerebral atherosclerosis in Hong Kong Chinese. Severity in intracranial and extracranial vessels. Stroke. 1993 Jun;**24**(6):779-786

[28] Keo HH, Baumgartner, Hirsch AT, Duval S, Steg PG, Pasquet B, Bhatt DL, Roether J, REACH Registry Investigators. Carotid plaque and intima-media thickness and the incidence of ischemic events in patients with atherosclerotic vascular disease. Vascular Medicine. 2011 Oct;**16**(5):323-330

[29] Tanimoto S, Ikari Y, Tanabe K, Yachi S, Nakajima H, Nakayama T, Hatori M, Nakazawa G, Onuma Y, Higashikuni Y, Yamamoto H, Tooda E, Hara K. Prevalence of carotid artery stenosis in patients with coronary artery disease in Japanese population. Stroke. 2005 Oct;**36**(10): 2094-2098

[30] Gu Y, Feng L, Xu Y, Zhao Y. Co-prevalence of carotid stenosis and coronary artery disease in Chinese patients with paroxysmal atrial fibrillation. The Journal of International Medical Research. 2014 Dec;**42**(6):1294-1300

[31] Chee KH, Tan KS. Impact of atrial fibrillation among stroke patients in a Malaysian teaching hospital. The Medical Journal of Malaysia. 2014 Jun;**69**(3):119-123

[32] O'Donnell MJ, Chin SL, Rangarajan S, Xavier D, Liu L, Zhang H, et al. Global and regional effects of potentially modifiable risk factors associated with acute stroke in 32 countries (INTERSTROKE): A case-control study. Lancet. 2016 Aug 20;**388**(10046):761-775

[33] Bekwelem W, Jensen PN, Norby FL, Soliman EZ, Agarwal SK, Lip GY, Pan W, Folsom AR, Longstreth WT Jr, Alonso A, Heckbert SR, Chen LY. Carotid atherosclerosis and stroke in Atrial fibrillation: The atherosclerosis risk in communities study. Stroke. 2016 Jun;**47**(6):1643-1646

[34] Chen LY, Leening MJ, Norby FL, Roetker NS, Hofman A, Franco OH, Pan W, Polak JF, Witteman JC, Kronmal RA, Folsom AR, Nazarian S, Stricker BH, Heckbert SR, Alonso A. Carotid Intima-media thickness and arterial stiffness and the risk of Atrial fibrillation: The atherosclerosis risk in communities (ARIC) study, multi-ethnic study of atherosclerosis (MESA), and the Rotterdam study. Journal of the American Heart Association. 2016 May;**20**:5(5)

[35] Li D, Wang ML, Li SM, Ling F. Distribution and risk factors of steno-occlusive lesions in patients with ischemic cerebrovascular disease. Zhonghua Yi Xue Za Zhi. 2008;**88**:1158-1162

[36] Bots ML, Breslau PJ, Briët E, de Bruyn AM, van Vliet HH, van den Ouweland FA, de Jong PT, Hofman A, Grobbee DE. Cardiovascular determinants of carotid artery disease. The Rotterdam Elderly Study. Hypertension. 1992 Jun; **19**(6 Pt 2):717-720

[37] Amarenco P, Lavallée PC, Labreuche J, Ducrocq G, Juliard JM, Feldman L, Cabrejo L, Meseguer E, Guidoux C, Adraï V, Ratani S, Kusmierek J, Lapergue B, Klein IF, Gongora-Rivera F, Jaramillo A, Mazighi M, Touboul PJ, Steg PG. Prevalence of coronary atherosclerosis in patients with cerebral infarction. Stroke. 2011 Jan;**42**(1):22-29

[38] Shen J, Zhang M, Sun M, Tang K, Zhou B. The relationship of miR-146a gene polymorphism with carotid atherosclerosis in Chinese patients with type 2 diabetes mellitus. Thrombosis Research. 2015 Dec;**136**(6):1149-1155

[39] Yoo HJ, Hwang SY, Hong HC, Choi HY, Seo JA, Kim SG, Kim NH, Choi DS, Baik SH, Choi KM. Association of metabolically abnormal but normal weight (MANW) and metabolically healthy but obese (MHO) individuals with arterial stiffness and carotid atherosclerosis. Atherosclerosis. 2014 May;**234**(1):218-223

[40] Harland J, Unwin N, Bhopal R, White M, Watson B, Laker M, Alberti KG. Low levels of cardiovascular risk factors and coronary heart disease in a UK Chinese population. Journal of Epidemiology and Community Health. 1997;**51**:636-642

[41] Nishimaru K, McHenry LC Jr, Toole JF. Cerebral angiographic and clinical differences in carotid system transient ischemic attacks between American Caucasian and Japanese patients. Stroke. 1984 Jan-Feb;**15**(1):56-59

2

Basics of Angiography for Peripheral Artery Disease

Yoshiaki Yokoi

Abstract

Angiography has been historically used to image the peripheral artery system and still remains the gold standard for diagnostic and endovascular treatment. There is no standardized method for lower limb artery angiography. In this chapter, the basic standard technique for angiography of peripheral artery is described from aortoiliac, femoropopliteal and below the knee arteries. To obtain a good image, adequate contrast dose and image size must be determined with the appropriate catheter. For puncture, echo-guided approach is becoming popular; each lab needs to have echo machine to minimize the vascular complication. In cases of renal dysfunction, CO_2 angiography is suited. However, care must be taken to deliver gas into arterial system and to know the merit and demerit of CO_2 angiography.

Keywords: peripheral artery, peripheral artery disease, contrast angiography, echo-guided puncture, CO_2 angiography

1. Angiography-suite for endovascular therapy of peripheral artery disease (PAD)

1.1. Detector size

High resolution, accurate imaging is the key to success in endovascular therapies. In recent years, most machines provide fairly good images. An important point is the detector size of the angiography machine. Some physicians still use a coronary lab for peripheral artery intervention, however, when considering the vessel length and area, at least a 30 cm detector is needed. In **Figure 1**, two types of detectors are shown.

In peripheral artery angiography, the 30 cm system on the left (INNOVA 3100, 30 cm, GE healthcare, Uppsala, Sweden) (**Figure 1A**) is basically used while the 20 cm coronary system (INNOVA IGS620, 20 cm, GE healthcare, Uppsala, Sweden) (**Figure 1B**) is too small for peripheral artery angiography. For example, the superficial femoral artery (SFA) is the longest vessel and difficult to visualize in its entirety. In **Figures 1** and **2**, two SFA short lesions are shown.

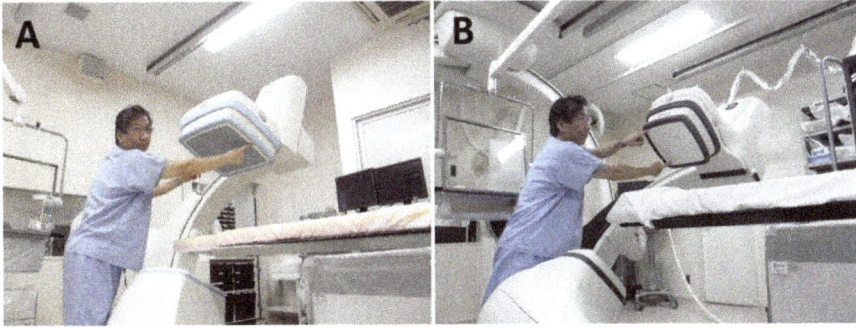

Figure 1. Detector size: (A) 30 cm × 30 cm, (B) 20 cm × 20 cm. In peripheral artery angiography, at least a 30 cm image size is needed. The 20 cm image size is too small for peripheral artery angiography.

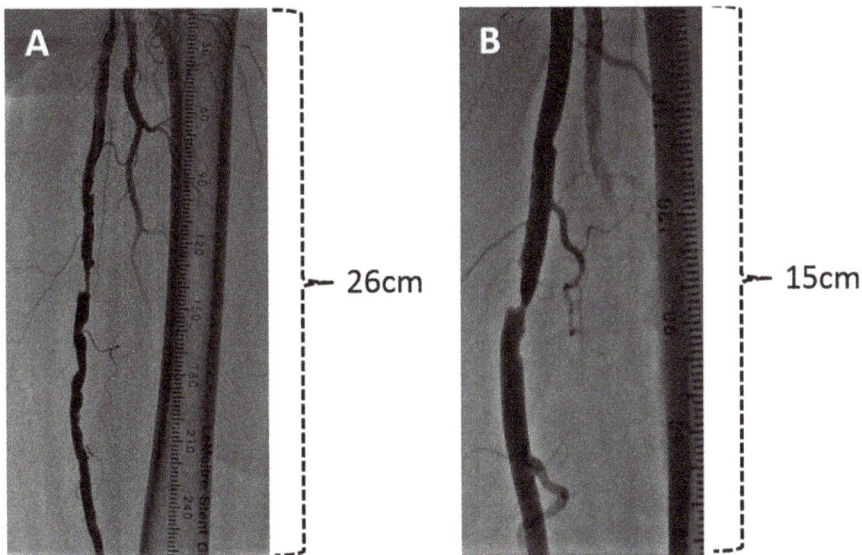

Figure 2. Image field of 20 cm and 30 cm detector in SFA. (A) In the 30 cm detector, about 26 cm of SFA is visualized. (B) In the 20 cm detector, only 13 cm of SFA is seen.

In the 30 cm panel, about 26 cm of the SFA can be visualized and intermediate stenosis around the culprit lesion (**Figure 2A**) can be discerned. On the other hand, the coronary detector could visualize only 13 cm of the SFA in 20 cm mode (**Figure 2B**). In a coronary lab, to visualize the SFA or below the knee (BK) arteries, the table is panned but a good static image of the lesion is difficult to obtain.

1.2. Extra monitor

In an angiographic suite, operators usually stand on the right side of the table. Most labs use one monitor and all medical staffs rely on this one screen. In right limb angiography via the left femoral artery approach, the operator who is standing on the right side has difficulty manipulating the catheter. In this situation, one operator needs to stand on the left side of the table to manipulate the catheter and hold the sheath. For this purpose, an extra-monitor should be installed (**Figure 3**).

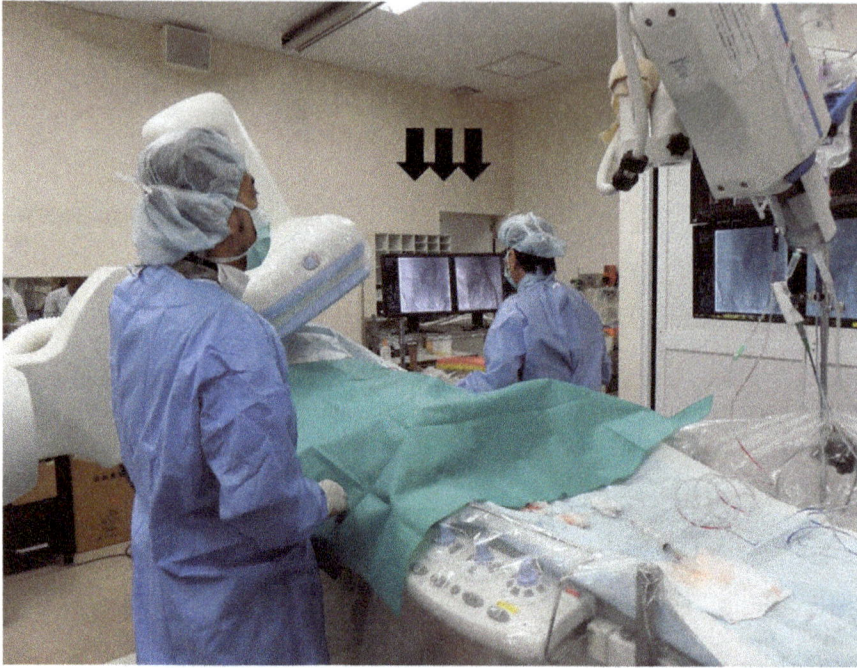

Figure 3. Extra-monitor. In right superficial artery (SFA) intervention, the main operator stands on the left side of the table watching the extra-monitor while the assisting operator watches the central monitor. Without moving the central image monitor, the main operator can manipulate the catheter from the left side.

A typical right superficial artery (SFA) intervention is shown in **Figure 3**. The main operator is standing on the left side of the table and watching the extra-monitor while the assisting operator keeps an eye on the central monitor. Without moving the central image monitor, the main operator is able to perform the procedure. This extra-monitor is useful in the left brachial approach as well. It is a convenient way to intervene in the right femoropopliteal artery or cross-over approach for right below the knee arteries. In the left below the knee artery procedure via the cross-over approach, the C-arm is rotated to the left side. The cranial side operator may not see the central image. In this situation, the extra monitor can be placed on the left cranial side.

1.3. Injector

For most of the small vessels in selective angiography, hand injection of the contrast dye is adequate. However, for optimal opacification of high-flow blood vessels like the aorta, the use of a power injector is mandatory. A constant and high volume of dye should be injected through an electronically calibrated power injector. There are two types of injectors: one is a conventional power injector and the other is an assisted device that introduces small or large amounts of dye by an injector attached to the catheter table. The contrast volume is adjusted manually so that even a small dose of dye can be injected. However, the space on the left side of the table is occupied by this assisted device. Thus, a conventional power injector mounted to the ceiling is preferable since it affords more space around the catheter table. Furthermore, the distance allows a significant reduction in radiation exposure during dye injection. With the assisted device, radiation exposure is difficult to prevent since the operator has to be beside the table during dye injection (**Figure 4**).

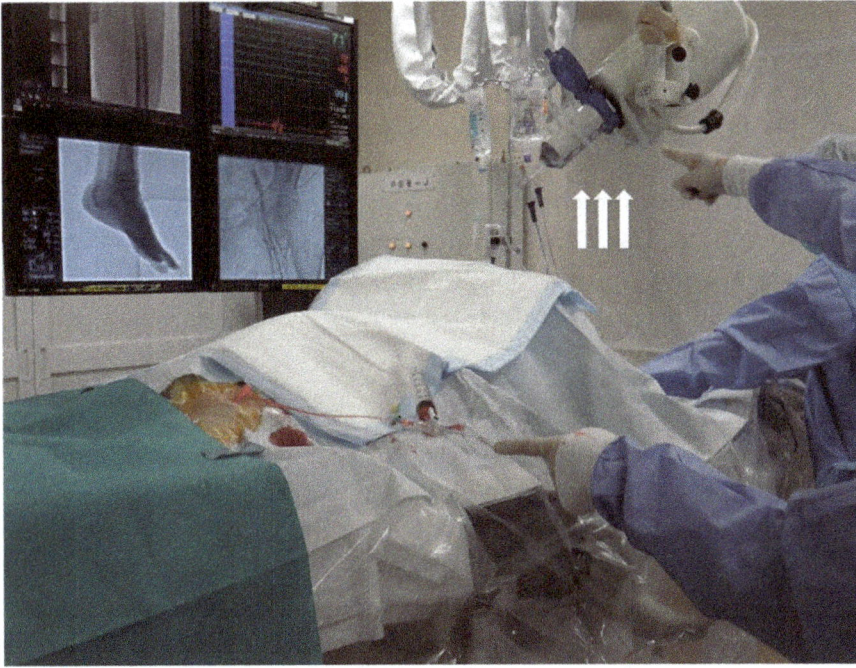

Figure 4. Power injector mounted to the ceiling. The ceiling-mounted injector allows more space around the catheter table.

1.4. Contrast dose

Contrast-related factors include the vascular access site, injection time duration, injection rate, contrast volume and dye concentration. The key factor is the injection rate. An increased rate of injection can induce a greater extent of vascular opacification but the safety and total volume of the contrast dose must be carefully monitored. The contrast volumes for opacification of the major arteries are shown in **Table 1**. These are the injection volumes mainly used in our catheter laboratory although the actual contrast volume depends on the patient's condition, the catheter size, amount of contrast and speed of injection. Therefore, the contrast dose should be individualized for each case.

Location	Catheter	Injection rate (ml/s)	Total volume (ml)
Aortoiliac	5Fr Pig tail	14–16	15–25
CFA-SFA-Pop A	4–5Fr MP	5–7	16–20
Run: CFA-BTK	4–5Fr MP	4	9–12
SFA	4–5Fr MP	4–5	8–10
Run: BTK	4Fr MP	3–4	10–12
BTK	4Fr MP	3–4	5–7
Below the ankle	4Fr MP	3–4	5–7

Table 1. Contrast injection rate and injection volume.

There is no universally agreed upon threshold in the degree of renal dysfunction beyond which intravascular iodinated contrast medium should not be administered. We use Visipaque 320 [2]. Contrast-induced nephropathy (CIN) is an infrequent adverse reaction to iodinated contrast agents [3]. In endovascular procedures, particular complex procedures are associated with CIN and larger doses of contrast are considered a risk factor. Thus, as a precaution against CIN, the use of contrast media at the lowest dosage possible is advised. To minimize the contrast dose, we dilute Visipaque 320 by adding 30 cc of saline solution in a 100 cc bottle. The key factor is the injection rate which indicates the amount of dye per second. In our experience, 1/3rd diluted contrast does not decrease image quality.

1.5. Radiation safety

Angiography machines which use fluoroscopy for endovascular work are equipped with pulsed fluoroscopy instead of continuous fluoroscopy and this, to a large extent, helps to reduce the radiation dose (three radiation pulse mode). During this procedure, both the patient and physician are exposed to a certain degree of radiation so that its dose needs to be minimized. Constant measurement of radiation doses in patients and personnel is vital. Above all, the shielding in the room is particularly important. We use a suspended ceiling shield as well as a floor installed shield (**Figure 5**). During digital subtraction angiography (DSA) imaging, other comedical staffs are outside the angiosuite. The main operator besides the patient is protected by a ceiling-mounted radiation shielding glass. After the procedure, radiation exposure levels must be routinely recorded and archived.

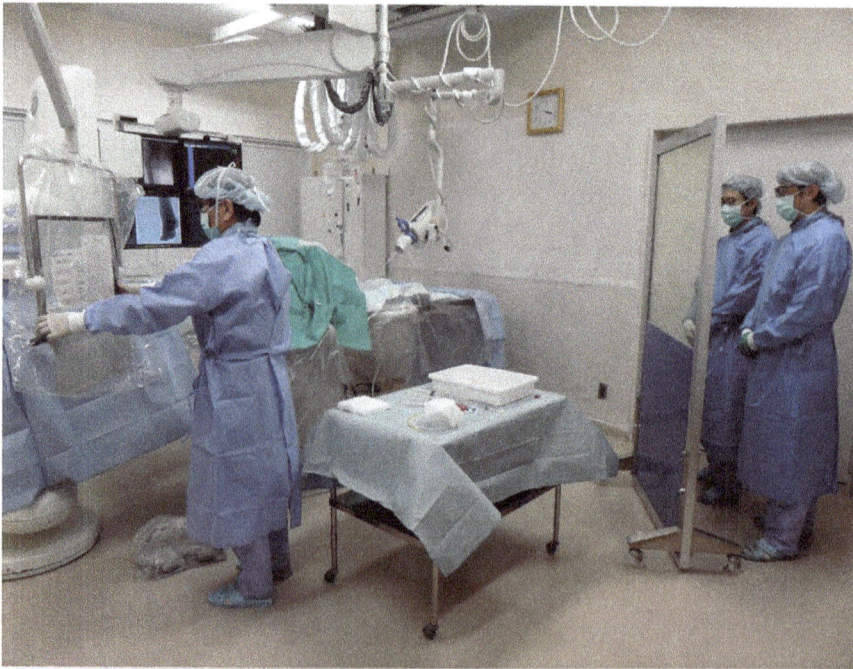

Figure 5. Radiation shield. Operator uses the ceiling-mounted radiation shield and the assistant is behind the shield during contrast injection.

2. Imaging techniques

2.1. Sheath

2.1.1. 4Fr sheath

The 4Fr sheath is mainly used for the antegrade femoral approach. For initial access, a 4Fr sheath is placed from the common femoral artery (CFA) to the SFA. The reason is that an antegrade puncture is technically more demanding and if we fail to make the puncture, the sheath can be withdrawn or repositioned. While keeping the 4Fr sheath in the profunda femoris artery (PFA), we can even place an additional 4Fr sheath into the CFA. The long 4Fr sheath is for below the knee work. However, it is easily kinked and there may be an increased risk of hematoma formation. In interventions below the knee arteries, most occlusion balloons accept the 4Fr sheath with the use of a 0.014 or 0.018 in. guidewires. And to minimize sheath size in the ipsilateral CFA approach, a 4Fr long sheath is ideal for patients with critical limb ischemia (CLI) (**Figure 6A**).

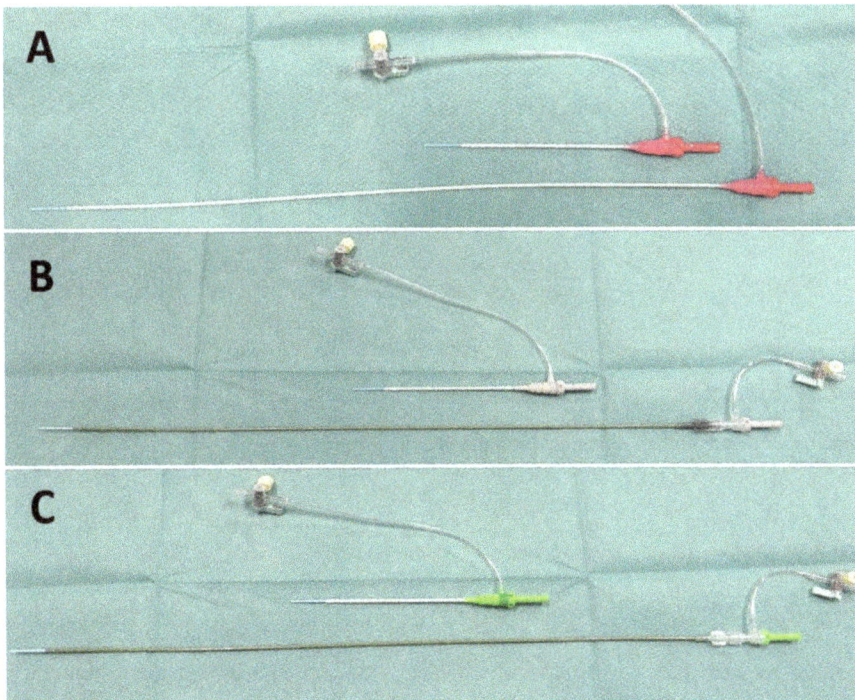

Figure 6. Sheath. (A) 4Fr sheath, (B) 5Fr sheath, (C) 6Fr sheath.

2.1.2. 5Fr sheath

In ad hoc interventions, we have standardized the 5Fr sheath for the initial retrograde CFA approach. When stent implantation is planned, we start with a 6Fr sheath. Either a 4Fr or 5Fr pigtail catheter can be used for aortography. With a 4Fr pigtail catheter, the amount of dye is limited to around 10–13 cc/s. To opacity the terminal aorta to both the iliac and common femoral arteries, the rate of injection should be 15–20 cc/s and this flow rate can be achieved with at least a 5Fr pigtail catheter. Introducer sheaths are used for all angiography and endovascular procedures. The 5Fr 45 cm cross-over sheath is used for either the retrograde or antegrade approach. In a contralateral SFA intervention, a 5Fr 45 cm crossover sheath is used. However, when stenting is performed, the sheath should be replaced with a 6Fr crossover sheath. In the antegrade approach for BK interventions, a 5Fr 45 cm crossover sheath gives more back-up support to intervene on the tibial arteries (**Figure 6B**).

2.1.3. 6Fr sheath

When an iliac artery stent is already planned, a 6Fr short sheath should be placed in a retrograde manner. In a cross-over approach, a 6Fr 45 cm cross-over sheath is employed. The advantage of the 6Fr system is that the closure device can be applied after the procedure. In some medical centers, the antegrade 6Fr short sheath is placed for SFA stenting. However, we do not routinely use the 6Fr sheath for antegrade work (**Figure 6C**) (**Table 2**).

Advantage	Disadvantage
Better wire control with short wire	Complication related to antegrade common femoral artery (CFA) puncture
Short distance to the lesion	Might miss proximal superficial femoral artery (SFA) lesion
Precise stent placement	Need caution of proximal end of stent
Access to below the knee arteries	Compression of ischemic side after procedure

Table 2. Advantage and disadvantage of ipsilateral antegrade approach.

2.2. Wires

2.2.1. 0.035 in. wire

There are three types of tips for the 0.035 wire. We do not use a regular J-tip Radifocus wire (Terumo, Tokyo, Japan) (**Figure 7A**). The initial wire is always a 1.5 mm J-type Radifocus wire (Terumo, Tokyo, Japan) (**Figure 7B**). The tip of this wire has a 1.5 mm round shape and is quite safe when the wire migrates into the small branches or other vessels. Once the guidewire crosses the lesion, we change to a regular 0.035 in. spring wire (**Figure 7C**). The Radifocus wire is slippery and is difficult to keep in place while regular spring wires tend to stay in place. Thus, for stability, the wire should be changed to a spring wire once the lesion is crossed. These three types of 0.035 in. wires should always be at hand.

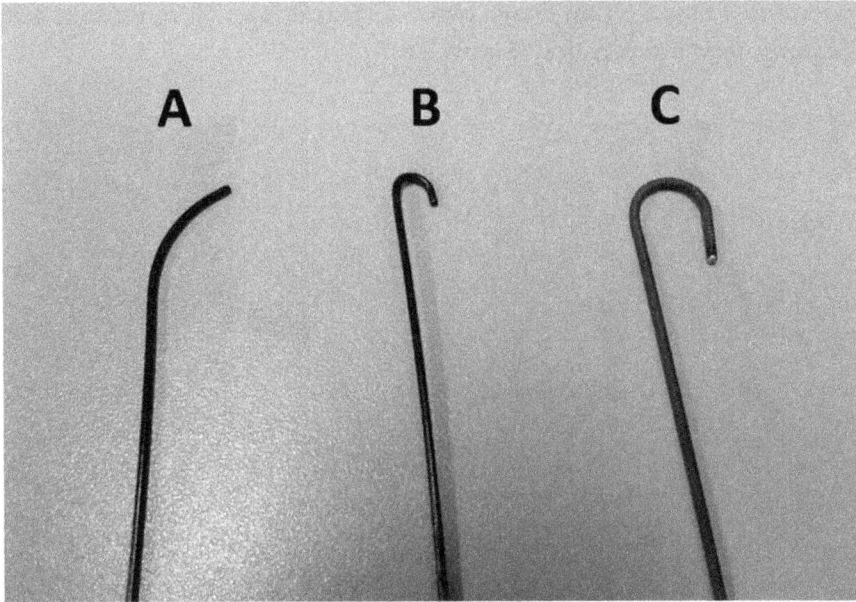

Figure 7. 0.035 in. guidewires. There are three types of tips for the 0.018 in. wire. We do not use regular a J-tip Radifocus wire (A). The initial wire is always a 1.5 mm J-type Radifocus wire (B). Once used to cross the lesion, it is exchanged to a 0.018 in. spring wire (C).

2.2.2. 0.018, 0.014 in. wires

Basically, we do not use the 0.018 in. wire as a regular wire. Chronic total occlusion (CTO), a 0.018 in. Treasure 12-g (Asahi Intec, Nagoya, Japan) wire is initially selected. It has a 12-g tip load and is best suited as a peripheral CTO wire. The V 18 (Boston Scientific, Cambridge, MA, USA) wire has a strong main shaft with a soft tip and can be used for cross-over ballooning or stent implantation. There are many 0.014 in. wires and their purposes vary. For below the knee artery work, the 0.014 in. wire is the basic wire used.

2.3. Digital subtraction angiography (DSA) vs. digital angiography (DA)

Digital subtraction angiography (DSA) has long been the gold standard for evaluation of atherosclerotic lesions in patients with PAD. Image quality has been further improved by replacing traditional image intensifiers with flat panel detectors so that regular digital angiography (DA) is now replacing DSA. When considering the high radiation doses, not all cases need imaging by DSA. Above all, critical limb ischemia is difficult to manage and some patients have difficulty staying still during injection of the contrast dye. Thus, adequate optimization with either DSA or DA should be employed to obtain accurate imaging of the diseased segments.

2.3.1. Aortoiliac artery

A typical DSA image of the iliac artery is shown in **Figure 8**. In the 30 cm image, we can see from the terminal aorta to both common femoral arteries (**Figure 8A**). In the 20 cm image, a clearer view can be seen (**Figure 8B**).

In our routine, we first take a 30 cm image by DSA (**Figure 9A**). Next, we take a 20 cm image by DA for the purpose of intervention (**Figure 9B**).

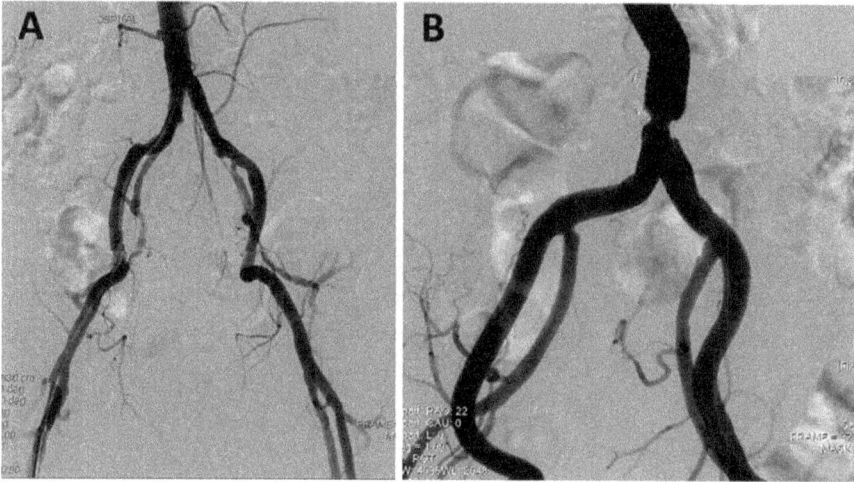

Figure 8. Iliac artery angiography, 30 cm vs. 20 cm image. (A) 30 cm image, we could see from the terminal aorta to both common femoral arteries. (B) 20 cm image, a clearer view is obtained.

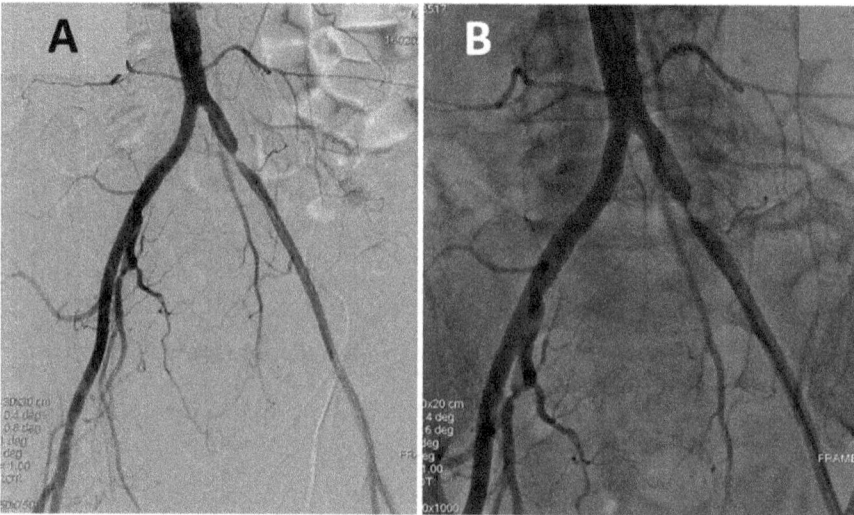

Figure 9. DSA vs. DA image of the iliac artery. (A) 30 cm image by DSA for diagnostic purposes. (B) 20 cm image by DA for interventions. DSA, digital subtraction angiography; DA, digital angiography.

DA is more practical for stent implantation since it provides the background image. In the aortoiliac artery segment, the image is hampered by bowel and gas movements. Aortoiliac artery angiography is basically taken by DSA, however, due to bowel and gas movements, the image is blurred (**Figure 10A**). In such a circumstance, we change to the DA image (**Figure 10B**). In **Figure 10**, a left common iliac aneurysm with distal stenosis can be seen; the DSA image is blurred while the DA image clearly reveals stenosis.

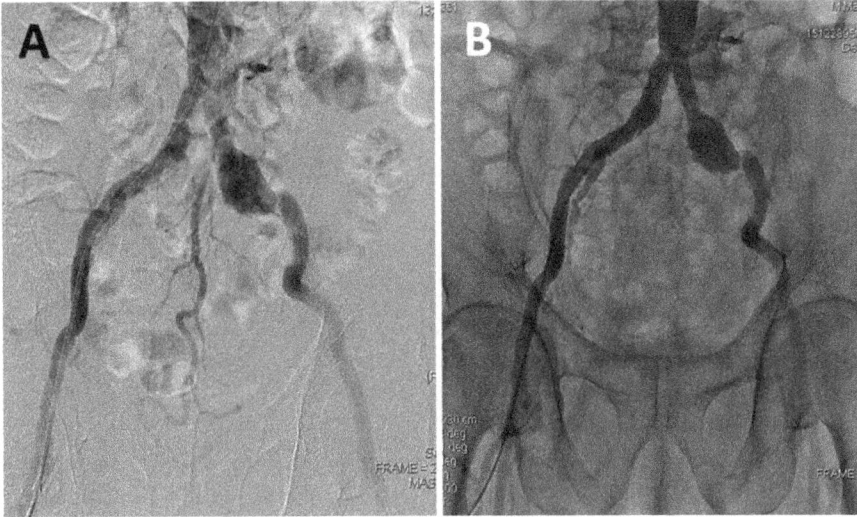

Figure 10. DSA vs. DA image of the iliac artery. (A) DSA image is blurred by bowel gas. (B) DA image shows clear image of left common iliac aneurysm with distal stenosis. DSA, digital subtraction angiography; DA, digital angiography.

2.3.2. Femoropopliteal artery

The initial angiographic image is the ipsilateral angled view. Either DSA or DA can provide a reasonable image (**Figure 11**), although the DSA image (**Figure 11A**) is shown to be better than the DA image (**Figure 11B**). In the DA image, the background is shown and can be used as reference (**Figure 11B**).

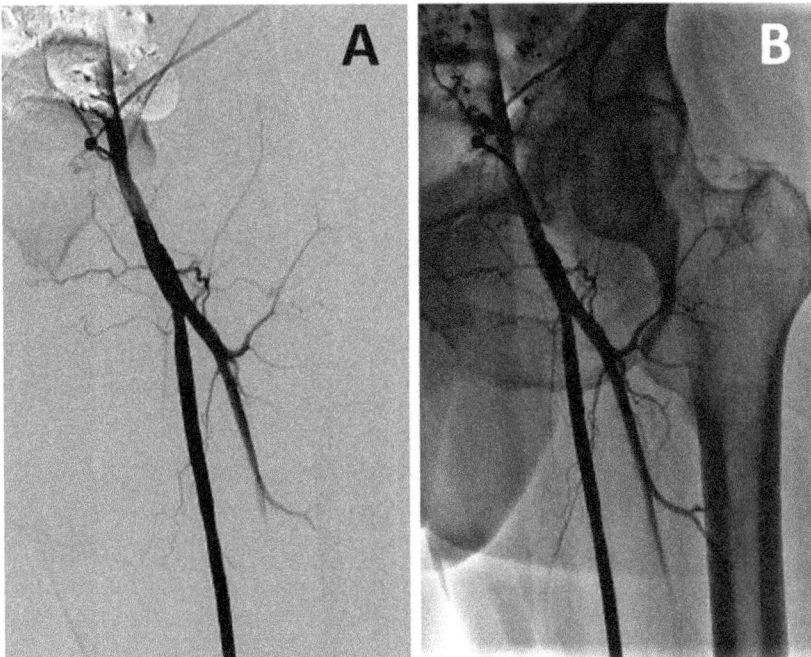

Figure 11. Proximal femoral artery. (A) DSA image for ipsilateral angled view of the left proximal femoral artery. (B) DA image shows the background and identifies bifurcation point.

A calcified lesion is often seen in the common femoral artery. In such cases, DSA provides a clearer view than the DA image (**Figure 12**). DSA clearly shows the calcified lesion (**Figure 12A**) while, in contrast, the lesion could not be determined in the DA image due to low contrast (**Figure 12B**).

For the SFA, we use either the DSA or DA image. For a calcified lesion, DSA is preferable (**Figure 13A**), but in most cases, DA provides a reasonably good image (**Figure 13B**).

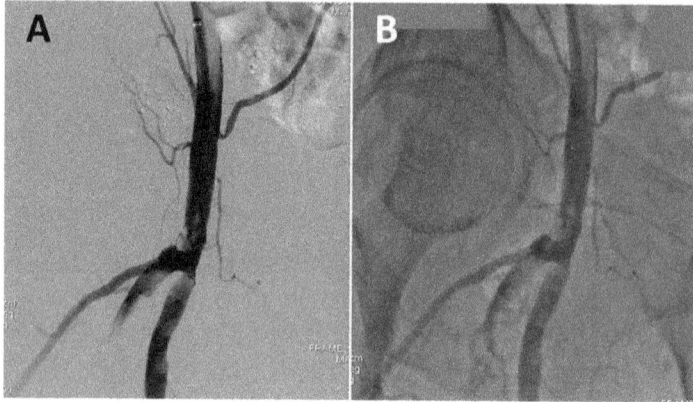

Figure 12. Calcified common femoral artery. (A) DSA clearly shows calcified lesion. (B) DA image could not determine lesion due to low contrast.

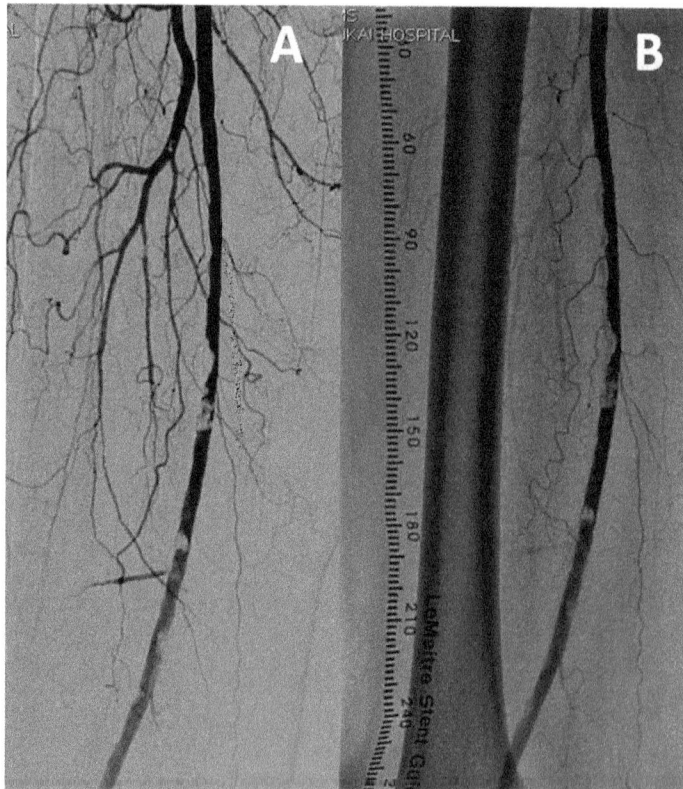

Figure 13. SFA angiography, DSA vs. DA. (A) DSA shows clearer image and branches are well seen. (B) DA gives reasonably good image.

In a SFA lesion, measurement of the lesion length is important to decide the interventional strategy and we prefer a DA image for the pre-interventional angiogram. The popliteal artery is located deep in the posterior fossa of the knee joint. Surrounded by a bony structure, the popliteal artery is very difficult to visualize by DA. Basically, a DSA image is taken for the popliteal artery (**Figure 14A**). In **Figure 14A**, tight stenosis of the mid-popliteal artery is well visualized with rich collateral circulation. In the DA view, stenosis is well observed but most of the collateral vessels are not visualized (**Figure 14B**).

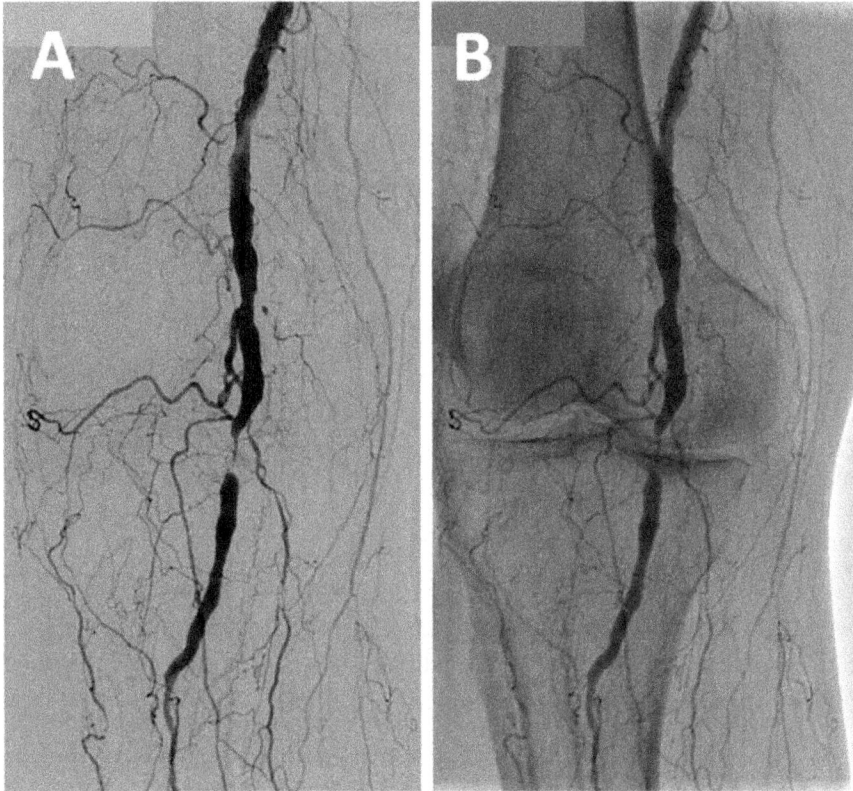

Figure 14. Popliteal artery angiography, DSA vs. DA. (A) Popliteal artery surrounded by bone and basically taken with DSA. (B) DA view shows well visualized stenosis but most collateral vessels unclear.

2.3.3. Below the knee arteries

Diseases of below the knee arteries are closely associated with critical limb ischemia (CLI) and detailed anatomical information is required to plan intervention. Compared to other limb arteries, angiography remains the imaging method of choice in most cases of CLI. How to take a good image is the cornerstone of successful endovascular therapy. DSA is a must for imaging of below the knee arteries. In **Figures 2–10**, comparisons of the DSA and DA images of the left proximal tibial arteries are shown. In the DSA image, posterior tibial artery occlusion is well observed (**Figure 15A**). On the other hand, the DA image failed to show the tibioperoneal trunk and occlusion of the posterior tibial artery (**Figure 15B**).

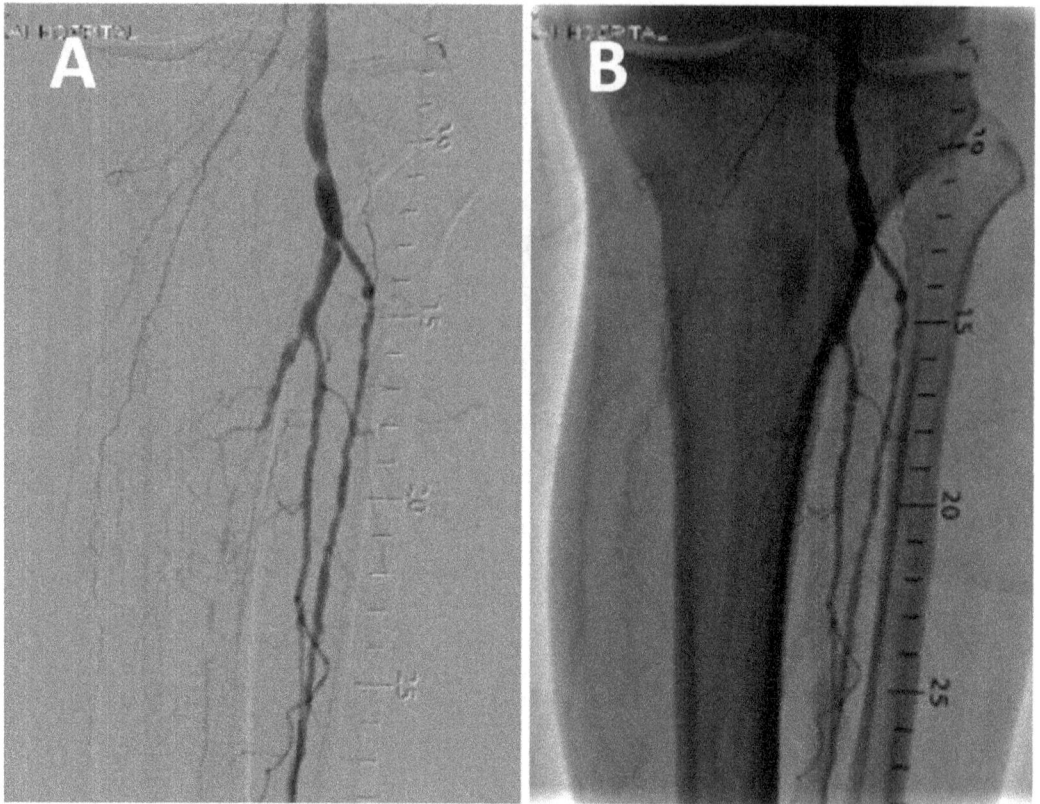

Figure 15. Proximal below the knee angiography, DSA (A) vs. DA (B).

A similar case of the left proximal below the knee artery is shown in **Figure 16**. In the DSA image, three tibial arteries are shown with multiple stenosis (**Figure 16A**). In the DA image, precise diagnosis cannot be made (**Figure 16B**).

Assessment of the distal tibial arteries is vital in evaluating below the ankle disease. Continuation from the anterior tibial artery to the dorsal artery and the posterior tibial artery to the planted artery must be clarified. However, due to the bony structure, the DA image could not show these distal tibial and below the ankle arteries (**Figure 17**). In **Figure 17A**, the planter artery is not clearly visualized in the DSA image. In the DA image, most of the vessels remain un-visualized (**Figure 17B**).

2.4. Basic angiography for PAD

2.4.1. Angiography from the terminal aorta to below the knee artery

In an angiographic approach for PAD diagnosis, we need to assess three segments of the lower limb artery, that is, the aortoiliac, femoropopliteal and below the knee arteries. In **Figure 18**, the basic angiography is shown. First, angiography of the aortoiliac artery was taken (**Figure 18A**). The second angiography is an ipsilateral view of the proximal femoral artery (**Figure 18B**). In the right leg, a 30° right anterior oblique (RAO) view was chosen to separate the proximal SFA and PFA. Third, angiography from the CFA to the distal below the ankle artery was taken by running the table (**Figure 18C**). After observing these three angiograms, we could assess in which segment stenosis or occlusion was located.

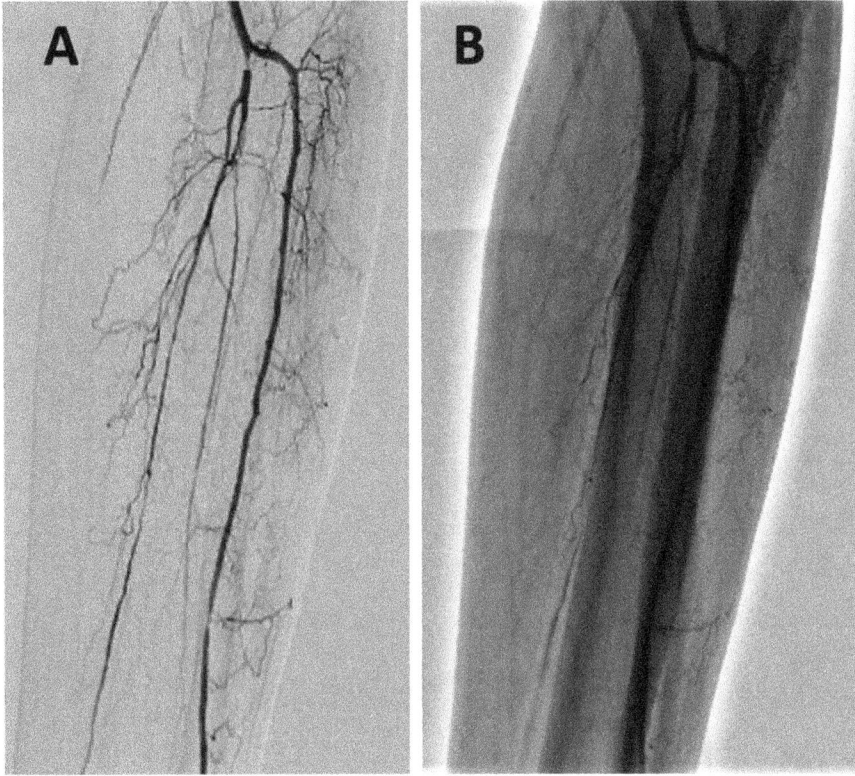

Figure 16. Mid-below the knee angiography, DSA (A) vs. DA (B).

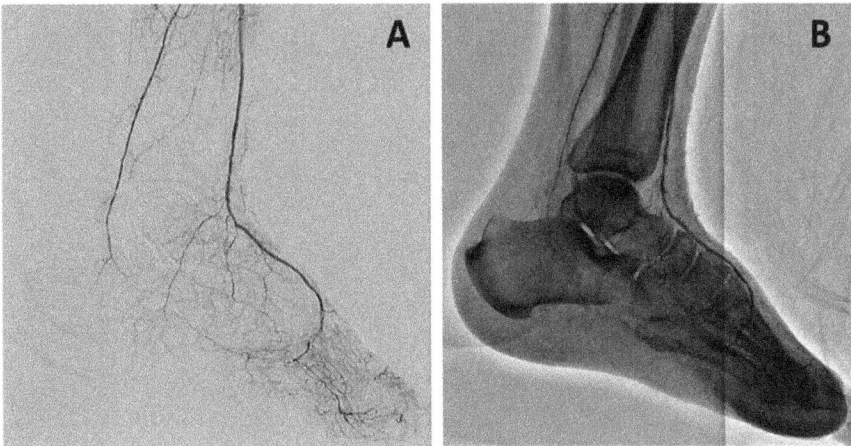

Figure 17. Below the ankle angiography, DSA (A) vs. DA (B).

A typical claudication with SFA disease is shown in **Figure 19**. Aortoiliac artery angiography showed no significant stenosis (**Figure 19A**). In the proximal femoral artery, there was no stenosis in the SFA and PFA (**Figure 19B**). Left limb angiography showed focal stenosis in the mid-SFA while the left anterior tibial artery was not visualized (**Figure 19C**). By using DA, left SFA angiography was taken and revealed focal tight stenosis in the mid-SFA (**Figure 19D**). This DA image was used as reference in interventional work (**Figure 19D**).

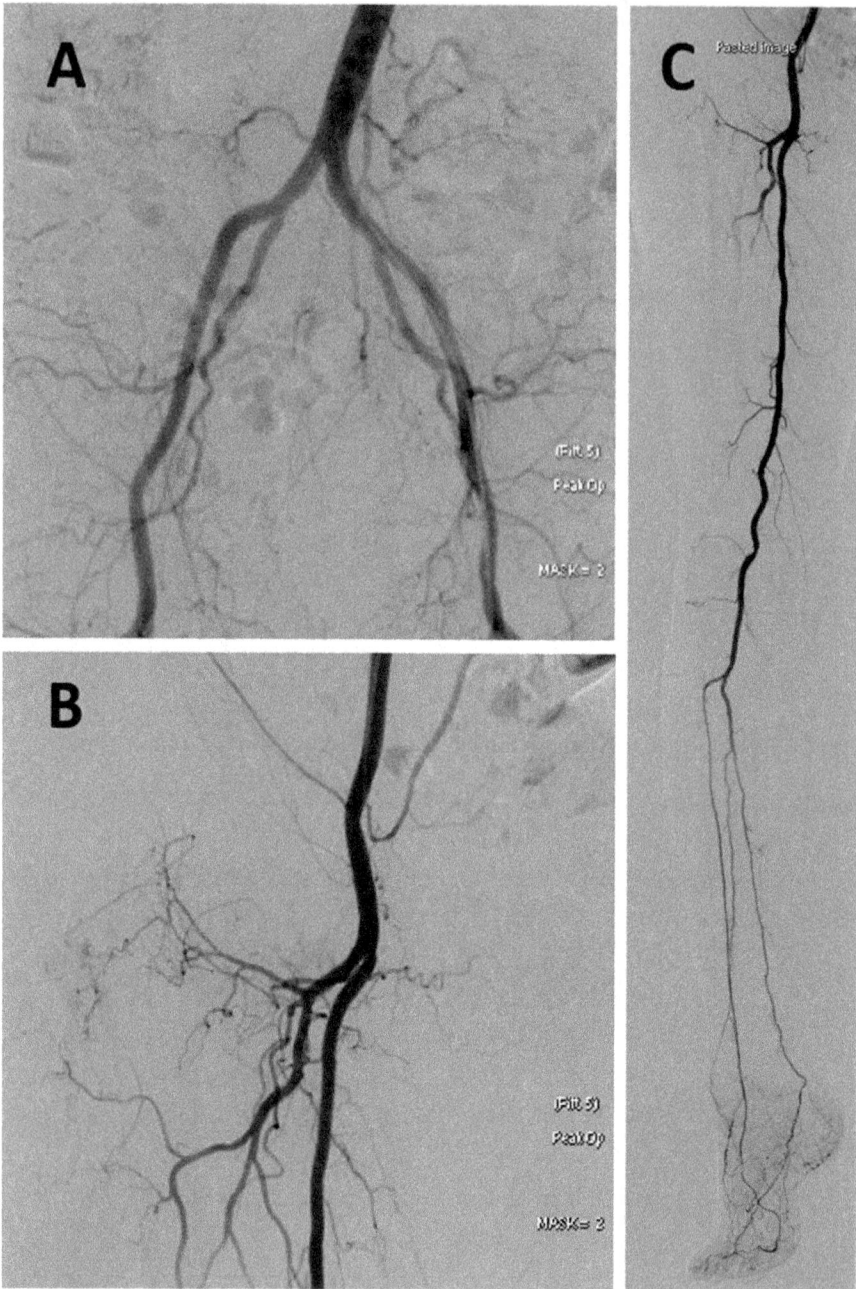

Figure 18. Basic lower limb artery angiography. (A) Aortoiliac artery angiography. (B) Proximal femoral artery by a 30° right anterior oblique view. (C) From the right common femoral artery to the distal below the ankle artery.

Figure 20 shows isolated below the knee artery disease. From the iliac to femoropopliteal artery level, no atherosclerotic changes could be observed (**Figure 20A** and 20B). A lesion is located in the right below the knee arteries. Below the knee arteries showed a stenotic lesion of the anterior tibial artery, and the posterior tibial artery and peroneal artery are occluded (**Figure 20C**). This type of lesion, that is, "isolated below the knee artery disease" is often found in patients with critical limb ischemia.

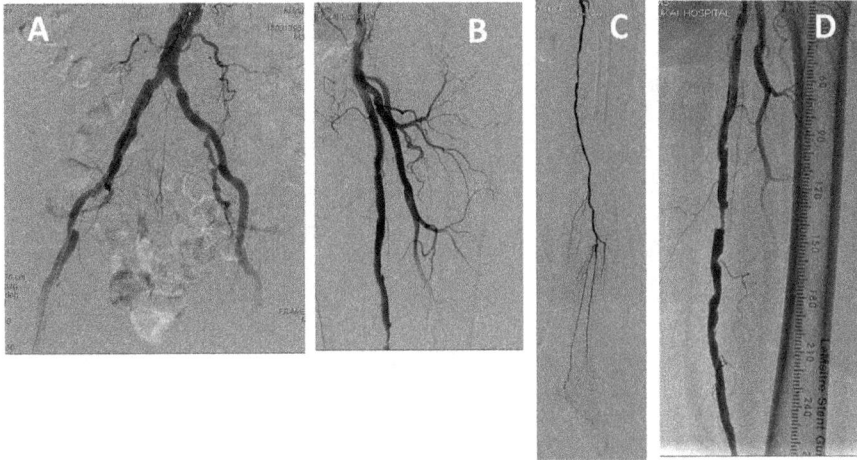

Figure 19. A typical claudication with SFA disease (A) Aortoiliac artery angiography showed no significant stenosis. (B) In the proximal femoral artery, there was nostenosis in the SFA and PFA. C: Left limb angiography showed focal stenosis in themid-SFA. (D) LeftSFA angiography revealed focal tight stenosis in the mid-SFA.

2.4.2. Magnification of images

The image size has two purposes: one is to see the whole vessel, for example, in the aortoiliac artery, visualization from the terminal aorta to both the right and left CFA (**Figure 21A**). The other is to better intervene on the target lesion utilizing appropriate magnification of the image size (**Figure 21B**). For wiring to this lesion, a 20 cm magnified image was taken and successful wiring was carried out using a 0.014 in. wire (**Figure 21B**).

In **Figure 22**, right SFA stent restenosis was visualized with a 30 cm image (**Figure 22A**). Moreover, using the 20 cm magnified mode, stent restenosis was well observed (**Figure 22B**).

In below the knee arteries, the whole image shows which vessels are diseased (**Figure 23A**). However, this running image does not give detailed information on the three tibial arteries. In the 30 cm image, the three proximal tibial arteries are well observed, and the peroneal and posterior tibial arteries are diffusely diseased (**Figure 23B**). The further magnified 20 cm image revealed that there is tight stenosis at the ostium of the right anterior tibial artery (**Figure 23C**).

2.4.3. Pre- and postinterventional image

Basically, all interventional work requires two images to be taken, that is, pre- and postintervention. These two images reveal the angiographic changes pre and post procedure. In **Figure 24A**, the femorofemoral bypass was occluded and a long total occlusion of the right iliac artery is seen. After successful recanalization and stenting, angiography of the exact same iliac artery was taken (**Figure 24B**).

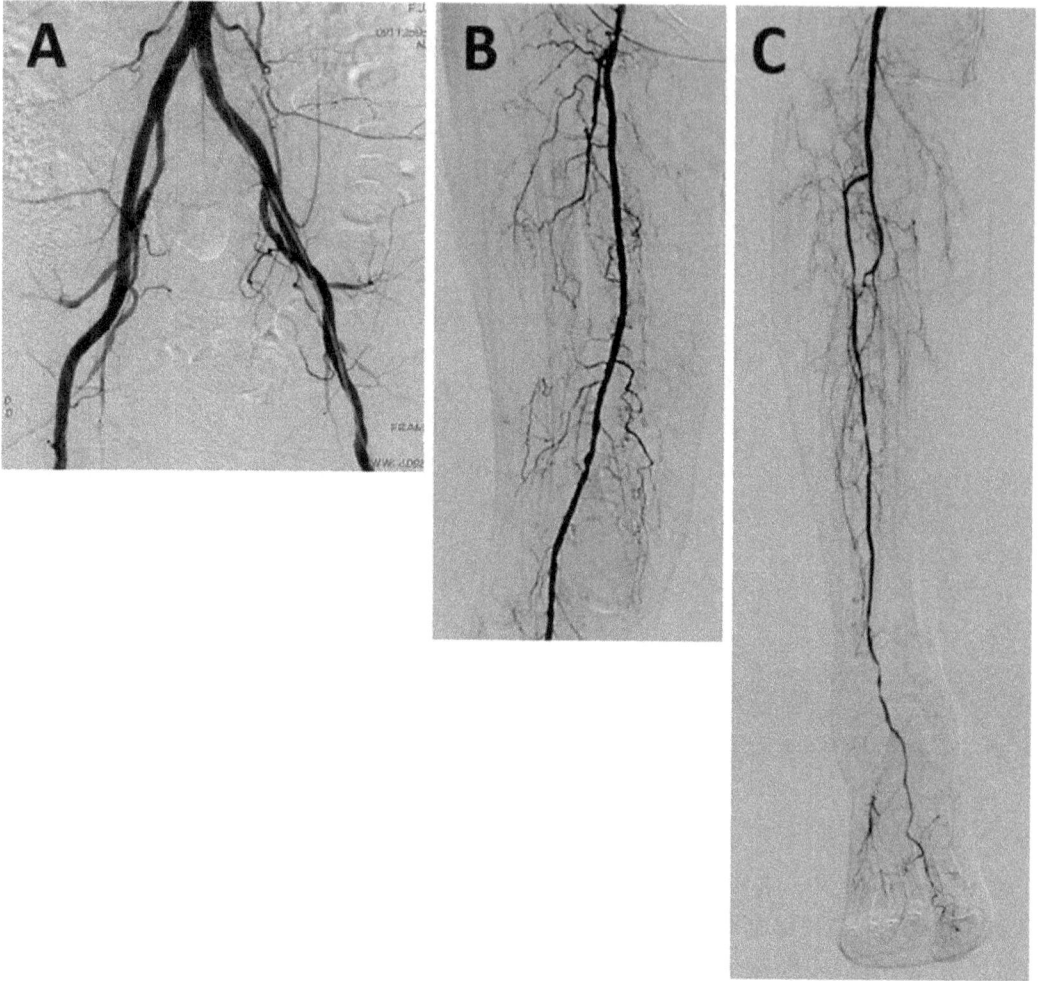

Figure 20. Basic lower limb artery angiography. Isolated below the knee artery disease. (A) Aortoiliac artery showed no disease. (B) Right femoropopliteal artery showed no disease. (C) Right below the knee arteries showed a stenotic lesion of the anterior tibial artery, and the posterior tibial artery and peroneal artery are occluded.

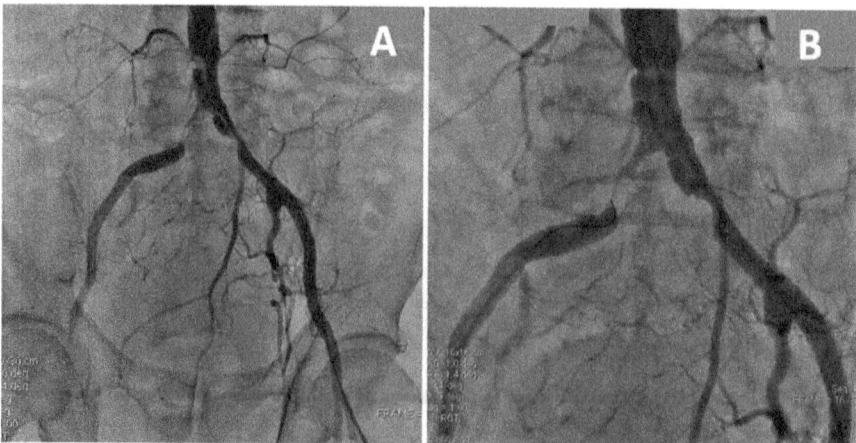

Figure 21. Iliac artery angiography, 30 cm (A) vs. 20 cm image (B).

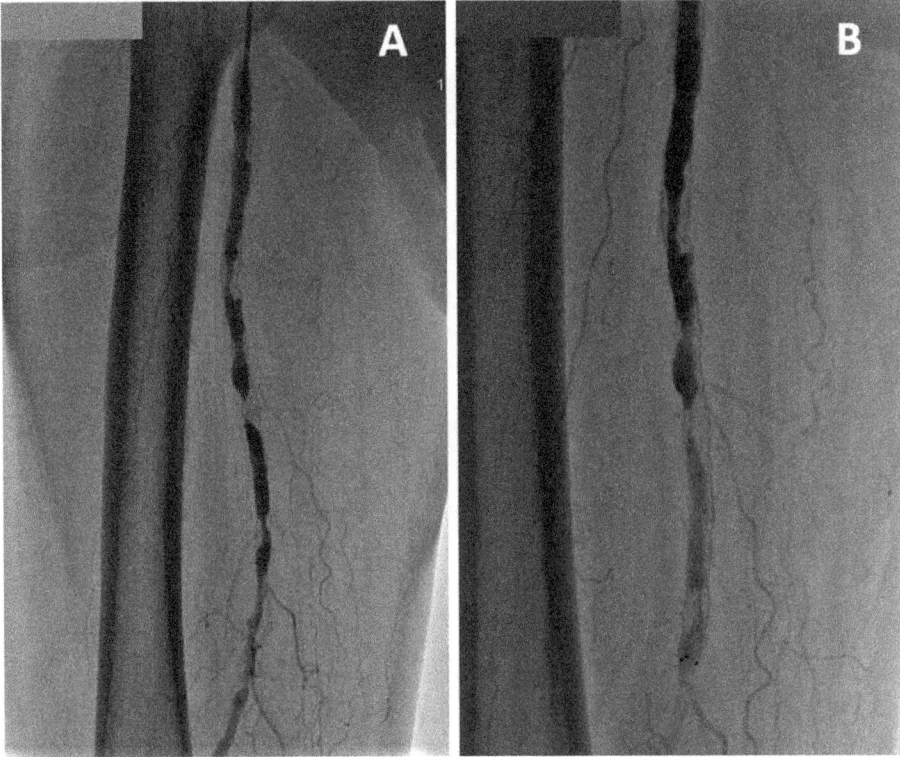

Figure 22. SFA angiography, 30 cm (A) vs. 20 cm image (B).

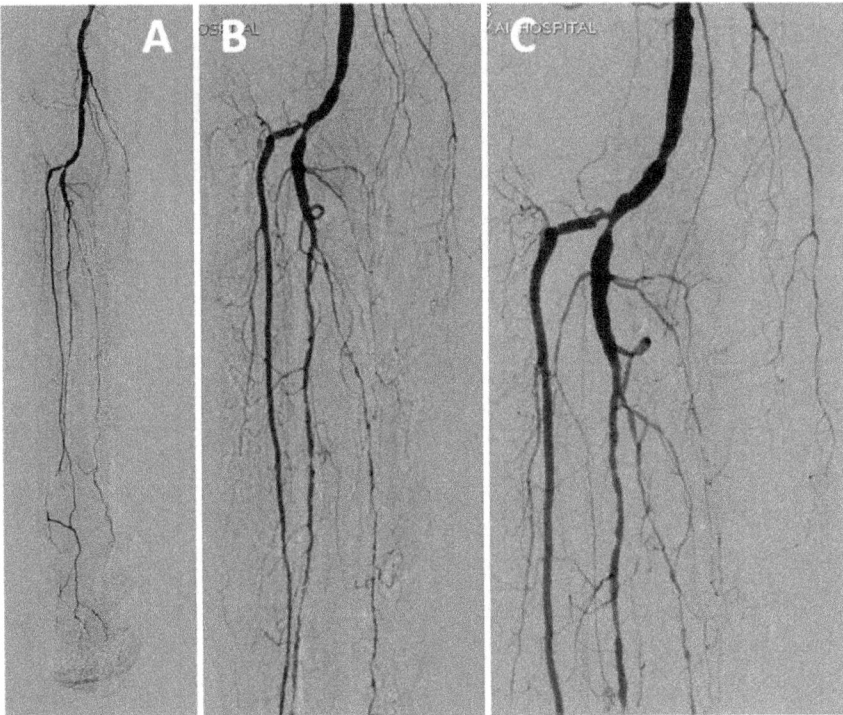

Figure 23. Below the knee angiography, 30 cm (A), 20 cm (B) and 16 cm images (C).

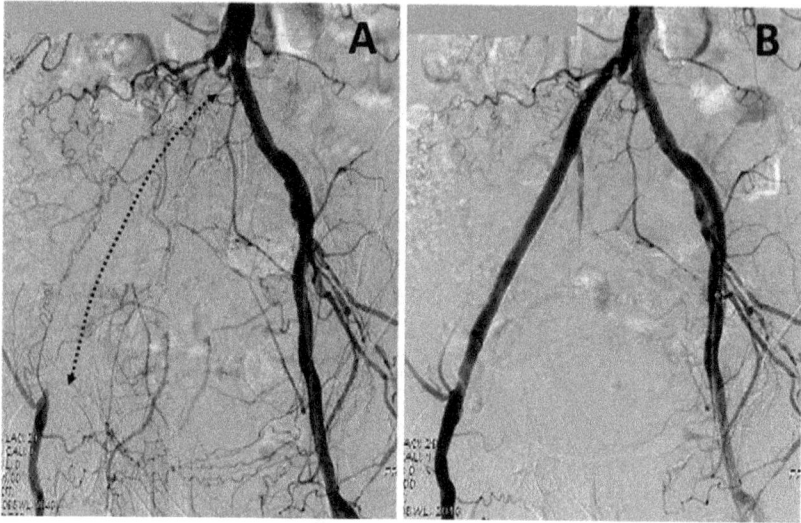

Figure 24. A case of right iliac artery occlusion. Pre (A) and post iliac artery angiography (B).

In **Figures 2–20**, typical left SFA occlusion was seen (**Figure 25A**). After balloon angioplasty, dissection and incomplete dilatation were observed (**Figure 25B**). Post stent angiography showed excellent dilatation of the left SFA lesion (**Figure 25C**). During the procedure, the table was frequently moved and oftentimes, post angiographic images were not taken in the different positions, giving a false impression of the postinterventional image.

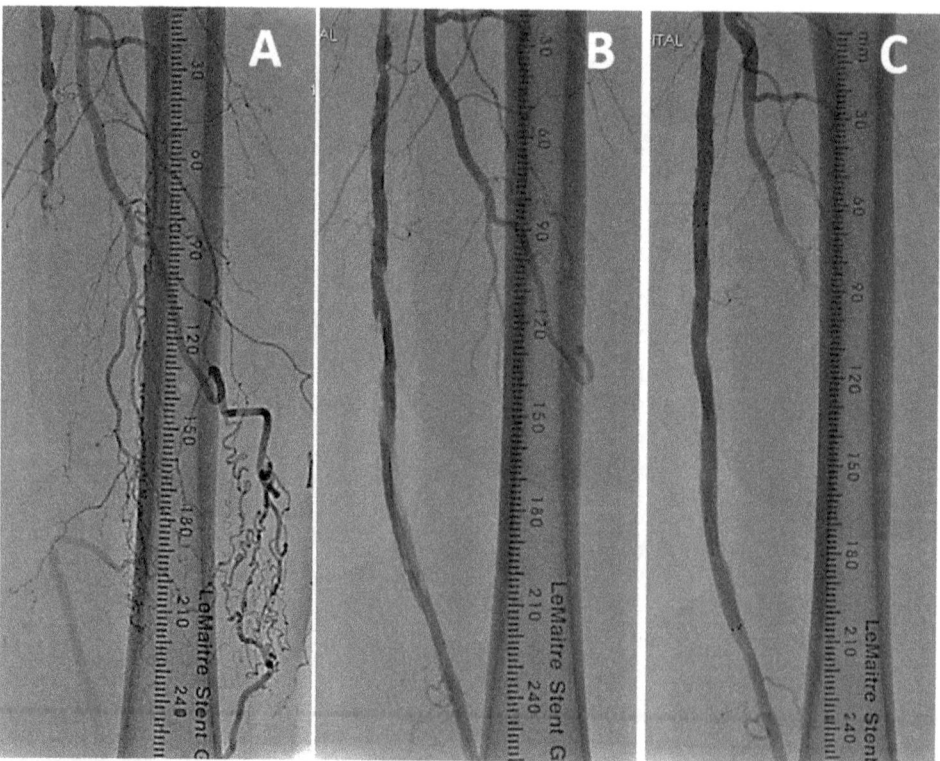

Figure 25. A case of SFA occlusion. Pre (A) and post SFA angiography (B).

3. Echo-guided puncture femoral artery puncture

The common femoral artery (CFA) remains the most widely accepted site for endovascular artery access. Vascular access site-related complications are a major cause of periprocedural morbidity among patients undergoing percutaneous endovascular intervention. In particular, patients with PAD may be more likely to have atherosclerosis affecting the CFA. Ultrasound guidance is an emerging trend for all percutaneous procedures and its use for femoral artery puncture has decreased vascular complications and improved first-pass success rates [4–6].

3.1. Retrograde common femoral artery puncture

The CFA is the main access site for angiography and interventional procedures. Among the various puncture sites, the retrograde CFA puncture is the most commonly employed and the basis of arterial punctures. We have described a safe and echo-guided technique for avoiding femoral access site complications.

3.1.1. Puncture point

The inferior border and upper border of the femoral head should be realized by fluoroscopy (**Figure 26A**). After checking the maximum arterial pulse (**Figure 26B**), Xylocaine is given 1 cm below the middle of the femoral head (**Figure 26C**).

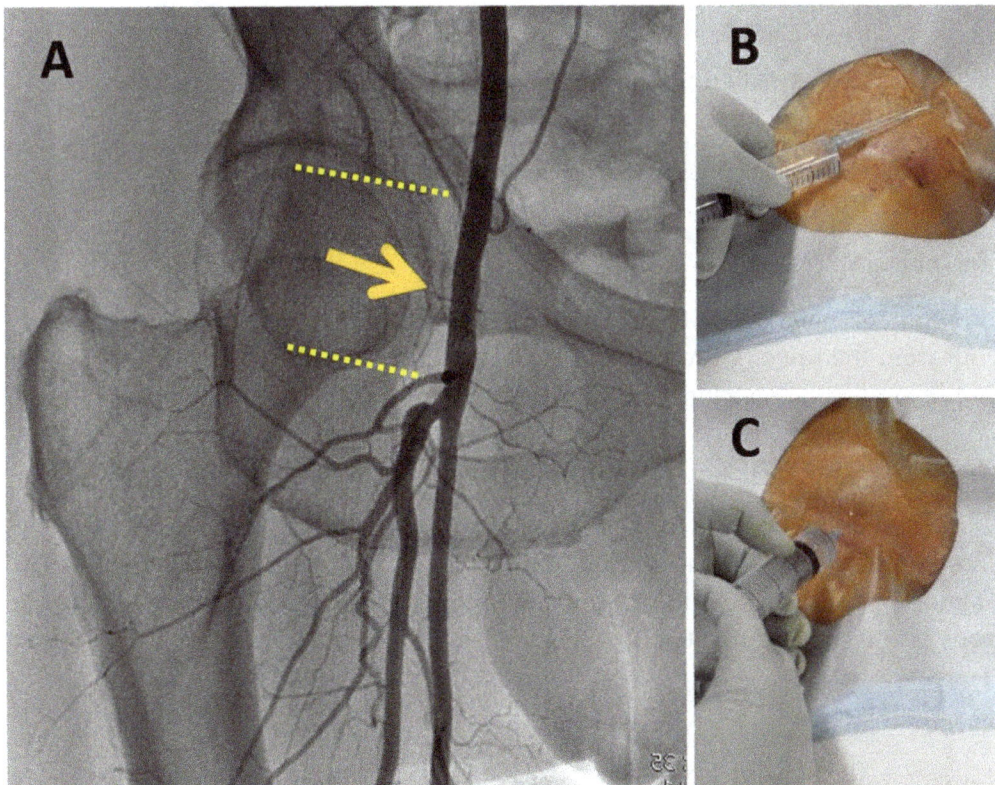

Figure 26. Puncture point of common femoral artery. (A) Realizing the inferior border and upper border of the femoral head by fluoroscopy. (B) Marking middle of femoral head. (C) Xylocaine to be given 1–2 cm below.

3.1.2. Preparation

A sheath and two types of wires were prepared. Once a puncture is performed, the wire should be ready to be inserted and if there is resistance, change to a different kind of wire is advised (**Figure 27**).

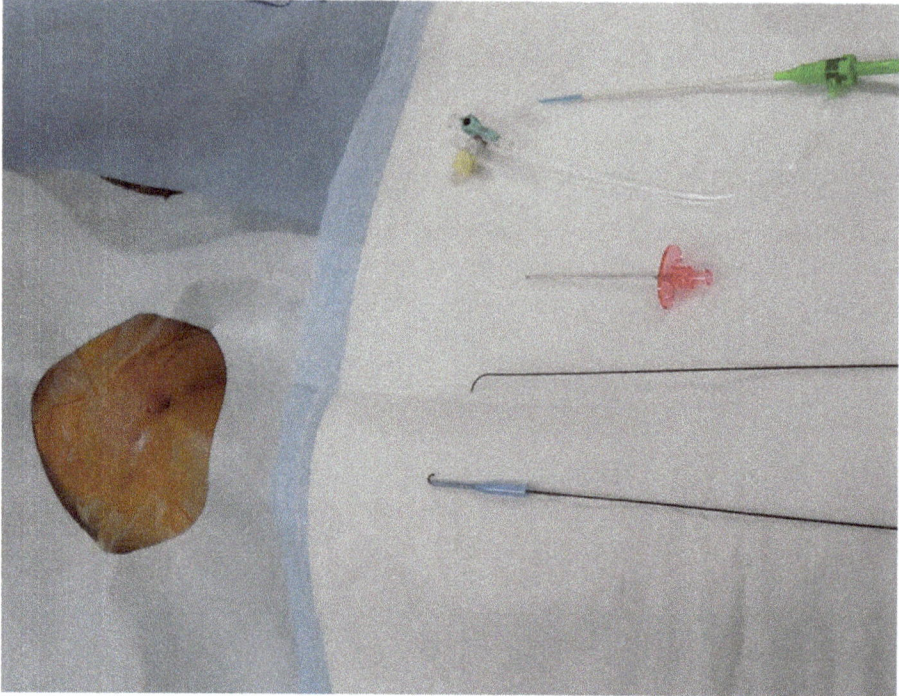

Figure 27. Preparation of sheath and two types of wire. Prepare sheath and two type wires close to puncture site. Once puncture completed, insert wire and if resistance encountered, change to different shape wire.

3.1.3. Echo scanning

For an echo-guided puncture (NEMIO MS, Toshiba, Tochigi, Japan), first, echo scanning was carried out from the upper CFA to proximal SFA (**Figure 28**). We could identify where the bifurcation is located. Either a long axis (**Figure 28A**) or short axis can be obtained (**Figure 28B** and **C**). A scan is basically made by a short-axis view. The ideal puncture site of the CFA can then be located (**Figure 28B**) and the bifurcation site can be identified (**Figure 28C**).

An echo image is best seen from the upper common femoral artery to the distal external iliac artery. When total reliance is on echo guidance, the puncture site locates higher than the middle femoral head. To avoid too low or high punctures, rechecking the puncture site by fluoroscopy is advised (**Figure 26A**).

3.1.4. Puncture

Arterial access was obtained with an 18-G needle (COOK Medical, Bloomington, Indiana) using the modified Seldinger technique. The needle was inserted at an angle of about 45° from the skin at a level just below the center of the femoral head. In viewing the short axis, the aim should be for the top of the vessel. During flash backs of blood, a gentle wire insertion must be made. When resistance is felt, change from a straight wire to round shaped wire is advised (**Figure 29**). When the plaque in the CFA is found, a normal CFA puncture site should be located. In **Figure 29A**, the long-axis view showed the plaque in the CFA.

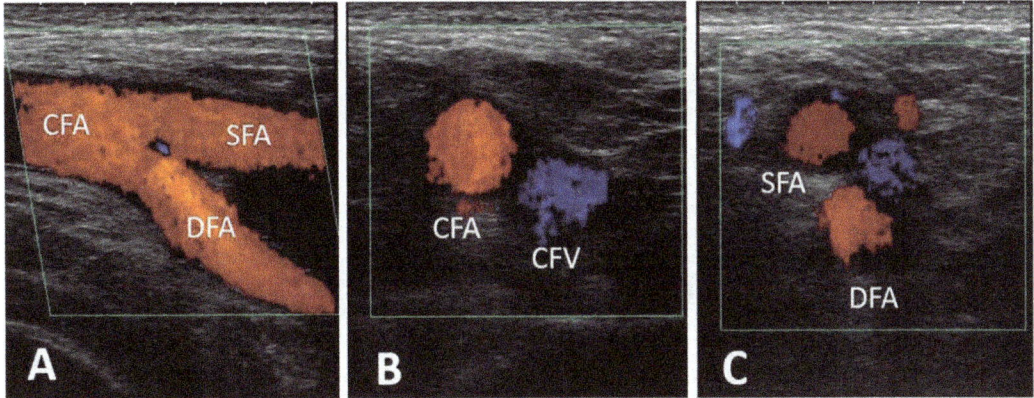

Figure 28. Color Doppler scanning from CFA to SFA and PFA. (A) Long-axis view of CFA and SFA. (B) Short-axis view of CFA. (C) Short-axis view of SFA and PFA. Using color Doppler, scan from upper CFA to SFA and PFA. Locate the ideal puncture site of CFA and identify the bifurcation point. CFA, common femoral artery; SFA, superficial femoral artery; PFA, profunda femoral artery.

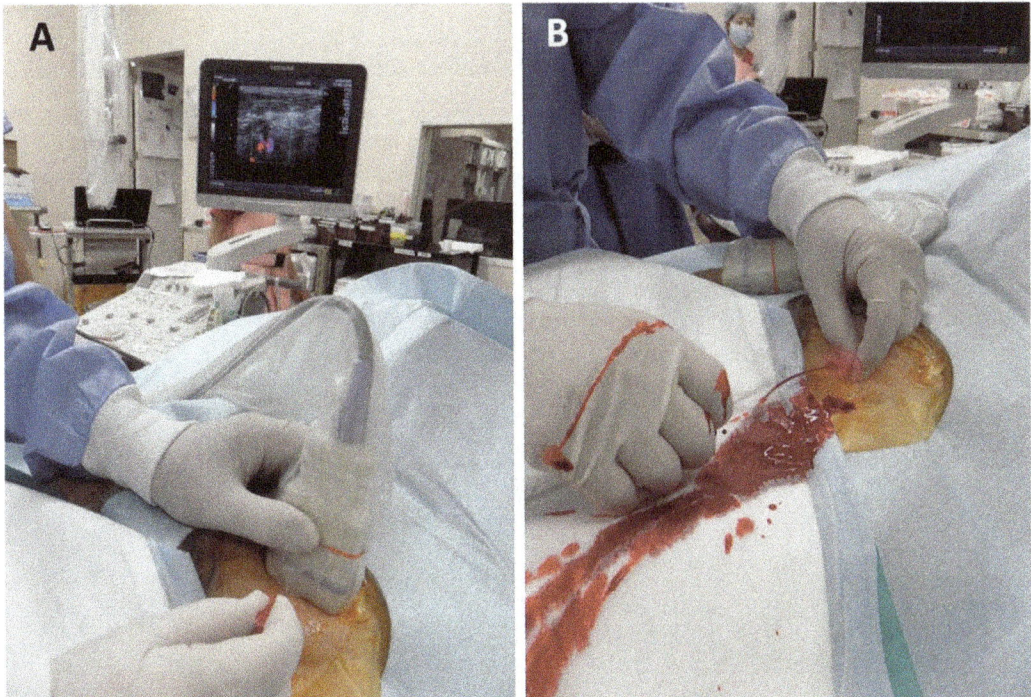

Figure 29. Puncture. (A) Echo guidance. (B) 18G needle puncture. In viewing short axis, aim for top of the vessel. During flash-back of blood, gentle wire insertion should be made. If resistance encountered, change straight wire to round shaped wire.

In this situation, a plaque free zone within the CFA should be located (**Figure 30B–D**).

In **Figure 31**, a puncture was made at the site of CFA disease and the wire went into false lumen, resulting in the total occlusion of the CFA.

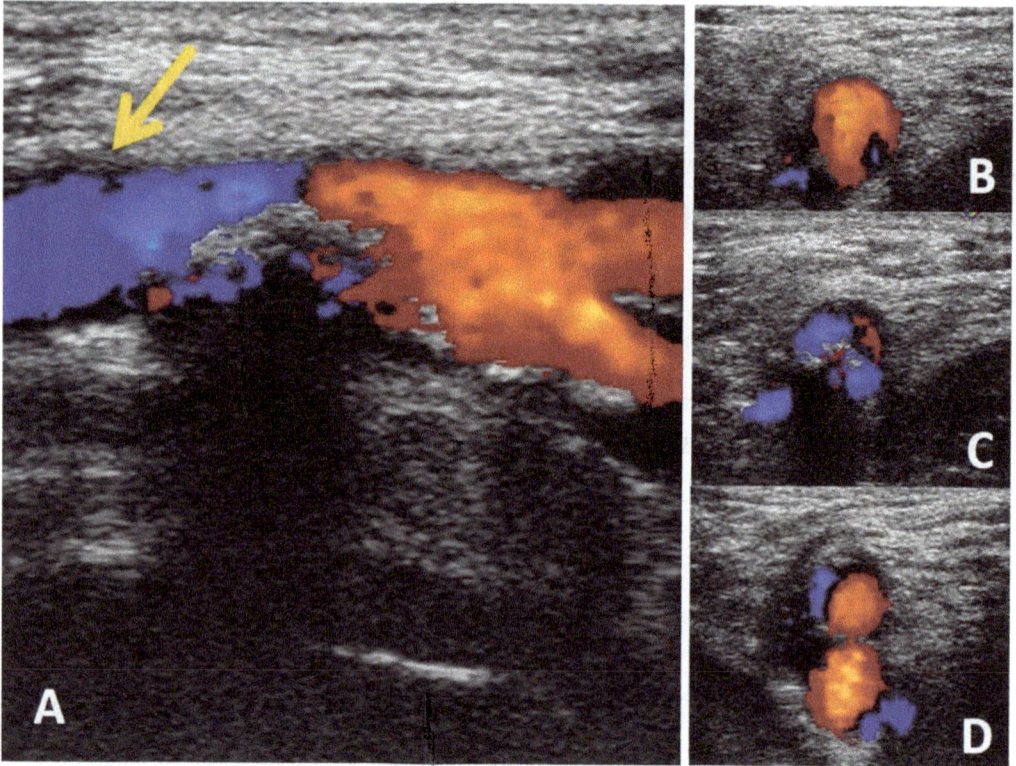

Figure 30. Presence of CFA plaque. (A) Long-axis view of CFA and SFA. Note CFA plaque. (B) Plaque free site of CFA in short axis. (C) Presence of plaque. Should not be punctured. (D) SFA and PFA level. When finding plaque in the CFA (A), should look for normal CFA puncture site. Must find plaque free zone within CFA. CFA, common femoral artery; SFA, superficial femoral artery; PFA, profunda femoral artery.

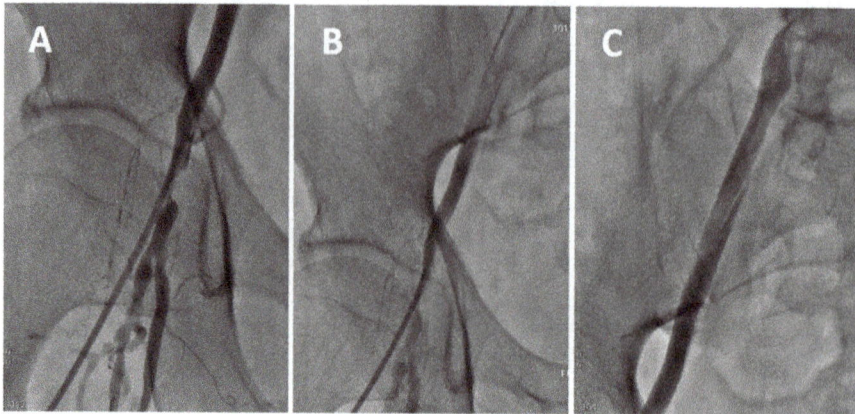

Figure 31. Puncture of common femoral artery plaque. (A) Puncture into CFA plaque. Creates false lumen. (B) TIMI 0 flow. (C) Dissection of iliac artery. Without knowledge of CFA disease, puncture was made. Wire went into false lumen and ended up in total occlusion of CFA.

3.2. Antegrade common femoral artery puncture

For treatment of femoropopliteal artery disease, the standard approach has been to access the contralateral common femoral artery (CFA). However, an ipsilateral, antegrade CFA approach has certain advantages. Compared to the contralateral approach, access to the lesion distance is short which in turn improves the responsiveness of the wire handling used to perform the intervention. In other clinical situations such as post aorto-bi-femoral surgical bypass, deployment of iliac kissing stents, post stent grafting and for aortoiliac occlusive disease, an antegrade approach is the method of choice to reach the lesion. The advantages and disadvantages are shown in **Table 2**.

The CFA is approximately 4–5 cm in length and arises from the external iliac artery (EIA) as it passes below the inguinal ligament. It then bifurcates into the PFA and SFA. An anatomical knowledge of the level of origin for the PFA is important in avoiding retroperitoneal bleeding, iatrogenic femoral arterial-venous fistula and/or formation of a pseudo aneurysm. The most lethal complication of femoral access remains retroperitoneal hemorrhaging due to a high puncture. Thus, the best first step toward reducing the incidence of retroperitoneal bleeding is to prevent high punctures.

3.2.1. Preparation of an antegrade puncture

As we perform in a retrograde puncture, two kinds of wires should be at hand. The initial sheath we place is always the 4Fr size sheath (**Figure 32**).

The main reason is, when obtaining access to the CFA fails, the sheath can be easily withdrawn or left in the PFA. Once placing the sheath in the SFA is successful, it can be changed to any sheath as desired. Pointing to the middle of the femoral head, local xylocaine should be given around the inguinal ligamentum (**Figure 33**).

Echo was applied in the same way. However, the proximal CFA to external iliac artery is well observed by echo and may result in a very high puncture site. Under fluoroscopic guidance with echo assistance, point to the middle of the CFA.

3.2.2. Puncture

A puncture should be made by aiming an imaginary line over the center of the femoral head. The maximum level of bifurcation should be at or below the inferior border of the femoral head (**Figure 34A**). In about 1/4th of cases, bifurcation locates in the CFA (**Figure 34B**). In **Figure 34B**, the bifurcation point is in the middle of the CFA and there is a short margin for the antegrade puncture site.

3.2.3. Two-wire technique

Even when the puncture site is above the bifurcation, the wire may go to the PFA. In this situation, we use a two-wire technique (**Figure 35**). If the wire goes to the PFA, the first step is to place a 4Fr sheath into the PFA. Two short 0.025 in. wires are inserted into the RFA (**Figure 35A**). Withdrawing the sheath, one 0.025 in. wire should be manipulated into the SFA

(**Figure 35B**). Once the SFA is accessed, leaving one wire in the PFA, the other wire should be advanced to the SFA (**Figure 35C**). After confirming the wire in the SFA, the other PFA wire is withdrawn and a 4Fr sheath should be placed into the SFA (**Figure 35D**). If the sheath comes out, it can be repositioned back into the PFA by a 0.025 in. wire.

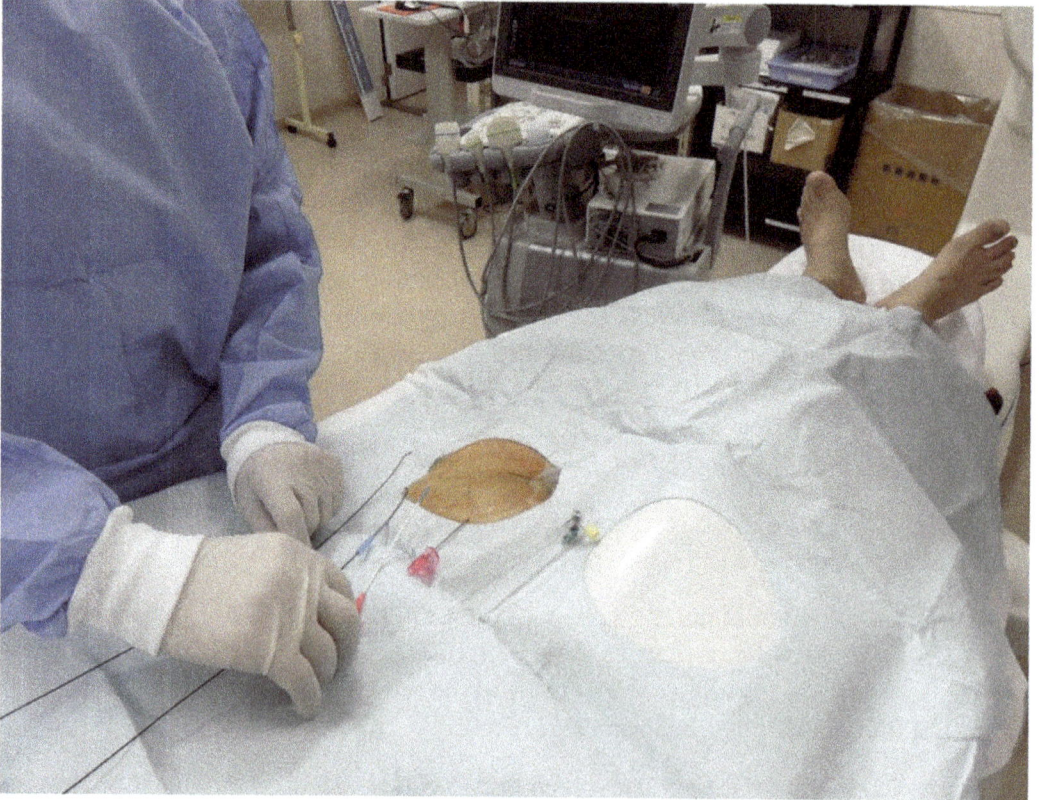

Figure 32. Preparation of antegrade puncture. 18G needle, 4Fr sheath and two kinds of wire at hand.

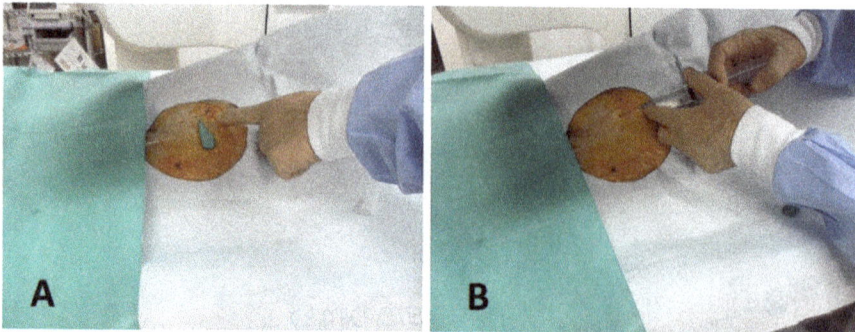

Figure 33. Antegrade puncture of common femoral artery. Puncture site. (A) Locate middle of femora; head. (B) Local xylocaine to be given at inguinal ligamentum.

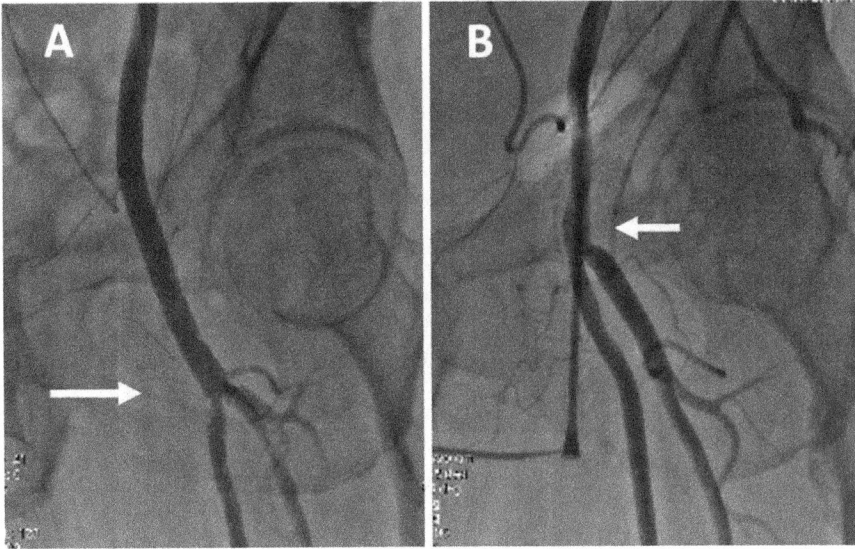

Figure 34. Bifurcation point of CFA to SFA. (A) Level of the bifurcation is below the inferior border of the femoral head. (B) The bifurcation point is in the middle of CFA and only short margin for ideal puncture sire. CFA, common femoral artery.

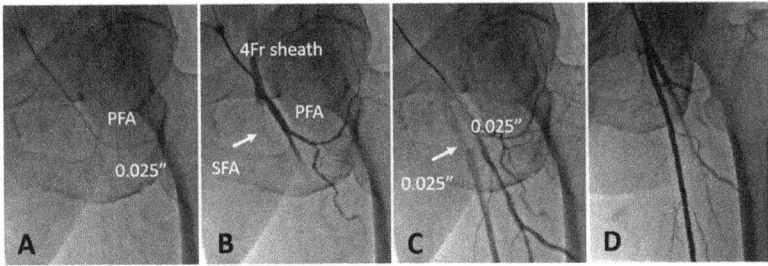

Figure 35. Two wire technique. (A) If wire goes to PFA, the first step is to place a 4Fr sheath into PFA. Two short 0.025 in. wires are inserted into PFA. (B) Withdrawing sheath, one 0.025 in. wire to find SFA leaving another wire in PFA (**Figure 10B**). (C) Once SFA obtained, wire advanced to SFA (**Figure 10C**). (D) After confirming wire in SFA, other PFA wire withdrawn and 4Fr sheath placed into SFA. SFA, superficial femoral artery; PFA, profunda femoral artery.

3.2.4. High bifurcation case

After surveying the CFA by echo, we may find high bifurcation of the SFA and PFA. In these cases, high puncture carries the risk of retroperitoneal bleeding. The puncture point should be in the range of the femoral head. In this situation, puncturing the SFA is one option. In **Figure 36,** there is high bifurcation and a CFA puncture is almost impossible. In this case, we decided to puncture the proximal SFA.

3.2.5. Sheath kinking

The angle of puncture should be more than 60° and almost vertical. After sheath insertion, care to avoid sheath kinking is advised. Once a hematoma is observed with sheath kinking, change to a larger size anti-kink sheath is necessary. In **Figure 37**, the initial 4Fr sheath was kinked (**Figure 37A**) and hematoma formation was detected. After the 4Fr sheath was replaced with a 6Fr sheath, the hematoma was stabilized (**Figure 37B**).

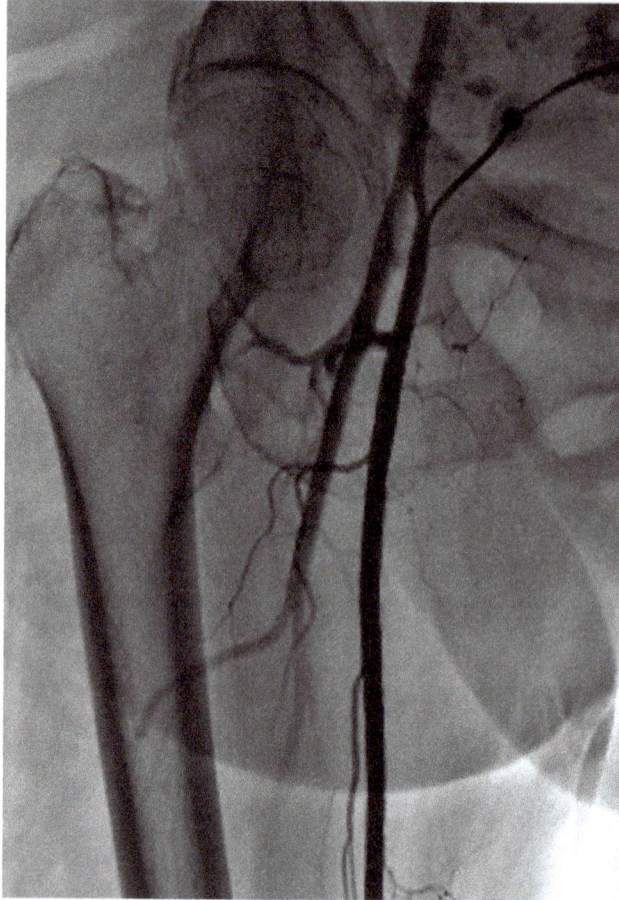

Figure 36. SFA puncture in high bifurcation case. After surveying CFA by echo, observed high bifurcation of SFA and PFA. In this situation, puncturing SFA is one option.

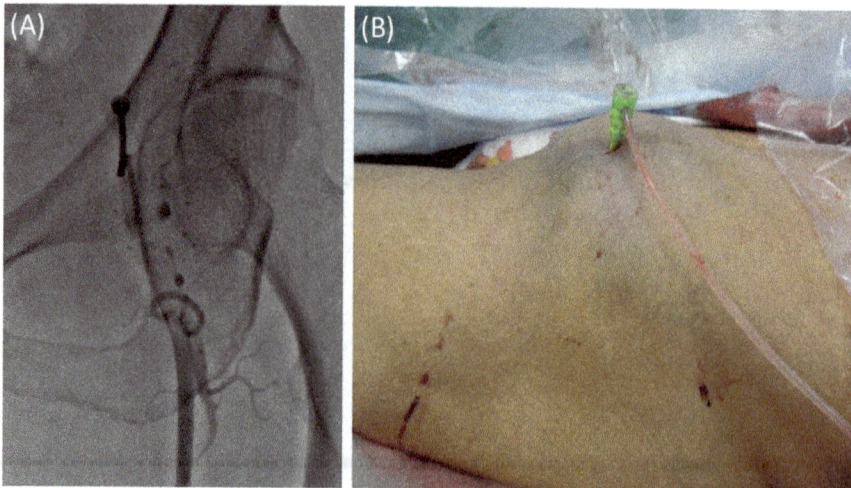

Figure 37. Sheath kinking during antegrade puncture. (A) Angle of puncture is more than 60° and almost vertical. After inserting sheath, observed sheath kinking. (B) 4Fr sheath replaced with 6Fr sheath and hematoma stabilized.

4. CO$_2$ angiography

The number of patients with chronic kidney disease (CKD) complicated with PAD is significantly increasing. In these patients, iodinated contrast may enhance the risk of contrast-induced nephropathy (CIN). CIN is an acute renal injury and may lead to irreversible loss of renal function. Carbon dioxide (CO$_2$) gas angiography is indicated for those with renal insufficiency and high-risk patients who are allergic to iodinated contrast material [7]. CO$_2$ is imaged using digital subtraction equipment with a CO$_2$ software program. Modern DSA equipment has a software program that allows integration of multiple images into a single composite image.

4.1. CO$_2$ delivery system

The system consists of a medical grade CO$_2$ gas cylinder with a regulator, a disposable sterile plastic tube with a bacteria-removal filter, and a 50-ml delivery syringe (**Figure 38**).

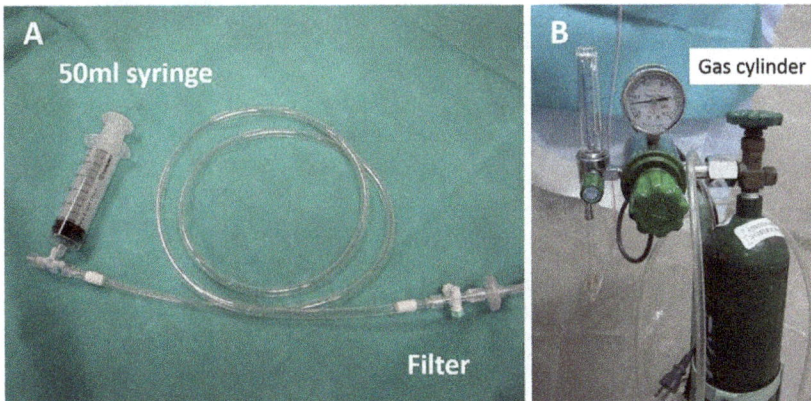

Figure 38. CO$_2$ delivery system. (A) A disposable, sterile plastic tube with a bacteria-removal filter and a 50-ml delivery syringe; (B) a medical grade CO$_2$ gas cylinder with a regulator.

Collection of CO$_2$ to the syringe and injection system should be separated to avoid erroneous gas injection to an artery (**Figure 39**).

The gas should be purged three to four times during collection to prevent room air contamination from the tube and delivery syringe in the circuit and then filled with gas at a stationary flow of 2 l/min. About 40 cc of aspirated gas was filled into the delivery syringe and 30–40 cm^3 of CO$_2$ gas was manually injected into the vessel leaving about 5 cm^3 in the injection syringe (**Figure 40**).

After gas injection, the remaining gas and blood were carefully aspirated into the syringe. Gas injections were spaced at least 30 s apart. Although we do not have experience in mechanical injection, manual injection is sufficient to inject 30–40 cc of CO$_2$. However, the safety of injecting large amounts of CO$_2$ is not guaranteed [8]. If a patient complains of abdominal pain, further CO$_2$ injection should be avoided. And if the angiogram shows a slow flow, further CO$_2$ delivery by syringe should also be stopped (**Table 3**).

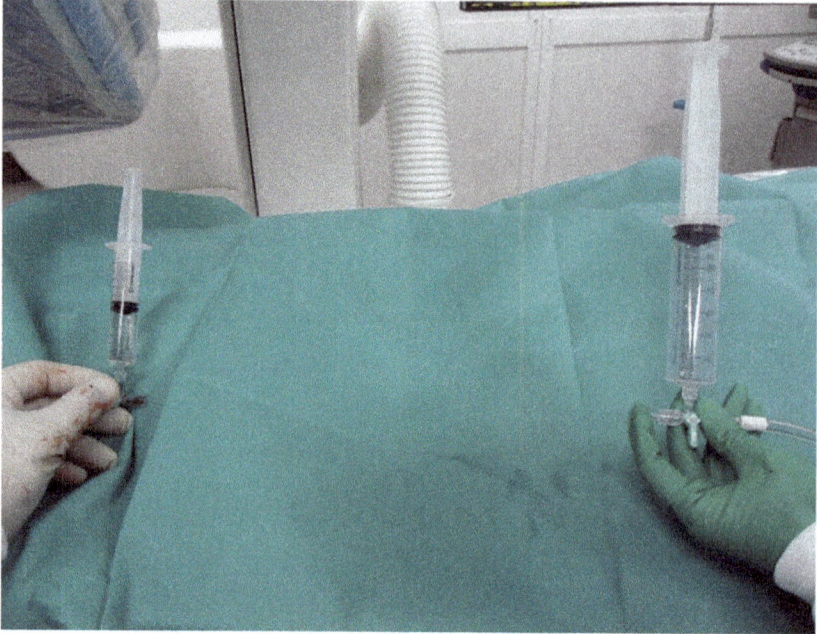

Figure 39. Separate system between CO_2 suction and injection. Collection of CO_2 to syringe (left) and injection system (right) should be separated to avoid erroneous gas injection to artery.

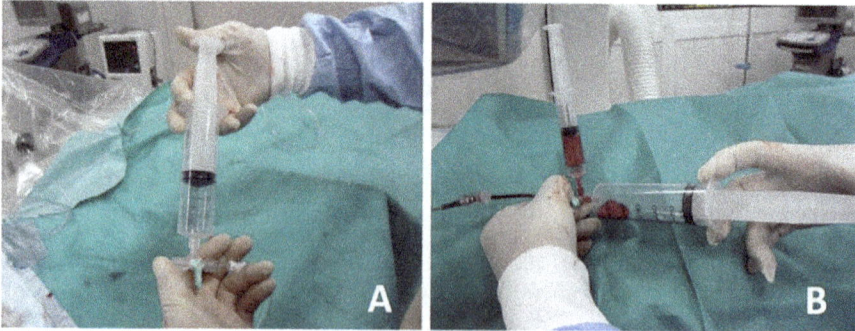

Figure 40. Infusion and injection of CO_2 gas by 50 cc syringe. (A) Gas was purged 3–4 times during collection to exclude room air contamination from the tube and delivery syringe in circuit. Filled with gas at a stationary flow of 2 l/min. (B) 40 cc of aspirated gas filled into delivery syringe, 30–40 cm^3 of CO_2 gas manually injected into the vessel, leaving about 5 cm^3 in the injection syringe.

4.2. Iliac artery angiography by CO_2

The iliac artery is a large sized vessel and its inflow is the larger abdominal aorta. Moreover, there are two internal iliac arteries and two femoral arteries. CO_2 angiography requires displacement of all or most of the blood to achieve adequate images. Due to such anatomical reasons, the iliac artery is not well suited for CO_2 angiography. In **Figure 41A**, CO_2 was administered from a 5Fr pigtail catheter at the terminal aorta and, in the left external iliac artery, CO_2 was unfilled and there appears to be stenosis. With contrast angiography, no stenotic lesion is seen in the left external iliac artery (**Figure 41B**).

- Make a separate system with CO_2 cylinder
- Average dose of CO_2 is about 30 ml by using 50 ml syringe
- Be sure complete air excretion
- Manual injection not a mechanical injection
- If patient complains of abdominal pain, avoid further injection
- When a slow flow are observed, avoid an further CO_2 injection

Table 3. Setup of CO_2 delivery system and CO_2 injection.

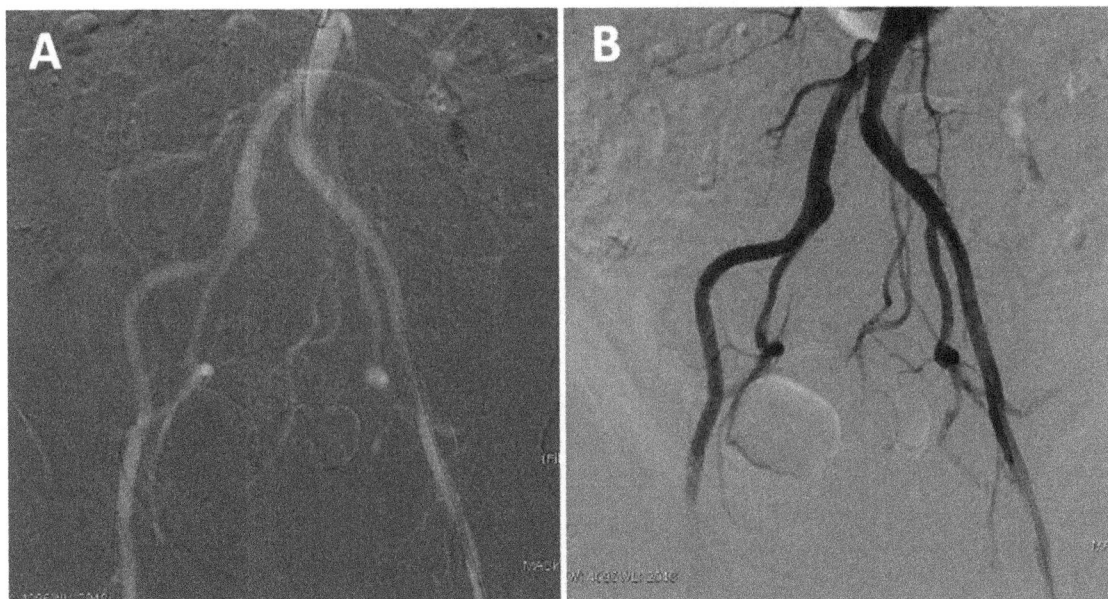

Figure 41. Iliac artery angiography by CO_2 and DSA. (A) CO_2 administered from 5Fr pigtail catheter at the terminal aorta, in left external iliac artery, CO_2 unfilled and stenosis suspected. (B) In DSA, no stenotic lesion in left external iliac artery observed.

In **Figure 42A**, total occlusion of the left external iliac artery is observed. CO_2 injection from the terminal aorta shows chronic total occlusion (CTO) of the left external iliac artery. To confirm CTO, a crossover sheath was positioned at the left common iliac artery and CO_2 injection was repeated at a right anterior oblique (RAO) projection of 30° (**Figure 42B**). In this angiogram, CTO is clearly visualized and the left common femoral artery is well observed via the collateral flow from the deep circumflex artery. In CO_2 angiography of the iliac artery, the angiogram is hampered by bowel and gas movements.

In **Figure 43A**, the left iliac artery is not seen, but contrast angiography shows a clear picture of the entire iliac arteries (**Figure 43B**).

Generally speaking, when the iliac artery is not well visualized by CO_2 angiography, increasing the volume of CO_2 in the iliac abdominal aorta might be considered. However, there are important visceral vessels and the risk of various complications due to the injection of gas in these vessels must also be considered.

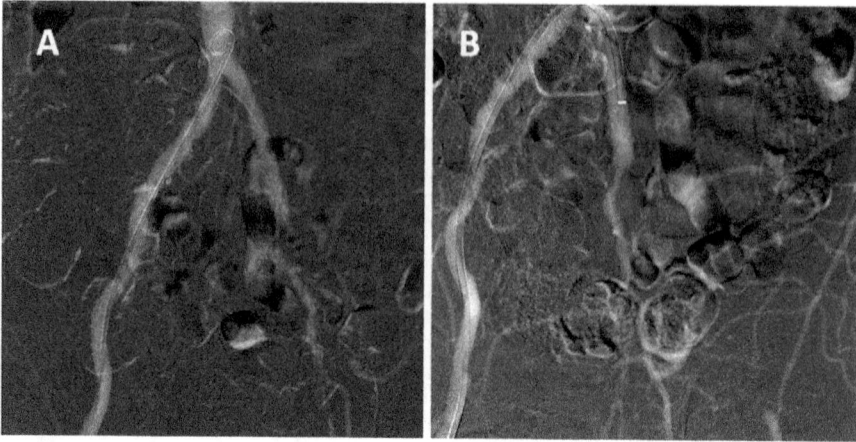

Figure 42. Left external iliac artery occlusion by CO_2 angiography. (A) CO_2 injection from terminal aorta in AP view. Total occlusion of left external iliac artery. (B) CO_2 injection from left common iliac artery by RAO 30.

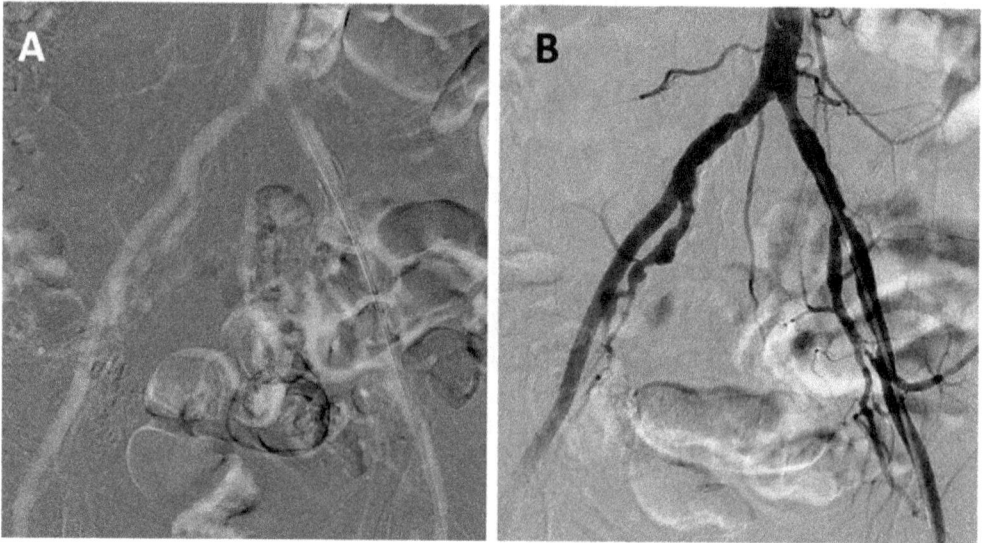

Figure 43. Bowel gas in iliac artery angiography. (A) In CO_2 angiography, left external iliac artery is hampered by bowel gas. (B) DSA shows a clear picture of whole iliac arteries.

4.3. Femoropopliteal artery angiography by CO_2

Visualization by CO_2 angiography is best suited for the femoropopliteal artery segment. The main reason is that the superficial femoral artery (SFA) is a straight vessel with small branches. The vessels sizes are about 4–7 mm and could easily be filled by CO_2 gas. In **Figure 44**, there are three kinds of SFA angiograms for the same patient. Digital angiography enabled visualization of the background (**Figure 44A**) while DSA could obtain the highest quality angiogram (**Figure 44B**). CO_2 angiography has poor visibility of small distal branches. However, it could visualize SFA fairly well and can be used as a substitute for contrast angiography (**Figure 44C**).

Similarly, the popliteal artery could be well observed even with the CO_2 angiogram (**Figure 45**).

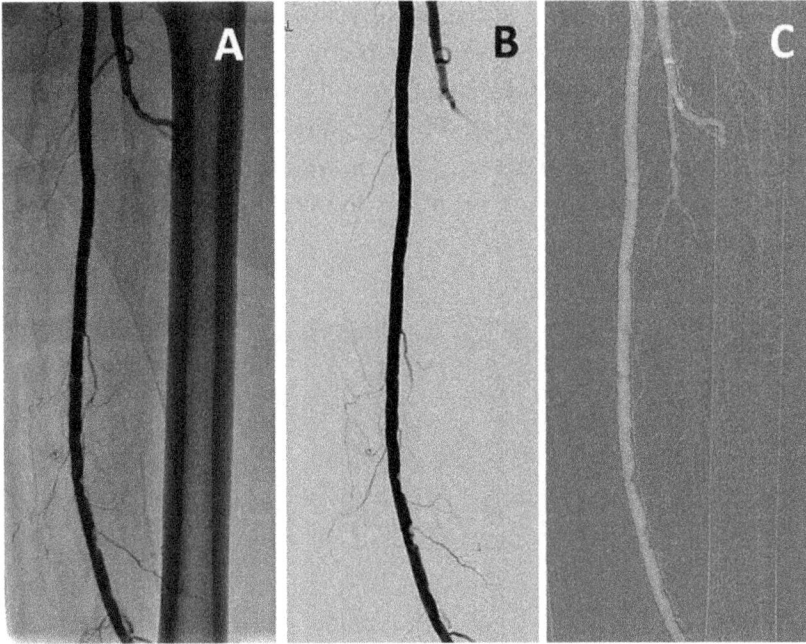

Figure 44. SFA angiography by digital, DSA and CO_2. (A) Digital angiography could visualize background to be used as reference. (B) DSA obtained most accurate image. (C) CO_2 angiography cannot replace digital angiography, but can be used as a substitute for contrast angiography.

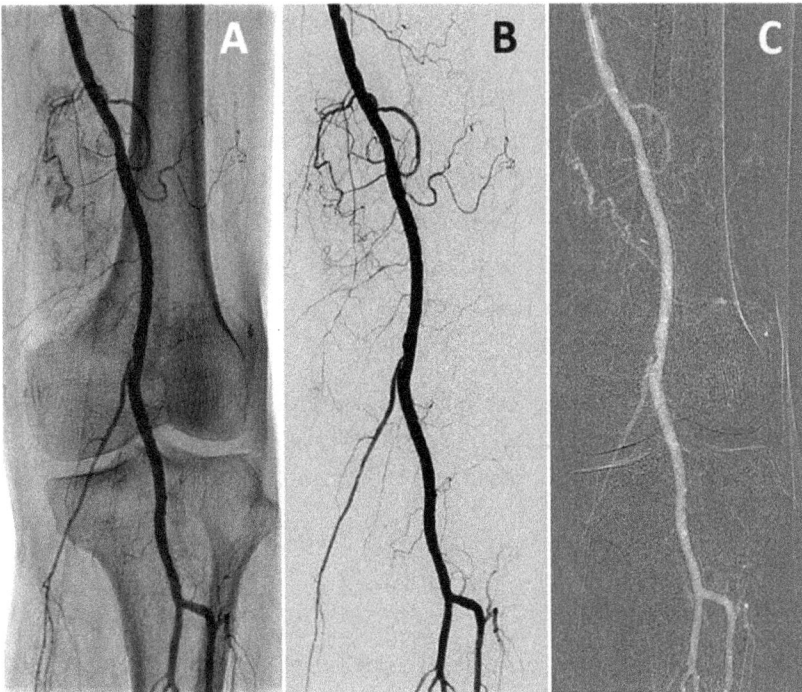

Figure 45. Popliteal artery angiography by digital, DSA and CO_2. (A) Digital angiography could visualize background to be used as reference. (B) DSA obtained most accurate image. (C) CO_2 angiography obtained similar image to DSA.

In the DA angiogram, distal SFA is not well visualized compared to the DSA image (**Figure 45A**). In fact, a perfect image was obtained by DSA (**Figure 45B**). The CO_2 angiogram shows a fairly clear picture of the distal SFA and popliteal artery (**Figure 45C**) while the right femoropopliteal artery was visualized by CO_2 (**Figure 46**). In proximal SFA, separation between the SFA and deep femoral artery (DFA) is well observed (**Figure 46A**). In the mid-SFA, no stenosis is seen (**Figure 46B**). In the distal SFA and popliteal artery, moderate stenosis is detected (**Figure 46C**).

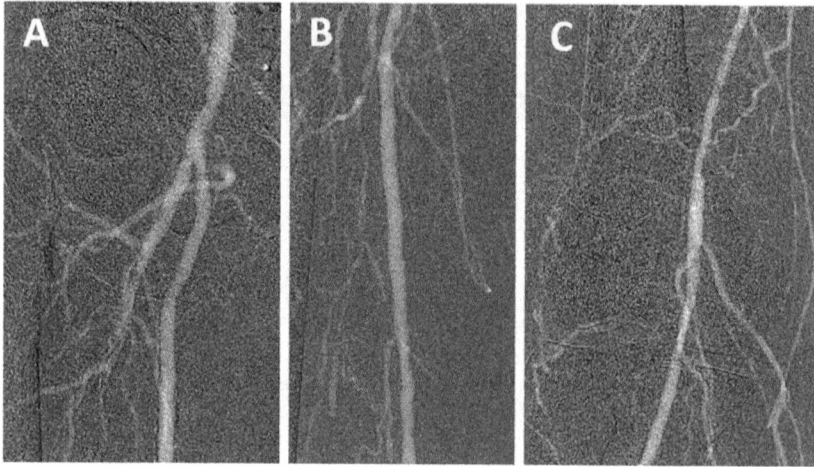

Figure 46. CO_2 angiography for right femoropopliteal artery. (A) In proximal SFA, separation between SFA and deep femoral artery (DFA) is well shown by RAO view. (B) In mid-SFA, there is no stenosis. (C) In distal SFA and the popliteal artery, there is moderate stenosis.

Comparisons between CO_2 angiography and digital angiography for the diseased SFA are shown in **Figures 47** and **48**. Stenosis is seen in the distal SFA in **Figure 47**. Both CO_2 (**Figure 47A**) and DA images (**Figure 47B**) could identify distal SFA stenosis.

The totally occluded left SFA was well visualized by CO_2 angiography (**Figure 48A**). Although DSA shows a clearer image with a rich collateral network (**Figure 48B**), the CO_2 image can also be used for interventional work.

The CTO of the left SFA was intervened using CO_2 angiography (**Figure 49**) in a patient with stage 4 CKD. The CO_2 angiogram showed typical CTO of the SFA (**Figure 49A**). After successful wiring, balloon angioplasty was performed (**Figure 49B**). Contrast was only used in the final angiogram (**Figure 49C**).

4.4. Below the knee angiography by CO_2

CO_2 angiography cannot be applied in below the knee (BK) work. The arterial vessel size below the knee is between 1.5 and 3 mm in diameter and the accuracy of CO_2 angiography is insufficient. Above all, in BK cases, most of the patients have critical limb ischemia and cannot tolerate large amounts of gas injection. In **Figure 50**, proximal right below the knee angiography was performed by CO_2 (**Figure 50A**) and DSA (**Figure 50B**). In the CO_2 angiogram, stenosis of the peroneal trunk could be seen; however, the right anterior tibial artery and posterior tibial artery are not well visualized when compared to DSA.

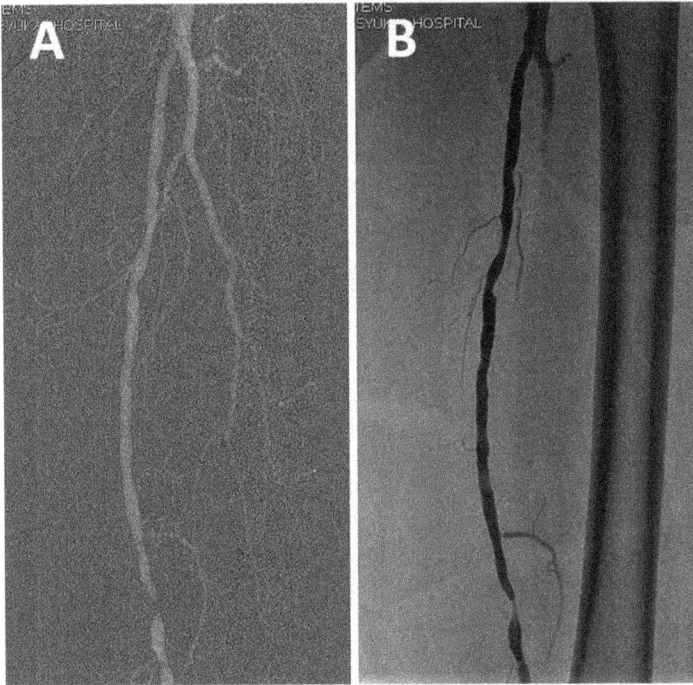

Figure 47. Left SFA stenosis by CO_2 and digital angiography. (A) CO_2 angiography shows moderate stenosis in mid SFA and tight stenosis in distal SFA. (B) Digital angiography confirmed these two lesions. Image quality is similar between CO_2 and digital angiography.

4.5. Problems of CO_2 angiography

CO2 angiography can be performed with minimal or no contrast media and can be used on CKD patients. However, CO2 angiography carries several potential risks (8). Gas delivery into the vessel is basically contraindicated. Moreover, erroneous injection of excessive volumes may result in catastrophic clinical consequences. There are many reports about transient lower limb pain and transient abdominal pain. Fujihara et al. have conducted a multi-center prospective CO_2 study and have reported that two patients (2%) developed CO_2-related non-occlusive mesenteric ischemia which resulted in death. These non-occlusive mesenteric ischemia cases were caused by the trapping of CO_2 gas in the celiac, superior and/or inferior mesenteric arteries [8]. The quality of CO_2 angiography is still not clear enough in the iliac artery and should not be employed in below the knee arteries. It should be used for the femoropopliteal artery although, even in the femoropopliteal artery, precise lesion evaluation may be difficult in some cases. Other complementary modalities such as surface echo, IVUs and/or pressure measuring should also be employed to confirm lesion severity (**Table 4**).

In treating claudication, safety is the first priority so that CO_2 use may be limited for most patients except those who have anaphylaxis to iodinated contrast media.

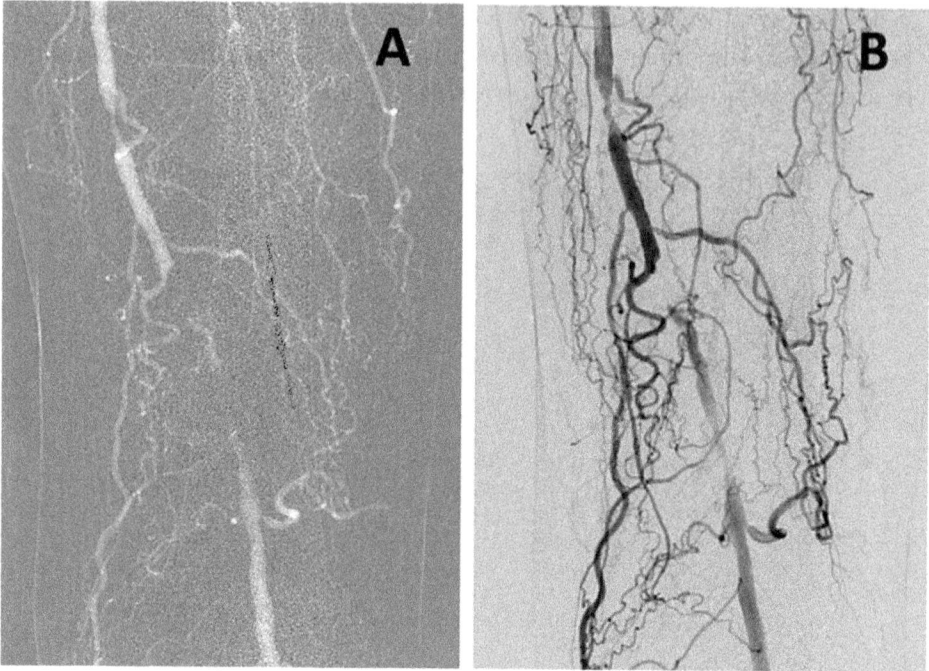

Figure 48. Left SFA occlusion by CO_2 and DSA. (A) CO_2 angiography shows totally occluded left SFA. (B) DSA shows clearer image with more collateral visualization.

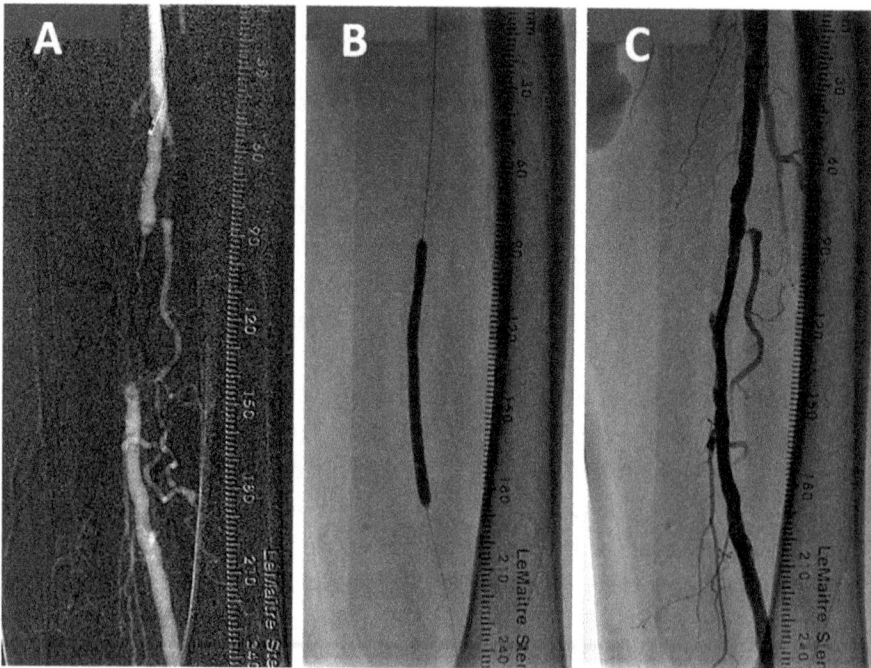

Figure 49. Left SFA CTO intervention by CO_2 angiography. (A) CO_2 angiography showed typical SFA CTO. (B) After wiring, balloon angioplasty was performed. (C) Contrast used only in final angiogram.

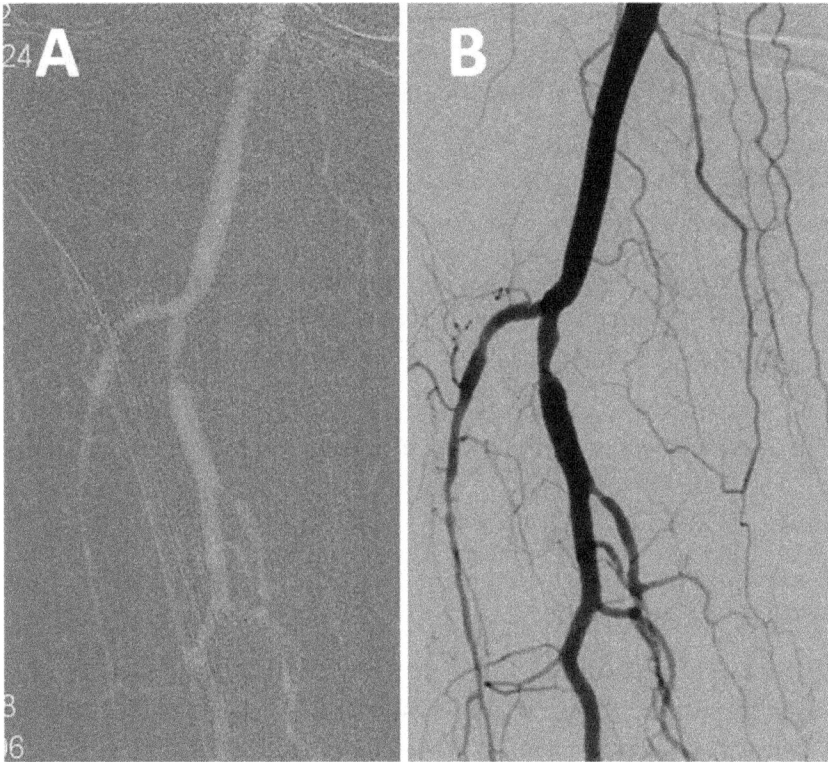

Figure 50. Below the knee angiography by CO_2 and DSA. (A) Proximal below the arteries by CO_2 angiography. Stenosis of peroneal trunk could be seen, otherwise, unable to identify right anterotibial and posterior tibial artery. (B) DSA shows detail of proximal below the knee arteries with small branches.

- Cause abdominal pain and leg pain
- Poor quality angiogram in iliac artery by bowel gas and movement
- Not applicable to below knee artery
- Rapid transition to venous circulation
- Risks of cerebral infarction
- Risk of nonobstructive mesenteric ischemia

Table 4. Problems of CO_2 angiography.

Author details

Yoshiaki Yokoi

Address all correspondence to: smtyokoi@gmail.com

Kishiwada Tokushukai Hospital, Osaka, Japan

References

[1] Grynne BH, Nossen JO, Bolstad B, Borch KW. Main results of the first comparative clinical studies on Visipaque. Acta Radiol Suppl. 1995;399:265–70.

[2] Nicola R, Shaqdan KW, Aran K, Mansouri M, Singh A, Abujudeh HH. Contrast-induced nephropathy: identifying the risks, choosing the right agent, and reviewing effective prevention and management methods. Curr Probl Diagn Radiol. 2015;44(6):501–4.

[3] Gedikoglu M, Oguzkurt L, Gur S, Andic C, Sariturk U, Ozkan C. Comparison of ultra-sound guidance with the traditional palpation and fluoroscopy method for the common femoral artery puncture. Catheter Cardiovasc Interv. 2013;82(7):1187–92

[4] Lo RC, Fokkema MT, Curran T, Darling J, Hamdan AD, Wyers M, Martin M, Schermerhorn ML. Routine use of ultrasound-guided access reduces access site-related complications after lower extremity percutaneous revascularization. J Vasc Surg. 2015;61(2):405–12.

[5] Fujihara M, Haramitsu Y, Ohshimo K, Yazu Y, Izumi E, Higashimori A, Yokoi Y. Appropriate hemostasis by routine use of ultrasound echo-guided transfemoral access and vascular closure devices after lower extremity percutaneous revascularization. Cardiovasc Interv Ther. 2016. [Epub ahead of print] PubMed PMID: 27430637.

[6] Cho KJ. Carbon dioxide angiography: scientific principles and practice. Vasc Specialist Int. 2015;31(3):67–80.

[7] Kawasaki D, Fujii K, Fukunaga M, Masutani M, Nakata A, Masuyama T. Safety and efficacy of endovascular therapy with a simple homemade carbon dioxide delivery system in patients with ileofemoral artery diseases. Circ J. 2012;76(7):1722–8.

[8] Fujihara M, Kawasaki D, Shintani Y, Fukunaga M, Nakama T, Koshida R, Higashimori A, Yokoi Y. Endovascular therapy by CO_2 angiography to prevent contrast-induced nephropathy in patients with chronic kidney disease: a prospective multicenter trial of CO_2 angiography registry. Catheter Cardiovasc Interv. 2015;85:870–7.

3

Genetics in Peripheral Artery Disease

Amir-Houshang Shemirani, Katalin Szilvia Zsóri,
András Jávor and Zoltán Csiki

Abstract

Besides traditional risk factor, it has been proved that genetics and gene–environment interaction have a possible independent role in the development and progression of peripheral arterial disease (PAD). Knowledge about such genetic factors will increases our understanding about pathophysiologic mechanisms of PAD and could facilitate the therapeutic approaches. Human genetics has gone through an advanced improvement and it increases our chance to acquire better diagnostic and therapeutic approaches. In this chapter, we try to provide an update on the genetics of PAD, which is mostly about genome-wide association studies, linkage analyses, heritability, candidate gene studies, and epigenetics. Finally, we discuss challenges and future developments of researches in PAD genetics.

Keywords: peripheral arterial disease, genetics, genome-wide association study, linkage analyses, heritability, candidate gene studies, epigenetics

1. Introduction

Common cause of PAD is atherosclerosis. Besides environmental risk factors (e.g., smoking, gender, age), some heritable risk factors are described for atherosclerosis. These are included hyperlipidemia, hypertension and diabetes mellitus. A reliable genetic marker could identify those individuals with PAD and accelerate their treatment. Besides, finding new genetic targets uncover new insights to the pathophysiology of PAD, and consequently new target for the cure. Earlier studies suggested heritability of PAD [1–4]. One study on monozygotic and dizygotic pairs revealed that with the similar environmental risk factors 48% variability of Ankle brachial Index (ABI) could be explained by additive genetic effects [2]. GENOA study

(Genetic Epidemiology Network of Arteriopathy) and the Framingham Offspring cohort study also found heritability in ABI variations [3, 4]. The degree of genetic variations on the PAD, regardless of the influences of other risk factors, remains to be revealed.

2. Genetic studies

Table 1 demonstrates comparisons between different genetic tests.

2.1. Linkage analysis

Genetic linkage analysis has the power to identify parts of genome that contain genes that could be inherited together. In this kind of genetic study, low resolution genome scanning investigates for genetic markers (microsatellites and Single nucleotide polymorphisms-SNPs) and that are pass to the next generation with the phenotype of interest. The results express in logarithm of the odds (LOD). Positive LOD indicates that co-segregation of two genetic markers is more likely, and negative LOD favors that likelihood less likely. It is advisable to consider LOD more than three statistically significant [5]. Next step is then to map neighboring region of the genome with tied association between genetic marker and phenotype.

Three studies demonstrated relation between different loci and PAD [3, 6]. First Gudmundsson and colleagues [6], identified a locus as "PAOD1" on chromosome 1p31 (LOD = 3.93; $p = 1.04 \times 10^{-5}$) conferring susceptibility to PAD even after nullifying the effects of diabetes mellitus, hypertension and hyperlipidemia. Interestingly, the genes responsible for PAOD1 did not identified which is not surprising based on the difficulties for analyzing genetic background of a complex disease such as PAD. Another study demonstrated the association of ankle-brachial index (ABI) with 250 microsatellite markers on chromosomes 1p, 6q, 7q, and 10p in 1310 African Americans and on chromosomes 3p and 3q in 796 non-Hispanic whites [3]. This study was also unable to demonstrate any evidence of linkage to the PAD trait.

Genetic test type	Advantages	Disadvantages
Single gene/panel gene sequencing	Cost; no off-target incidental findings	Low sensitivity
Oligonucleotide microarray	High resolution, good copy number detection	No detection of balanced rearrangements
Genome sequencing	Full coverage of DNA sequence	Cost, turnaround time, analytical challenges, inaccurate for SNPs with lower frequency
GWAS	novel marker finding	high participants number
Linkage	studying different areas across the genome, analyzing multiple genetic markers at the same time	It needs a high participants number with several affected generations, less helpful for complex disorders

Table 1. Comparison of different genetic tests for PAD genetics analysis.

Although, linkage analysis does not require specific candidate gene and scans full genome, it did not show promising results. That could be related to lack of large family pedigrees and polygenic nature of PAD. Linkage analysis cannot identify the genetic contributions arise from many genes each with small effect sizes.

2.2. Genome-wide association study

In this observational study, a genome-wide set of genetic variants (SNPs) can be screened in a large cohorts of patients. This approach determines the associations between SNPs and specific phenotype compared to control individuals. Unlike linkage analysis, GWAS has the ability to detect modest genotypic effects.

In one study rs10757278 SNP at 9p21 was found to be associated with PAD (OR = 1.14, p = 6.1 × 10^{-5}), but exclusion of known CAD cases from sample sets reduced the effect of this variant significantly (OR = 1.09, p = 0.075) [7]. Another similar study showed an association between 9p21 SNP (rs 1,333,049) with severity and prevalence of PAD [8]. A Japanese study on 785 PAD and 20,134 control individuals found rs9584669 in IPO5/RAP2A related protein 2A (OR = 0.58, p = 6.78 × 10^{-14}), rs6842241 in endothelin receptor type A (ENDRA gene; p = 5.32 × 10^{-9}), and rs2074633 in histone deacylase 9 (HDAC9 gene; p = 8.43 × 10^{-8}) loci with susceptibility to PAD [9]. Thorgeirsson et al. identified a common variant (rs1051730) in the nicotinic acetylcholine receptor gene cluster on chromosome 15q24 with higher risk for PAD (OR = 1.19, P = 1.4 × 10^{-7}) [10]. A GWAS study found rs7025486 at 9q33 associated with PAD (OR = 1.14, p = 3.9 × 10^{-5}) [11]. An investigation performed on 699 PAD and 1540 Japanese controls identified rs1902341-A to have a strong association with PAD (OR = 1.31, p = 4.7 × 10^{-7}) [12]. A recent meta-analysis with a total of 41,692 participants of European ancestry demonstrated that rs10757269 at 9p21 had the strongest association with ABI and achieved genome-wide significance (p = 2.46 × 10^{-8}) [13].

After above mentioned meta-analysis, one study investigated 537,872 SNPs in 1641 PAD and 1604 control individuals in The Electronic Medical Records and Genomics consortium (eMERGE)-based GWAS of PAD [14]. They revealed that rs653178 in the ATXN2-SH2B3 locus was significantly associated with PAD (OR = 1.22, p = 6.46 × 10^{-7}). Another outcome of this study was that neither loci was linked to PAD after investigation of prior known SNPs related to PAD. eMERGE analyses of PAD GEWAS results could not reveal any strong associations between SNPs and PAD by investigating of mitochondrial SNPs and haplogroups in 1652 PAD and 1629 control individuals [15].

2.3. Candidate gene studies

This kind of study focuses on differences in allele frequency of a known specific variant between cases and controls among unrelated individuals. With ability for finer mapping of the causal variant, association studies demonstrate greater power to detect modest genetic effects. Generally, search of insertions, deletions, and individual SNPs among cases and controls points out to genes to be associated with the development of atherosclerosis and changes in various vascular biology pathways such as lipid metabolism [16], hemostasis [17–21], homocysteine [22–24], inflammation [25, 26], angiotensin converting enzyme [27], leukocyte adhesion [28], platelet activation and aggregation [29, 30], endothelial function [31, 32], and smooth muscle cell migration. A recent meta-analysis of around 50,000 SNPs and across about 2100 genes found only three SNPs associated with ABI or PAD [33]. They demonstrated that rs2171209 in SYTL3 (p = 6.02 × 10^{-7}) (originally linked to lipoprotein (a)) and rs290481 in TCF7L2 (p = 7.01 × 10^{-7}) (linked to diabetes mellitus type 2) were significantly associated with ABI and CYP2B6 (p = 4.99 × 10^{-5}) (linked to smoking behavior) was associated to PAD.

2.4. Epigenetics

By definition, epigenetics is a science of long-lived or even hereditary modification of gene function without alteration of DNA sequence. In epigenetics, DNA could go through methylation, histone post-translational modifications, or microRNAs (miRNA), long non-coding RNA (lncRNA) mechanisms [34, 35]. miRNAs are small (≈22 nucleotides) single-stranded RNAs that inhibit translation of mRNA after binding to a target gene. Each miRNA can regulate several genes, because they do not require 100% base pair match. lncRNAs defined as more than 200 nucleotide long transcripts with function other than translation to protein.

Epigenetic changes have been described in association with some PAD risk factors [36, 37]. Hyperhomocysteinemia induces DNA methylation and could contribute to development and progression of PAD [36]. DNA hypomethylation caused by smoking has been reported [37].

Most of the epigenetic studies relevant to PAD are currently about miRNAs. There are two approaches to explore the role of miRNA in PAD. They have involved either a small number of candidate intracellular miRNA which are known for their role in vascular diseases or the measure of a large cluster of miRNAs by microarrays. A miRNA SYBR Green Real-Time PCR assessed the alteration of miR-130a, miR-27b and miR-210 expression in PAD [38]. A whole-genome miRNA transcriptome profiling revealed downregulation of 12 miRNAs in PAD compared to controls [39]. Later, the same research group detected significant down-regulation of miR-15a, miR-196b, and let-7e and upregulation of miR-411 in 40 PAD and 40 control individuals [40].

Alterations in mitochondrial DNA (mtDNA) were proposed as a pathway for myopathy in PAD [41]. Mitochondrial dysfunction could be as a result of bouts of ischemia in these patients which causes damage to mitochondrion (mitochodriopathy).

2.5. Whole genome/exome sequencing

While massively parallel sequencing has not been performed on PAD patients specifically, some results from researches on atherosclerosis could be attributed to PAD. In one study, exonic regions of two persons with the early atherosclerosis were sequenced with next gen-eration sequencing platform, and they revealed a rare missense mutation (Scr818Cys) in

INO80D, a subunit of the human INO80 chromatin remodeling complex [42]. INO80 complex is involved in cardiovascular physiology and development [43]. Another study repeated this result in two patients with aortic hypoplasia, diffuse atherosclerosis, and PAD.

2.6. Mendelian randomization

This epidemiologic study design incorporates genetic results into epidemiologic methods. Mendelian randomization studies offer evidence for causal relations between risk factors and disease outcome.

Mendelian randomization has been used to examine the relations between polymorphisms of specific genes and the prevalence of coronary heart disease or myocardial infarction [44]. Recently, it is demonstrated that each standard deviation (SD, 2.76 points) increase in body mass index (BMI)-composite genetic risk score was associated with 0.43 in BMI and an odds ratio for PAD of 1.17 [45].

3. Discussion

As multiple atherogenic pathways are involved in the pathophysiology of PAD, a profound monogenic effect is unlikely [46]. Environmental influences such as age, smoking, sport, ethnicity, and diabetes mellitus status besides genetic effects could vary the outcome for this disease. GWAS results are not comprehensive. It could be due to modest effect of susceptible variants. To power GWAS analysis, large sample sizes are needed. GWAS results so far revealed limited results. Two linkage studies did not demonstrate breakthrough to identify significant mechanisms behind inheritance of PAD. SNPs association studies have provided weak and/or conflicting findings results. Next generation sequencing and epigenetics seem to provide some promising future. Whole-genome or exome sequencing or NGS-based RNA-sequencing has identified new causative links between new genes and PAD. It is imperative to merge deep sequencing data of the DNA findings with epigenetic data to find more interesting results. This is challenging as these methods produce huge amount of data to analyze. Environmental-Wide Association Study demonstrates gene-by-environment interactions. This new method to study inter-relation between environment and genomics was a topic in ascertaining causality in type II diabetes mellitus [47]. They showed that the pesticide heptachlor epoxide was associated with type II diabetes mellitus. This new method has some places in gene-environment studies in PAD.

In the future, we may apply personalized medicine on the basis of genetic analysis and treat the patient by specific therapeutic agents.

Author details

Amir-Houshang Shemirani[1]*, Katalin Szilvia Zsóri[1], András Jávor[2] and Zoltán Csiki[3]

*Address all correspondence to: shemirani1@gmail.com

1 Faculty of Medicine, Clinical Laboratory Research Division, Laboratory Medicine, University of Debrecen, Debrecen, Hungary

2 Debrecen University, Debrecen, Hungary

3 Faculty of Medicine, Institute of Internal Medicine, University of Debrecen, Debrecen, Hungary

References

[1] Allison MA, Criqui MH, McClelland RL, Scott JM, McDermott MM, Liu K, et al. The effect of novel cardiovascular risk factors on the ethnic-specific odds for peripheral arterial disease in the multi-ethnic study of atherosclerosis (MESA). Journal of the American College of Cardiology. 2006;**48**:1190-1197. DOI: 10.1016/j.jacc.2006.05.049

[2] Carmelli D, Fabsitz RR, Swan GE, Reed T, Miller B, Wolf PA. Contribution of genetic and environmental influences to ankle-brachial blood pressure index in the NHLBI twin study. American Journal of Epidemiology. 2000;**151**:452-458. DOI: 10.1093/oxfordjournals.aje.a010230

[3] Kullo IJ, Turner ST, Kardia SL, Mosley Jr TH, Boerwinkle E, de Andrade M. A genome-wide linkage scan for ankle-brachial index in African American and non-Hispanic white subjects participating in the GENOA study. Atherosclerosis. 2006;**187**:433-438. DOI: 10.1016/j.atherosclerosis.2005.10.003

[4] Murabito JM, Guo CY, Fox CS, D'Agostino RB. Heritability of the ankle-brachial index: The Framingham offspring study. American Journal of Epidemiology. 2006;**164**:963-968. DOI: 10.1093/aje/kwj295

[5] Lander E, Kruglyak L. Genetic dissection of complex traits: Guidelines for interpreting and reporting linkage results. Nature Genetics. 1995;**11**:241-247. DOI: 10.1038/ng1195-241

[6] Gudmundsson G, Matthiasson SE, Arason H, Johannsson H, Runarsson F, Bjarnason H, et al. Localization of a gene for peripheral arterial occlusive disease to chromosome 1p31. American Journal of Human Genetics. 2002;**70**:586-592. DOI: 10.1086/339251

[7] Helgadottir A, Thorleifsson G, Magnusson KP, Gretarsdottir S, Steinthorsdottir V, Manolescu A, et al. The same sequence variant on 9p21 associates with myocardial infarction, abdominal aortic aneurysm and intracranial aneurysm. Nature Genetics. 2008;**40**:217-224. DOI: 10.1038/ng.72

[8] Cluett C, McDermott MM, Guralnik J, Ferrucci L, Bandinelli S, Miljkovic I, et al. The 9p21 myocardial infarction risk allele increases risk of peripheral artery disease in older people.

Circulation. Cardiovascular Genetics. 2009;**2**:347-353. DOI: 10.1161/CIRCGENETICS. 108.825935

[9] Matsukura M, Ozaki K, Takahashi A, Onouchi Y, Morizono T, Komai H, et al. Genome-wide association study of peripheral arterial disease in a Japanese population. PLoS One. 2015;**10**:e0139262. DOI: 10.1371/journal.pone.0139262

[10] Thorgeirsson TE, Geller F, Sulem P, Rafnar T, Wiste A, Magnusson KP, et al. A variant associated with nicotine dependence, lung cancer and peripheral arterial disease. Nature. 2008;**452**:638-642. DOI: 10.1038/nature06846

[11] Gretarsdottir S, Baas AF, Thorleifsson G, Holm H, den Heijer M, de Vries JP, et al. Genome-wide association study identifies a sequence variant within the DAB2IP gene conferring susceptibility to abdominal aortic aneurysm. Nature Genetics. 2010;**42**:692-697. DOI: 10.1038/ng.622

[12] Koriyama H, Nakagami H, Katsuya T, Sugimoto K, Yamashita H, Takami Y, et al. Identification of evidence suggestive of an association with peripheral arterial disease at the OSBPL10 locus by genome-wide investigation in the Japanese population. Journal of Atherosclerosis and Thrombosis. 2010;**17**:1054-1062

[13] Murabito JM, White CC, Kavousi M, Sun YV, Feitosa MF, Nambi V, et al. Association between chromosome 9p21 variants and the ankle-brachial index identified by a meta-analysis of 21 genome-wide association studies. Circulation. Cardiovascular Genetics. 2012;**5**:100-112. DOI: 10.1161/CIRCGENETICS.111.961292

[14] Kullo IJ, Shameer K, Jouni H, Lesnick TG, Pathak J, Chute CG, et al. The ATXN2-SH2B3 locus is associated with peripheral arterial disease: An electronic medical record-based genome-wide association study. Frontiers in Genetics. 2014;**5**(166). DOI: 10.3389/fgene. 2014.00166

[15] Abrantes P, Rosa A, Francisco V, Sousa I, Xavier JM, Oliveira SA. Mitochondrial genome association study with peripheral arterial disease and venous thromboembolism. Atherosclerosis. 2016;**252**:97-105. DOI: 10.1016/j.atherosclerosis.2016.07.920

[16] Resnick HE, Rodriguez B, Havlik R, Ferrucci L, Foley D, Curb JD, et al. Apo E genotype, diabetes, and peripheral arterial disease in older men: The Honolulu Asia-aging study. Genetic Epidemiology. 2000;**19**:52-63. DOI: 10.1002/1098-2272(200007)19:1<52:: AID-GEPI4>3.0.CO;2-M

[17] Vazquez F, Rodger M, Carrier M, Le Gal G, Reny JL, Sofi F, et al. Prothrombin G20210A mutation and lower extremity peripheral arterial disease: A systematic review and meta-analysis. European Journal of Vascular and Endovascular Surgery. 2015;**50**:232-240. DOI: 10.1016/j.ejvs.2015.04.033

[18] Bayoglu B, Arslan C, Tel C, Ulutin T, Dirican A, Deser SB, et al. Genetic variants rs1994016 and rs3825807 in ADAMTS7 affect its mRNA expression in atherosclerotic occlusive peripheral arterial disease. Journal of Clinical Laboratory Analysis. 2017. DOI: 10.1002/ jcla.22174

[19] Renner W, Koppel H, Brodmann M, Pabst E, Schallmoser K, Toplak H, et al. Factor II G20210A and factor V G1691A gene mutations and peripheral arterial occlusive disease. Thrombosis and Haemostasis. 2000;**83**:20-22

[20] Lee AJ, Fowkes FG, Lowe GD, Connor JM, Rumley A. Fibrinogen, factor VII and PAI-1 genotypes and the risk of coronary and peripheral atherosclerosis: Edinburgh artery study. Thrombosis and Haemostasis. 1999;**81**:553-560

[21] Fowkes FG, Connor JM, Smith FB, Wood J, Donnan PT, Lowe GD. Fibrinogen genotype and risk of peripheral atherosclerosis. Lancet. 1992;**339**:693-696

[22] Sabino A, Fernandes AP, Lima LM, Ribeiro DD, Sousa MO, de Castro Santos ME, et al. Polymorphism in the methylenetetrahydrofolate reductase (C677T) gene and homocysteine levels: A comparison in Brazilian patients with coronary arterial disease, ischemic stroke and peripheral arterial obstructive disease. Journal of Thrombosis and Thrombolysis. 2009;**27**:82-87. DOI: 10.1007/s11239-007-0172-z

[23] Sofi F, Lari B, Rogolino A, Marcucci R, Pratesi G, Dorigo W, et al. Thrombophilic risk factors for symptomatic peripheral arterial disease. Journal of Vascular Surgery. 2005;**41**:255-260. DOI: 10.1016/j.jvs.2004.11.015

[24] Todesco L, Angst C, Litynski P, Loehrer F, Fowler B, Haefeli WE. Methylenetetrahydrofolate reductase polymorphism, plasma homocysteine and age. European Journal of Clinical Investigation. 1999;**29**:1003-1009

[25] Pola R, Flex A, Gaetani E, Flore R, Serricchio M, Pola P. Synergistic effect of –174 G/C polymorphism of the interleukin-6 gene promoter and 469 E/K polymorphism of the intercellular adhesion molecule-1 gene in Italian patients with history of ischemic stroke. Stroke. 2003;**34**:881-885. DOI: 10.1161/01.STR.0000062346.70983.DF

[26] Cesari M, Penninx BW, Newman AB, Kritchevsky SB, Nicklas BJ, Sutton-Tyrrell K, et al. Inflammatory markers and onset of cardiovascular events: Results from the health ABC study. Circulation. 2003;**108**:2317-2322. DOI: 10.1161/01.CIR.0000097109.90783.FC

[27] Renner W, Pabst E, Paulweber B, Malaimare L, Iglseder B, Wascher TC, et al. The angiotensin-converting-enzyme insertion/deletion polymorphism is not a risk factor for peripheral arterial disease. Atherosclerosis. 2002;**165**:175-178

[28] Brevetti G, Schiano V, Chiariello M. Cellular adhesion molecules and peripheral arterial disease. Vascular Medicine. 2006;**11**:39-47. DOI: 10.1191/1358863x06vm645ra

[29] Cassar K, Bachoo P, Ford I, Greaves M, Brittenden J. Platelet activation is increased in peripheral arterial disease. Journal of Vascular Surgery. 2003;**38**:99-103

[30] Fontana P, Gaussem P, Aiach M, Fiessinger JN, Emmerich J, Reny JL. P2Y12 H2 haplotype is associated with peripheral arterial disease: A case-control study. Circulation. 2003;**108**:2971-2973. DOI: 10.1161/01.CIR.0000106904.80795.35

[31] Flex A, Gaetani E, Angelini F, Sabusco A, Chilla C, Straface G, et al. Pro-inflammatory genetic profiles in subjects with peripheral arterial occlusive disease and critical limb ischemia. Journal of Internal Medicine. 2007;**262**:124-130. DOI: 10.1111/j.1365-2796.2007.01791.x

[32] Fatini C, Sticchi E, Sofi F, Said AA, Pratesi G, Pulli R, et al. Multilocus analysis in candidate genes ACE, AGT, and AGTR1 and predisposition to peripheral arterial disease: Role of ACE D/−240T haplotype. Journal of Vascular Surgery. 2009;**50**:1399-1404. DOI: 10.1016/j.jvs.2009.07.075

[33] Wassel CL, Lamina C, Nambi V, Coassin S, Mukamal KJ, Ganesh SK, et al. Genetic determinants of the ankle-brachial index: A meta-analysis of a cardiovascular candidate gene 50K SNP panel in the candidate gene association resource (CARe) consortium. Atherosclerosis. 2012;**222**:138-147. DOI: 10.1016/j.atherosclerosis.2012.01.039

[34] Allis CD, Jenuwein T. The molecular hallmarks of epigenetic control. Nature Reviews Genetics. 2016;**17**:487-500. DOI: 10.1038/nrg.2016.59

[35] Man HS, Yan MS, Lee JJ, Marsden PA. Epigenetic determinants of cardiovascular gene expression: Vascular endothelium. Epigenomics. 2016;**8**:959-979. DOI: 10.2217/epi-2016-0012

[36] Krishna SM, Dear A, Craig JM, Norman PE, Golledge J. The potential role of homocysteine mediated DNA methylation and associated epigenetic changes in abdominal aortic aneurysm formation. Atherosclerosis. 2013;**228**:295-305. DOI: 10.1016/j.atherosclerosis.2013.02.019

[37] Tsaprouni LG, Yang TP, Bell J, Dick KJ, Kanoni S, Nisbet J, et al. Cigarette smoking reduces DNA methylation levels at multiple genomic loci but the effect is partially reversible upon cessation. Epigenetics. 2014;**9**:1382-1396. DOI: 10.4161/15592294.2014.969637

[38] Li T, Cao H, Zhuang J, Wan J, Guan M, Yu B, et al. Identification of miR-130a, miR-27b and miR-210 as serum biomarkers for atherosclerosis obliterans. Clinica Chimica Acta. 2011;**412**:66-70. DOI: 10.1016/j.cca.2010.09.029

[39] Stather PW, Sylvius N, Wild JB, Choke E, Sayers RD, Bown MJ. Differential microRNA expression profiles in peripheral arterial disease. Circulation. Cardiovascular Genetics. 2013;**6**:490-497. DOI: 10.1161/CIRCGENETICS.111.000053

[40] Stather PW, Sylvius N, Sidloff DA, Dattani N, Verissimo A, Wild JB, et al. Identification of microRNAs associated with abdominal aortic aneurysms and peripheral arterial disease. The British Journal of Surgery. 2015;**102**:755-766. DOI: 10.1002/bjs.9802

[41] Pipinos II, Swanson SA, Zhu Z, Nella AA, Weiss DJ, Gutti TL, et al. Chronically ischemic mouse skeletal muscle exhibits myopathy in association with mitochondrial dysfunction and oxidative damage. American Journal of Physiology. Regulatory, Integrative and Comparative Physiology. 2008;**295**:R290-R296. DOI: 10.1152/ajpregu.90374.2008

[42] Shameer K, Klee EW, Dalenberg AK, Kullo IJ. Whole exome sequencing implicates an INO80D mutation in a syndrome of aortic hypoplasia, premature atherosclerosis, and arterial stiffness. Circulation. Cardiovascular Genetics. 2014;7:607-614. DOI: 10.1161/CIRCGENETICS.113.000233

[43] Han P, Hang CT, Yang J, Chang CP. Chromatin remodeling in cardiovascular development and physiology. Circulation Research. 2011;108:378-396. DOI: 10.1161/CIRCRESAHA.110.224287

[44] Yamada Y, Ichihara S, Nishida T. Molecular genetics of myocardial infarction. Genomic Medicine. 2008;2:7-22. DOI: 10.1007/s11568-008-9025-x

[45] Huang Y, Xu M, Xie L, Wang T, Huang X, Lv X, et al. Obesity and peripheral arterial disease: A Mendelian randomization analysis. Atherosclerosis. 2016;247:218-224. DOI: 10.1016/j.atherosclerosis.2015.12.034

[46] Lusis AJ, Mar R, Pajukanta P. Genetics of atherosclerosis. Annual Review of Genomics and Human Genetics. 2004;5:189-218. DOI: 10.1146/annurev.genom.5.061903.175930

[47] Patel CJ, Bhattacharya J, Butte AJ. An environment-wide association study (EWAS) on type 2 diabetes mellitus. PLoS One. 2010;5:e10746. DOI: 10.1371/journal.pone.0010746

4

Nonatherosclerotic Peripheral Artery Disease

Osami Kawarada

Abstract

Nonatherosclerotic peripheral artery disease (NAPAD) remains underappreciated compared to atherosclerotic peripheral artery disease. However, under- or misdiagnosis of NAPAD can potentially lead to serious adverse outcomes. There is a broad spectrum of disorders including vasculitis, thrombophilia, and other vascular anatomical or functional disorders in the context of NAPAD. This section briefly overviews vascular imaging, mainly invasive angiography, to optimize the management of NAPAD.

Keywords: awareness, nonatherosclerosis, peripheral artery disease

1. Introduction

Nonatherosclerotic peripheral artery disease (NAPAD) remains underappreciated compared to atherosclerotic peripheral artery disease (APAD) due to its low prevalence. Despite common symptoms such as claudication, rest pain, and tissue loss, most clinicians are unfamiliar with the diagnosis of NAPAD. NAPAD should be suspected clinically in younger patients, and in older patients with few atherosclerotic risk factors, few atherosclerotic features, or unusual lesion distributions. There is a broad spectrum of pathophysiologies in NAPAD, with the most common being arterial wall abnormalities, abnormal external and internal forces, spasm, vasculitis, and thrombophilia [1]. Under- or misdiagnosis of NAPAD can lead to serious adverse outcomes that, with awareness of its distinctive symptoms and signs, may be avoided or minimized [2–5]. Thus, this section briefly overviews vascular imaging, mainly invasive angiography, to optimize the management of NAPAD.

2. Workup for differential diagnosis

When there is a high clinical index of suspicion of NAPAD, the combination of blood examination (biochemical and serological tests) and vascular imaging is an integral part of the differential diagnosis process (**Figure 1**).

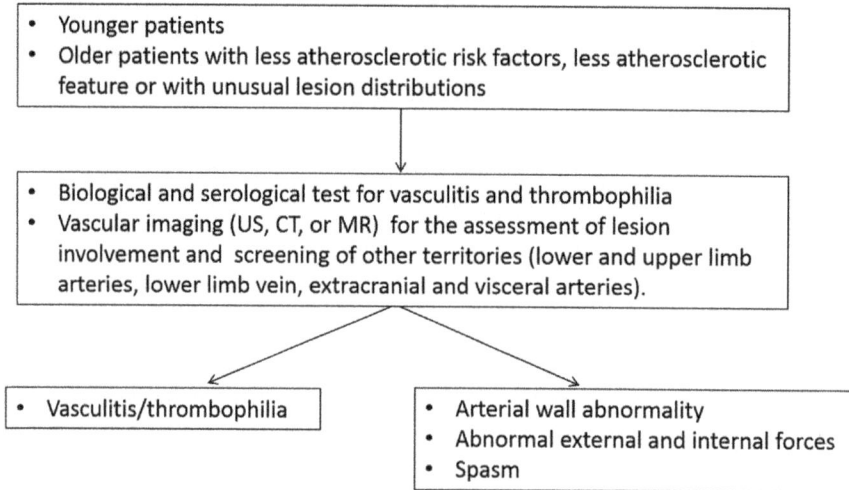

```
┌─────────────────────────────────────────────────────────────────┐
│ • Younger patients                                                │
│ • Older patients with less atherosclerotic risk factors, less     │
│   atherosclerotic feature or with unusual lesion distributions    │
└─────────────────────────────────────────────────────────────────┘
                              │
                              ▼
┌─────────────────────────────────────────────────────────────────┐
│ • Biological and serological test for vasculitis and thrombophilia│
│ • Vascular imaging (US, CT, or MR) for the assessment of lesion   │
│   involvement and screening of other territories (lower and upper │
│   limb arteries, lower limb vein, extracranial and visceral       │
│   arteries).                                                      │
└─────────────────────────────────────────────────────────────────┘
             ↙                                 ↘
┌────────────────────────────┐   ┌──────────────────────────────────┐
│ • Vasculitis/thrombophilia │   │ • Arterial wall abnormality        │
└────────────────────────────┘   │ • Abnormal external and internal   │
                                  │   forces                           │
                                  │ • Spasm                            │
                                  └──────────────────────────────────┘
```

Figure 1. Approach to diagnosis of nonatherosclerotic peripheral artery disease.

In combination with vascular imaging, the assessment of macrocirculation by the ankle-brachial index is important. Furthermore, in regard to microcirculation assessment, either skin perfusion pressure (SPP) or transcutaneous oxygen pressure (TcPO$_2$) can be applied in patients with critically ischemic limbs. Limb ischemia in younger patients warrants a high clinical suspicion of NAPAD. Even in older patients, most cases of NAPAD may be underdiagnosed or misinterpreted as an atherosclerotic condition.

3. Arterial wall abnormalities

3.1. Fibromuscular dysplasia

Fibromuscular dysplasia (FMD) is a noninflammatory disease that produces arterial narrowing, aneurysms, dissection, and occlusion. Although the cause is unknown, 90% of cases occur in females [6], most frequently in the renal and carotid arteries, followed by the mesenteric artery. Although lower extremity arteries are less commonly affected, FMD is one of the most significant causes of NAPAD [4, 7]. Pathologically, FMD can mainly be classified into three types, that is, intimal, medial, and perimedial. Angiographic classification identifies the multifocal type with multiple stenoses and the so-called "string-of-beads" appearance, the tubular type, and the focal type. The "string-of-beads" sign that is frequently associated with the medial type is the most indicative of FMD, while the tubular and focal types may mimic atherosclerotic lesions [8] (**Figure 2**).

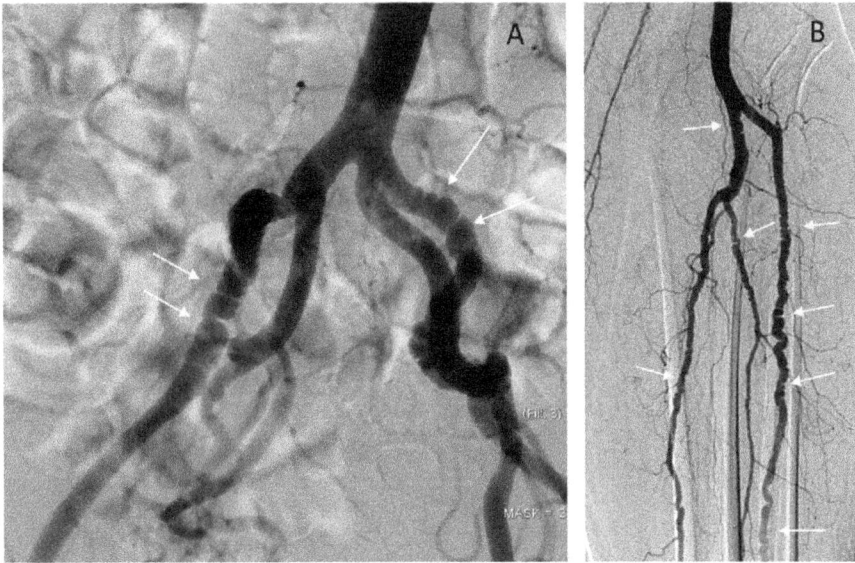

Figure 2. Fibromuscular dysplasia. (A) String-of-beads appearance in bilateral external iliac arteries (arrows). (B) Multiple string-of-beads appearances in the left crural artery (arrows).

There are isolated reports of FMD mimicking vasculitis such as polyarteritis nodosa, Takayasu's arteritis (TA), and other disorders such as Ehlers-Danlos's syndrome, Alport's syndrome, and pheochromocytoma [9].

3.2. Adventitial cystic disease

Adventitial cystic disease is characterized by a collection of mucin in the adventitial layer, typically in the popliteal artery. In rare cases, the external iliac artery or femoral artery can be affected. This disorder is typically observed in middle-aged persons, with a male-to-female ratio of 5–15:1 [4, 10]. Duplex ultrasound is considered a reasonable first-line method to diagnose adventitial cystic disease. Although stenotic lesions may develop into occlusion, the angiographic findings show a smooth, eccentric, and extrinsically narrowed appearance (**Figure 3**).

3.3. Midaortic syndrome

Coarctation of the aorta is mostly located just distal to ligament arteriosum. Midaortic syndrome (MAS) is a rare condition characterized by coarctation of the abdominal aorta or distal descending thoracic aorta and thought to arise from an embryonic development disorder [2]. It is essential to differentiate MAS such as involvement of the abdominal aorta from other causes in large-vessel vasculitis. In addition to idiopathic MAS, the association of MAS with neurofibromatosis, FMD, mucopolysaccharidosis, Alagille syndrome, and William's syndrome could be a genetic etiology. Others include tuberous sclerosis, retroperitoneal fibrosis, moyamoya disease, congenital rubella syndrome, epidermal nevus syndrome, and autosomal dominant supravalvar aortic stenosis syndrome [11, 12]. The most common anatomic type of MAS is suprarenal (60%), followed by intrarenal (25%) and infrarenal (15%) (**Figure 4**).

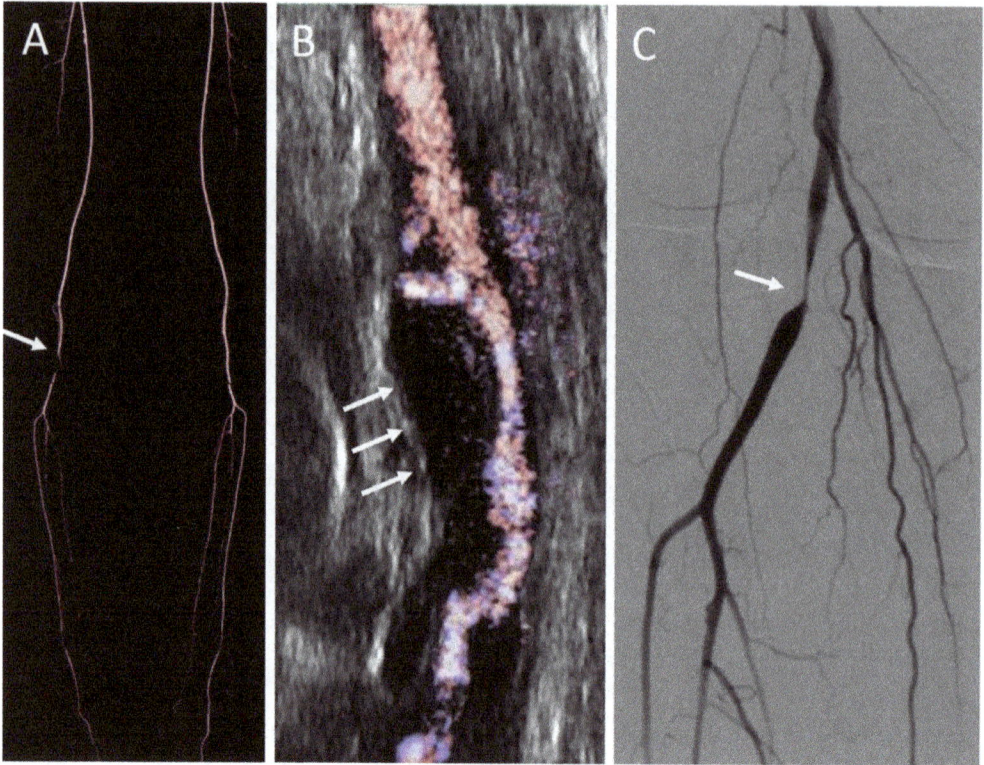

Figure 3. Adventitial cystic disease. (A) A 70-year-old male presenting moderate claudication. Enhanced CT shows focal stenosis in the midsegment of the right popliteal artery (arrow). (B) Ultrasonography revealed a low-echoic cystic lesion along the vessel wall causing significant stenosis in the popliteal artery (arrows). (C) Angiography could confirm focal stenosis in the right popliteal artery (arrow).

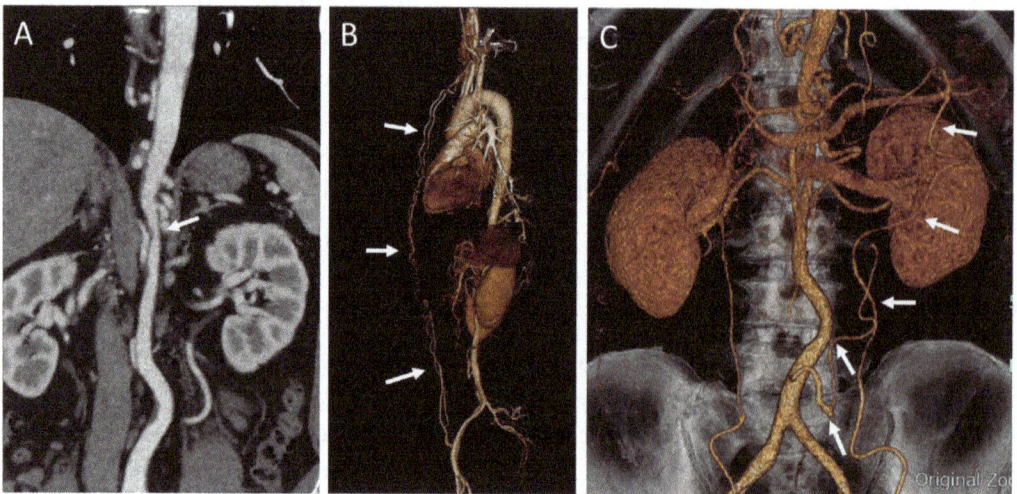

Figure 4. Idiopathic midaortic syndrome. A 51-year-old male presenting renovascular hypertension. Although the ABI was 0.70/0.67 (right/left), intermittent claudication was absent. (A) Enhanced CT showing suprarenal abdominal aortic coarctation below the origin of the superior mesenteric artery (arrow). (B) Lateral view demonstrates Winslow's pathway which is a collateral vessel developing from the subclavian arteries, internal thoracic (mammary) arteries, superior epigastric arteries, inferior epigastric arteries into the external iliac arteries (arrows). (C) Anteroposterior view AP view reveals the Arc of Riolan which is a mesenteric meandering artery between the superior and inferior mesenteric arteries (arrows).

It is usually discovered during workups for hypertension in children. Renal vessels, mesenteric vessels, or both may also be affected to varying degrees. According to previous reports, if the syndrome is left untreated, the majority of patients will die from complications of severe hypertension and ischemia by the age of 40 because of myocardial infarction, heart failure, intracranial hemorrhage, or aortic rupture [13, 14]. Recent study suggests that good long-term outcomes of MAS can be obtained by medical management [15]. Intermittent claudication might be an uncommon clinical presentation compared to manifestation of hypertension.

4. Abnormal external and internal forces

4.1. Endofibrosis

Endofibrosis typically involves the narrowing of the external iliac artery in young athletes such as cyclists, runners, triathletes, and skaters [16]. The disorder is characterized by intimal thickening and subsequent narrowing of the artery by collagen fibers, fibrous tissue, and smooth muscle proliferation [17]. The pathogenesis is presumed to involve repetitive vessel stretching during extreme hip flexion, external compression by psoas muscle hypertrophy, repeated vessel kinking during exercise, and shear stress during high cardiac output. This disorder is progressive and may lead to occlusion, frequently occurring (85%) unilaterally on the left. In addition to the external iliac artery (85%), the common femoral artery (5%) and superficial femoral artery (<5%) can be affected [4]. Since no specific angiographic findings are observed, a high clinical suspicion of this disorder is required for diagnosis and proper treatment.

4.2. Popliteal artery entrapment

Popliteal artery entrapment can be caused by compression of the popliteal artery in the popliteal fossa by adjacent or surrounding musculotendinous structures and ligaments. This disorder can occur bilaterally (30–67%) and is predominant in young males, although cases of elderly patients up to the age of 70 have been reported [4, 18]. The condition may become evident when the popliteal artery is abnormally positioned, or in cases of fibrous bands or abnormal muscle insertions or slips. There are six types of entrapment based on the anatomical compression of the popliteal artery [1]. Computed tomography (CT) angiography or magnetic resonance (MR) angiography may be useful techniques for identifying the structures causing external compression of the artery (**Figure 5**). Angiography may also reveal medial or occasionally lateral displacement of the popliteal artery if it is still patent. However, the position of the popliteal artery may be normal if the compression is due to the plantaris or popliteus muscles. In addition, pre-stenotic or post-stenotic dilatation can be associated with this disorder (**Figure 5**). Although popliteal artery narrowing induced by extension of the knee and dorsiflexion of the foot may support the diagnosis of this condition, there is some concern regarding the potential for false-positive results since popliteal artery compression can occur with active plantar flexion even in healthy individuals [19].

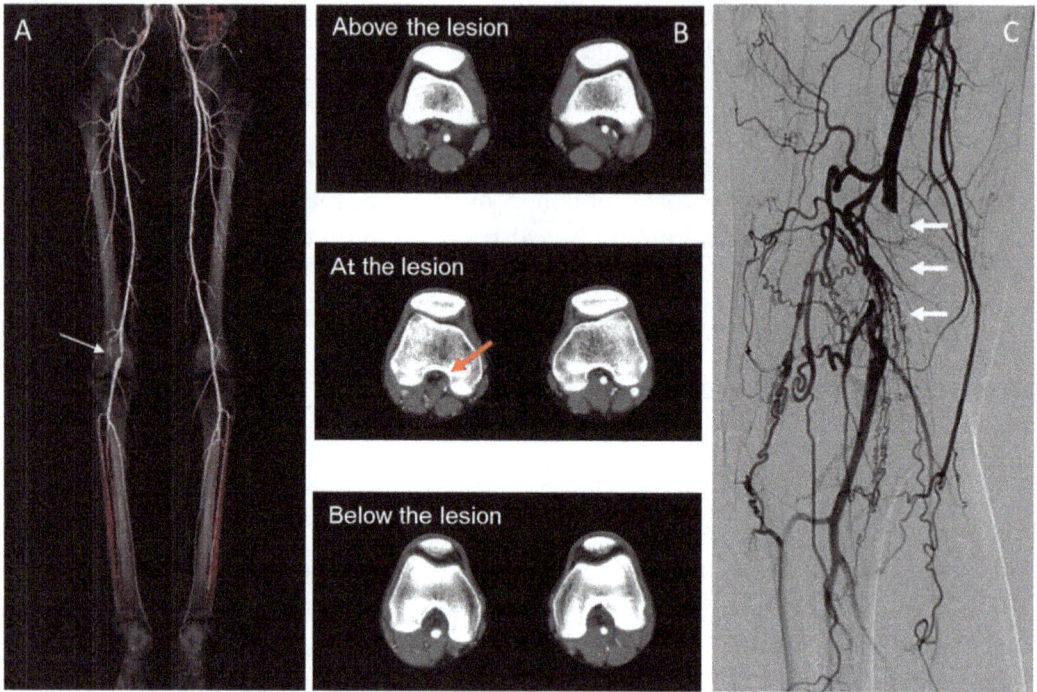

Figure 5. Popliteal artery entrapment syndrome. A 30-year-old male presenting moderate claudication. (A) Enhanced CT revealed tight stenosis and post-stenotic dilatation in the right popliteal artery (arrow). (B) Horizontal view of the CT showing compressed popliteal artery by the surrounding muscle (arrow). (C): Subsequent angiography revealed the progression to occlusion (arrows).

4.3. Adductor canal outlet syndrome

Adductor canal outlet syndrome involves the compression of the distal superficial femoral artery by the adductor canal. It is most commonly reported in runners and skiers, who present with exercise-induced intermittent claudication symptoms and paresthesias. Symptoms are typically chronic but can progress to occlusion and cause acute limb ischemia due to thrombus. This condition may be rare but it is possible relationship to acute intimal injury and thrombosis should be considered in order to save limbs that may otherwise be lost [20–22].

4.4. Other conditions

Other conditions including neoplasma, pseudoxanthoma elasticum, and Baker's cyst can cause lower limb ischemia [4].

5. Vasospasm

Vasospasm can occur even in the lower extremity arteries. There are a variety of causes, including idiopathic or certain vasospastic agents (e.g., ergotamine, cocaine, marijuana, and amphetamine) [23, 24]. The characteristic findings of drug-induced vasospasm are bilateral, symmetric, and abrupt narrowing of any segment of a lower limb artery. Vasospasm can be resolved by discontinuing the offending drug or administering vasodilators (**Figure 6**).

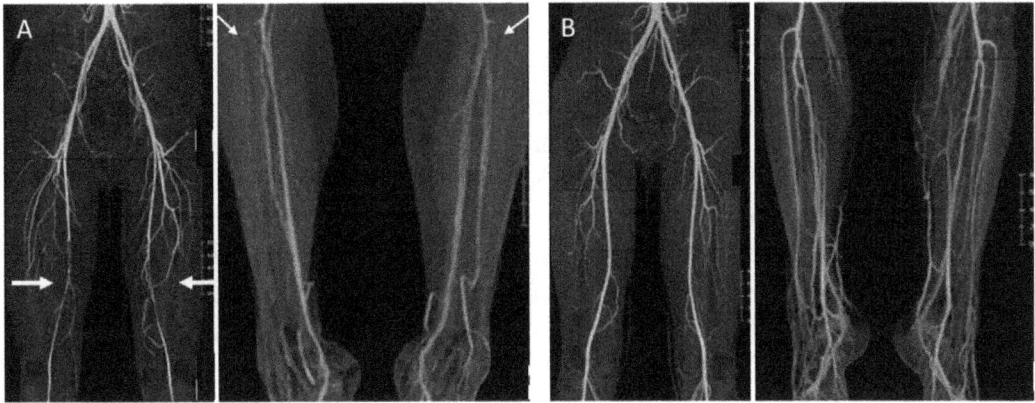

Figure 6. Idiopathic vasospasm (Ref. 24). A 28-year-old male presenting claudication with subsequent acute limb ischemia. (A) Diagnostic enhanced CT angiogram showing tight narrowings in the bilateral femoropopliteal segments (large arrows) and disruptions in the bilateral anterior tibial arteries (small arrows). Also, the proximal segment in the superficial femoral artery seems to be spastic. (B) After initiation of medical treatment during hospitalization, complete recovery of the disruptive lesions is observed though the crural arteries are superimposed on the veins.

6. Vasculitis

Vasculitis may confuse clinicians since it comprises a heterogeneous group of disorders characterized by inflammation and necrosis of blood vessels. However, the key to diagnosis when considering the possible presence of some type of vasculitis is to employ a multidisciplinary approach that involves rheumatologists as well as vascular specialists. Based on the size of the arteries involved and the underlying cause, vasculitis can be categorized as large vessel, medium vessel, or small vessel. The effects of vascular damage including arterial narrowing, thrombosis, or aneurysm formation become prominent over the course of these conditions. Invasive angiography is the gold standard for detecting such lesions and can be used to measure the trans-lesional pressure gradient. However, there are some concerns regarding invasive angiography for vasculitis. First, sheath or catheter insertion may cause vascular injury in the presence of active inflammation. Second, the potential exists for hypersensitivity reactions to the contrast dye as well as contrast nephropathy and volume overload. Moreover, invasive angiography does not provide any information on changes in vasculitis activity.

Takayasu's arteritis and giant cell arteritis (GCA) are typical large- and medium-vessel vasculitis that affect the aorta and its main branches, including the subclavian, carotid, vertebral, renal, mesenteric, and iliac arteries. The affected aortoiliac arteries may cause lower limb ischemia. Behcet's disease and Buerger's disease are representative conditions affecting various-sized arteries and venous systems. Medium-vessel vasculitis mainly comprise polyarteritis nodosa, anti-neutrophil cytoplasmic antibodies (ANCA)-related vasculitis (granulomatosis with polyangiitis (GPA), microscopic polyangiitis, and eosinophilic granulomatosis with polyangiitis), and Kawasaki disease. Assessment of the patient's clinical background and systemic examination are indispensable for the diagnosis of this vasculitis. They can also potentially emerge in an atypical vascular bed for each disorder, mimicking other types of vasculitis [25].

6.1. Takayasu's arteritis

This inflammatory vasculitis of large and medium elastic arteries, also called nonspecific aortitis, is characterized pathologically by giant cell infiltration and granuloma formation. Destruction of the entire vascular wall and progressive adventitial fibrosis can cause stenosis or dilatation that can be complicated with superimposed calcification at the chronic stage. This disorder is typically but not exclusively observed in young women of Asian or Latin descent. It primarily affects the aorta, its major branches, and the pulmonary arteries, including but not limited to the brachiocephalic, carotid (common carotid), vertebral, subclavian (proximal subclavian), renal, iliac, femoral, and coronary arteries. Clinically, it usually first presents in the second or third decade, but can occur at older ages. Many patients initially complain of fever, arthralgias, and malaise. Although the most common symptom of TA is arm claudication, observed in greater than 60% of cases, aortoiliac artery involvement can result in lower limb ischemic symptoms, and even the femoral artery may be involved [26, 27].

There are no serological tests to identify TA. The diagnosis of TA is based on clinical findings in the presence of compatible vascular imaging abnormalities (**Table 1**) [1].

1990 criteria for the classification of Takayasu arteritis
1. Age at disease onset <40 years
2. Claudication of extremities
3. Decreased brachial artery pulse
4. Difference of >10 mmHg in systolic blood pressure between arms
5. Bruit over subclavian arteries or abdominal aorta
6. Arteriogram abnormality (arteriographic narrowing or occlusion of the entire aorta, its primary branches, or large arteries in the proximal upper or lower extremities, not due to arteriosclerosis, fibromuscular dysplasia, or similar causes; changes usually focal or segmental)
Takayasu arteritis is defined clinically if at least three of these six criteria are present. The presence of any three or more criteria yields a sensitivity of 90.5% and a specificity of 97.8%.

Table 1. American College of Rheumatology diagnostic criteria for Takayasu arteritis.

Angiography can reveal the extent of luminal narrowing, with or without dilatation/aneurysm, in order to differentiate TA from other diseases. While CT angiography or MR angiography can provide the whole image alternative to angiography, measurement of the pressure gradients is one of the major advantages of invasive angiography (**Figure 7**). It can also provide opportunities for surgical or endovascular intervention. However, in terms of evaluating vessel wall thickening and edema, duplex US, CT, and MR are more informative than angiography.

6.2. Giant cell arteritis

Although giant cell arteritis is pathologically similar to TA, this type of vasculitis commonly affects the temporal artery. The disorder is observed in men and women of around 50 and older, and is particularly prevalent in patients aged 70 and older. The arteries potentially affected include the aorta and its branches, with a predilection for the distal subclavian, axillary, and proximal brachial arteries, as well as the branches of the carotid arteries, in particular the ophthalmic artery. Therefore, headaches, jaw claudication, and visual impairment can occur in addition to arm claudication. Also, a normal erythrocyte sedimentation rate (ESR) is more useful in excluding giant cell arteritis than an elevated ESR is in diagnosing this disease [1] (**Table 2**).

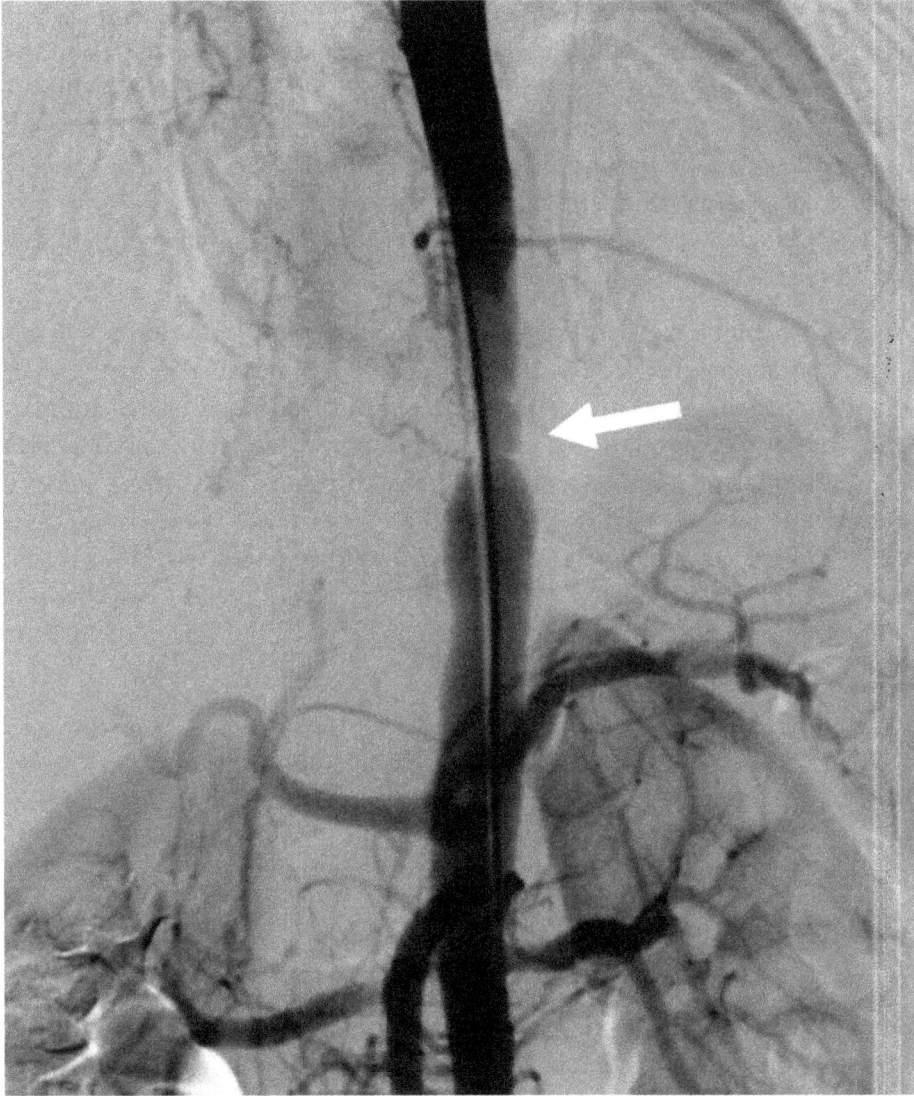

Figure 7. Takayasu arteritis. A 20-year-old female presenting mild claudication and renovascular hypertension. Invasive angiography revealed significant stenosis in the descending thoracic aorta (arrow). The pullback pressure gradient was 20 mmHg.

1990 criteria for the classification of giant cell arteritis

---

1. Age at disease onset <50 years
2. New headache
3. Temporal artery abnormality
4. Elevated erythrocyte sedimentation rate
5. Abnormal artery biopsy (biopsy specimen with artery showing vasculitis characterized by a predominance of mononuclear cell infiltration or granulomatous inflammation, usually with multinucleated giant cells)

Giant cell arteritis is defined clinically if at least three of these five criteria are present. The presence of any three or more criteria yields a sensitivity of 93.5% and a specificity of 91.2%.

Table 2. American College of Rheumatology diagnostic criteria for giant cell arteritis.

Lower limb arteries can also be affected by this disorder [28, 29]. According to positron emission tomography scan studies, the iliac artery was involved in 37% of cases and the femoral artery in 37% (subclavian artery 70%, axillary artery 40%) [30]. Other studies have reported that superficial femoral artery was involved in 33%, common femoral artery in 14%, internal iliac artery 11%, deep femoral artery in 6%, and popliteal artery in 6% of cases [4, 31–34]. US studies have also detected the involvement of distal lower limb arteries such as the femoropopliteal, tibial, and peroneal arteries [35]. It is sometimes challenging to differentiate lesions from atherosclerosis in older patients.

Findings of arteritis from a temporal artery biopsy can be supportive but not essential for a diagnosis. An accurate diagnosis of GCA requires a comprehensive approach that includes assessment of clinical manifestations, physical examination, laboratory studies, vascular imaging, and arterial biopsies. Positive temporal artery biopsies can occasionally be seen in other types of arteritis and the ESR may be normal in up to 10% of GCA patients so that cautious interpretation is required. Differential diagnosis of GCA should include brain disease, infectious disease, and malignant disease. It should be noted that other vasculitis such as polyarteritis nodosa or ANCA-related vasculitis may rarely present with temporal artery involvement. Polymyalgia rheumatic may also be included in this group of vasculitis as it is often regarded as one clinical entity with GCA.

Although angiography can confirm the extent of affected vessels, less invasive tools such as duplex US, CT angiography, and MR angiography should also be considered. In particular, CT is informative for the extent of calcification. The advantage of angiography is that it allows measurements of pressure gradients to identify hemodynamically significant lesions.

6.3. Behcet's disease

Vasculitis is observed in less than one-third of Behcet's disease cases. The etiology remains unclear and may involve both genetic and environmental factors. It can potentially be characterized by concomitant oral and genital ulcerations, skin lesions, uveitis, central nervous system, and gastrointestinal involvement. Approximately 80% of Behcet's disease patients have the human leukocyte antigen (HLA)-B51 allele. However, since no symptoms or laboratory findings are pathognomonic for Behcet's disease, diagnosis depends on the patient meeting a set of established clinical criteria. The major histopathological features of this disorder are predominantly perivascular inflammatory infiltrates and a tendency to thrombus formation in both veins and arteries of every size. In particular, venous disease is characteristic, including superficial phlebitis, varices, and thrombosis of the deep veins, vena cava, and cerebral sinuses. Large vessels frequently show luminal narrowing, aneurysm, or rupture. Medium and small vessels may also be affected [36, 37] (**Figure 8**).

6.4. Buerger's disease

Buerger's disease, also known as thromboangiitis obliterans (TAO), was first reported by Winiwarter in 1879, and later described in detail by Buergers in 1908 [38, 39]. Although the etiology remains unclear, this disorder is a segmental inflammatory disease typically affecting small- to medium-sized arteries of the upper and lower extremities, with occasional extension to the veins and nerves of the extremities [40–42]. Atypically, multiple large vessels can be affected [43]. This condition is more common in men than in women and is almost exclusively observed in patients who use tobacco so that it is widely recognized that tobacco is associated with the onset, progression, and recurrence of the disease. Symptoms can include claudication, rest pain, and ischemic tissue loss such as ulceration and gangrene. Unlike other vasculitis, inflammatory markers such as the ESR and C-reactive protein are typically normal. Angiography is often required to evaluate lesion extent and runoff conditions since there is the potential for over- or underestimation of the lesion with MR and CT imaging. Angiographic findings include segmental arterial occlusions of small- and medium-sized vessels while large arteries are typically spared (**Figure 9**) [44].

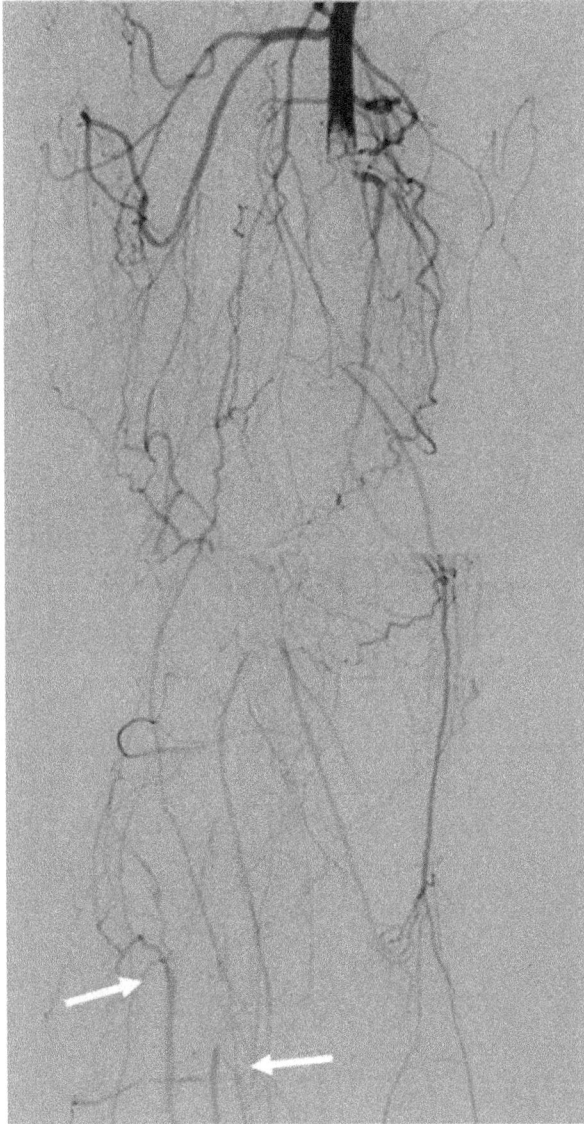

Figure 8. Behcet's disease. A 64-year-old male with a history of deep vein thrombosis and cerebral vein thrombosis presenting acute onset of rest pain and claudication in the right leg. Invasive angiography revealed right femorocrural occlusion. The proximal crural artery was reconstituted through the collateral vessels (arrows).

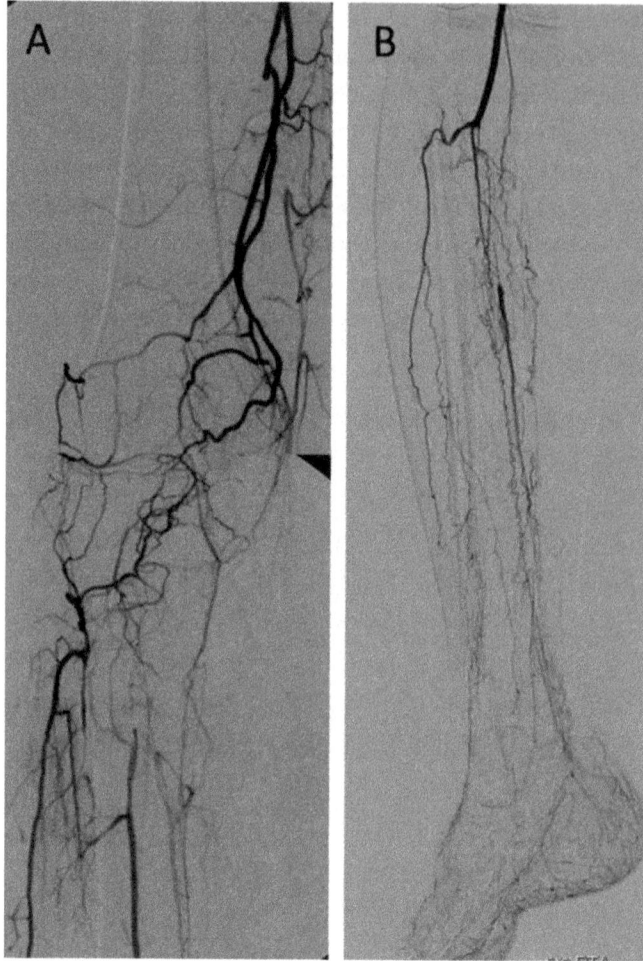

Figure 9. Buerger's disease. (A) Femorocrural occlusion beyond the right knee joint in a 38-year-old female presenting foot gangrene. (Ref. 44). (B) Crural artery occlusion in a 37-year-old male presenting right toe gangrene. Long total occlusions in the tibial arteries extending to the pedal arch.

The term "corkscrew" has recently been used to describe the appearance of collateral vessels in Buerger's disease patients. However, the original article attributes the corkscrew appearance to the recanalization of the affected native artery [45, 46]. Moreover, the corkscrew appearance is not pathognomonic for Buerger's disease as it may be seen in patients with other disorders including connective tissue disease. Thus, several different criteria have been proposed for the diagnosis of Buerger's disease (**Tables 3** and **4**) [40, 41].

- History of smoking
- Onset before age 50
- Infrapopliteal arterial occlusions
- Either arm involvement or phlebitis migrans
- Absence of atherosclerotic risk factors other than smoking

Table 3. Criteria of Buerger's disease by Shionoya [40].

- Age under 45
- Current or recent history of tobacco use
- Presence of distal extremity ischemia as indicated by claudication, pain at rest, ischemic ulcers, or gangrene, and documented by noninvasive vascular testing
- Exclusion of autoimmune diseases, hypercoagulable states, and diabetes mellitus
- Exclusion of a proximal source of emboli by echocardiography or arteriography
- Consistent arteriographic findings in the clinically involved and noninvolved limbs

Table 4. Criteria of Buerger's disease by Olin [41].

6.5. Other vasculitides

Other rare diseases, including Cogan's syndrome and relapsing polychondritis, can cause vasculitis of large- or medium-sized vessels. Small-vessel vasculitides include cryoglobulin-emic vasculitis, leukocytoclastic vasculitides such as Henoch-Schonlein purpura and isolated cutaneous leukocytoclastic vasculitis, and vasculitis secondary to systemic autoimmune disease, including rheumatoid arthritis, systemic lupus erythematosus (SLE), and scleroderma [30, 47]. It is worth noting that there is the possibility of atypical lesion distribution for any type of vasculitides (**Figures 10** and **11**).

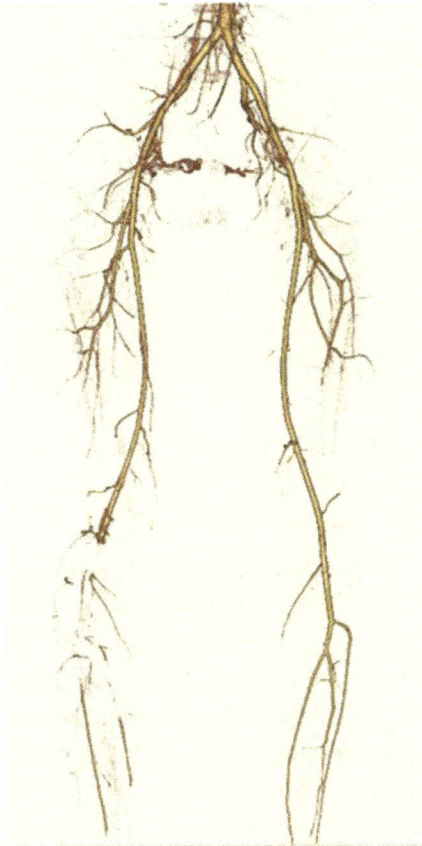

Figure 10. Systemic lupus erythematosus A 16-year-old female presenting claudication with subsequent acute limb ischemia as an initial clinical manifestation. Enhanced CT revealed severe femorocrural occlusion. Although the mid-tibial arteries were reconstituted, the distal tibial and pedal arteries were occluded.

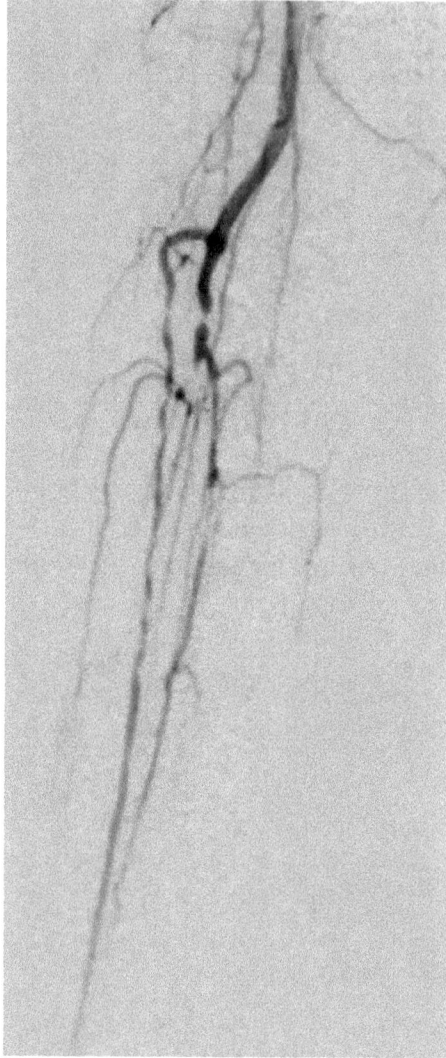

Figure 11. Scleroderma. An 80-year-old female presenting toe gangrene with a history of scleroderma. Invasive angiography showing multiple stenosis in the right crural artery.

For example, there have been case reports of large- or medium-vessel vasculitis in patients with rheumatoid arthritis, SLE and ANCA-related vasculitis [30, 47–62], and uncommon diseases including hypereosinophilic syndrome, Kimura disease, and angiolymphoid hyperplasia with eosinophilia can also mimic Buerger's disease [63–65]. Moreover, antiphospholipid syndrome (APS) can occur concomitantly with vasculitis secondary to systemic autoimmune disease (frequently SLE), and can develop into catastrophic APS [66–73] (**Figure 10**). Certain kinds of vasculitis can be complicated by thrombosis and potentially develop into thrombotic storm which has a devastating clinical course [74–77]. Radiation arteritis can occur years after high-dose radiotherapy for pelvic malignant disease. In such cases, stenotic or occlusive disease can be seen within the radiation field. Thus, with typical and atypical cases in mind, a careful diagnostic workup is vital for vasculitis.

7. Arterial thrombophilias

There are inherited and acquired disorders in which thrombosis develops in the arterial system. Inherited disorders include hyperhomocysteinemia/hyperhomocystinuria, antithrombin deficiency, protein S deficiency, and protein C deficiency, as well as gene polymorphisms such as Factor V Leiden. Acquired disorders are more common and can be caused by APS, malignancies, hormone therapy, and such myeloproliferative disorders as polycythemia vera, thrombocythemia, heparin-induced thrombocytopenia, and thrombotic thrombocytopenic purpura (**Figure 12**) [78].

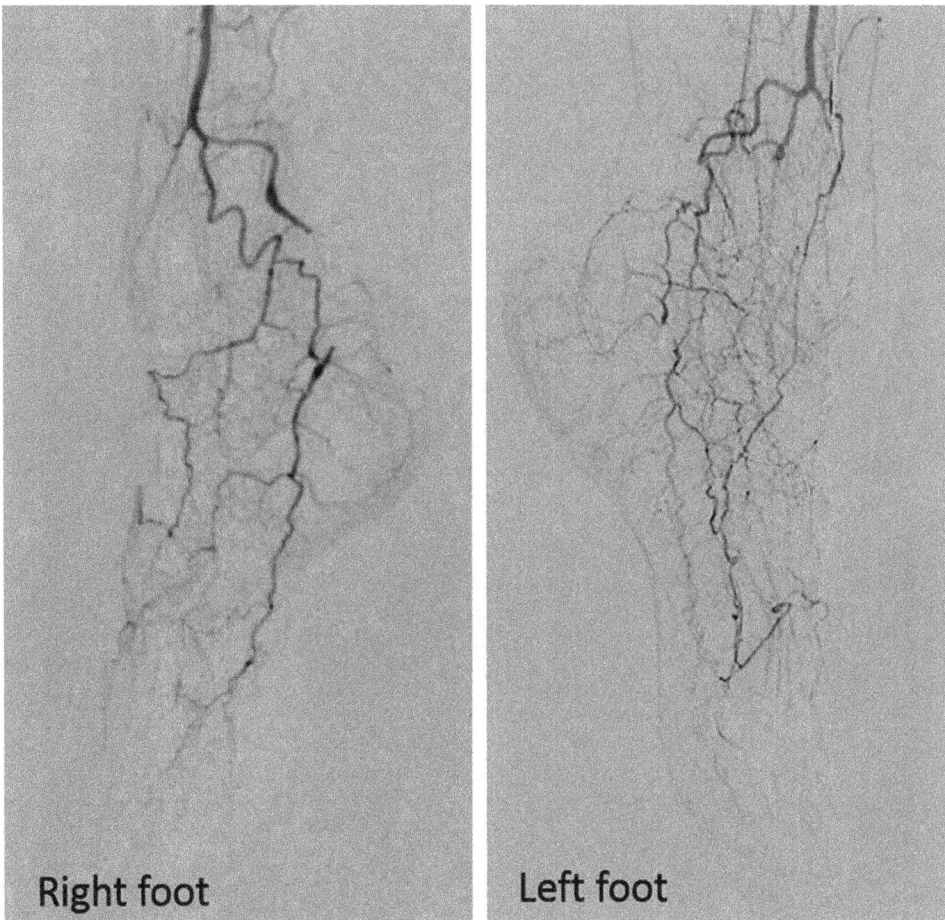

Figure 12. Primary antiphospholipid syndrome [78]. A 75-year-old female presenting symmetric peripheral gangrene in four limbs. Angiography shows the occlusions in the pedal arteries as well as the palmar arteries due to antiphospholipid syndrome.

Thrombosis can be seen in vasculitis [74, 79]. In particular, inflammation-induced thrombosis is considered to be a feature of certain kinds of vasculitis (systemic autoimmune diseases such as SLE, rheumatoid arthritis, and Sjogren's syndrome, and other vasculitis). Thus, primary or secondary APS concomitant with autoimmune diseases such as SLE can cause thrombosis and potentially develop into catastrophic APS [80–82].

8. Congenital variants

Congenital malformations of the iliofemoral arterial system are rare, but accurate diagnosis is essential to avoid unnecessary revascularization treatment. Congenital absence or hypoplasty of the common iliac artery, external iliac artery, and SFA has been reported [83, 84]. Congenital variants of the external iliac artery have been classified into three groups [85]: group 1, anomalies in the origin or course of the artery; group 2, hypoplasia or atresia compensated for by persistent sciatic artery (PSA); and group 3, isolated hypoplasia or atresia. Although group 1 may not be associated with lower limb ischemia and is most often discovered at autopsy, group 2, the so-called persistent sciatic artery, and group 3 are most likely to present with lower limb ischemia.

Above all, PSA is a popular variant. Failure of regression of the sciatic artery during fetal development is often associated with superficial femoral artery hypoplasia, and the PSA then provides the dominant arterial inflow to the lower limb. Therefore, there is continuation of the internal iliac artery into the thigh through the greater sciatic notch. This variant can cause not only acute lower limb ischemia due to thromboembolism but also chronic lower limb ischemia, with a high incidence of aneurysm formation and arteriosclerosis of the sciatic artery (**Figure 13**) [4, 86].

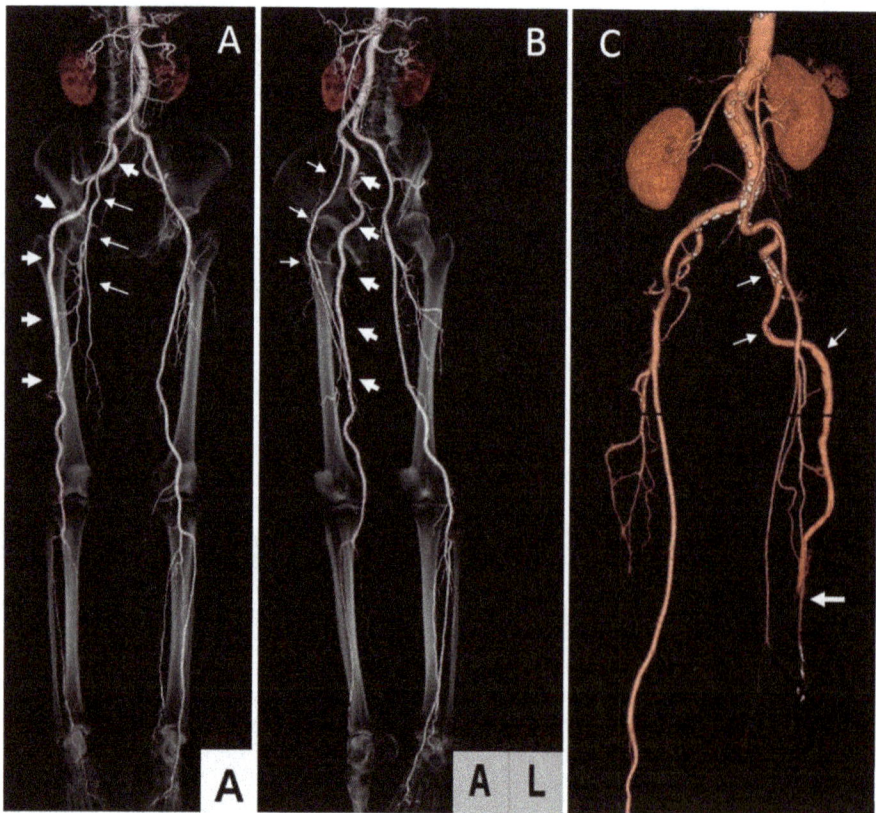

Figure 13. Persistent sciatic artery. (A, B) A 64-year-old male. Enhanced CT incidentally found persistent sciatic artery (large arrows) in the right. The right external iliac artery connects with the hypoplastic superficial femoral artery (small arrows). (C) A 60-year-old female presenting acute limb ischemia. The left external iliac artery connects with the hypoplastic superficial femoral artery whereas the persistent sciatic artery through the left internal iliac artery is the dominant blood supply (small arrows). The distal part of the sciatic artery is occluded due to thromboembolism (large arrow).

9. Embolism

Embolism can potentially cause manifestations of chronic lower limb ischemia, such as claudication and critical limb ischemia, but not acute limb ischemia in particular in the elderly population. Embolisms may have a number of sources including cardiac, aortic, and right-to-left shunts (paradoxical embolism from the venous circulation).

10. Vascular injury

Orthopedic surgery or trauma may cause lower limb ischemia because of dissection or thrombotic occlusion [87]. Additionally, pediatric cardiac catheterization using the transfemoral approach could be a cause of iliofemoral occlusion or stenosis due to thrombosis formation or intimal hyperplasia (**Figure 14**). This disorder may be asymptomatic until adulthood, but long-term uncorrected circulatory impairment can potentially cause limb growth retardation even in the absence of symptomatic evidence of ischemia [88–93].

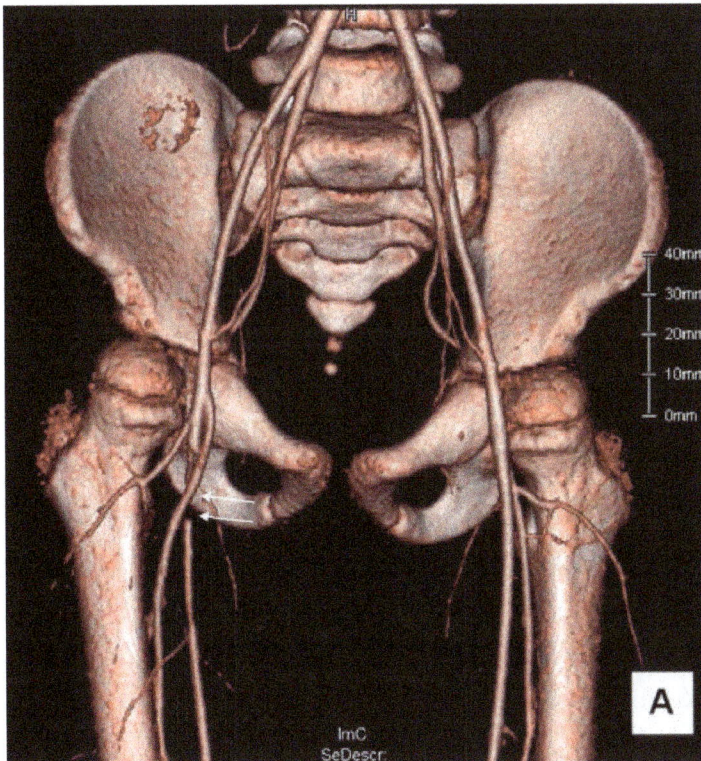

Figure 14. Vascular injury following catheterization. A 4-year-old boy experienced a pale foot on the right following catheterization. Enhanced CT revealed a short occlusion due to puncture site thrombosis in the proximal segment of the right superficial femoral artery (arrows).

11. Conclusions

This section is intended to focus on vascular imaging, mainly invasive angiography, for NAPAD. From a clinical standpoint, an increase in opportunities to experience the symptoms and signs of APAD heightens the importance of the differential diagnosis of NAPAD in daily practice. NAPAD cannot benefit from a one-size-fits-all approach compared to APAD. Thus, differentiation between NAPAD and APAD may be a challenging task but we clinicians need to increase our knowledge of the diversity of NAPAD so that such awareness can be translated into improved patient care.

Author details

Osami Kawarada

Address all correspondence to: kawarada.osami.hp@ncvc.go.jp

Department of Cardiovascular Medicine, National Cerebral and Cardiovascular Center, Osaka, Japan

References

[1] Sharma AM, Norton PT, Zhu D. Conditions presenting with symptoms of peripheral arterial disease. Semin Intervent Radiol. 2014; 31: 281–291.

[2] Weinberg I, Jaff MR. Nonatherosclerotic arterial disorders of the lower extremities. Circulation. 2012; 126: 213–222.

[3] Mintz AJ, Weinberg I. Nonatherosclerotic PAD: approach to exertional pain in the lower extremities. Curr Cardiol Rep. 2015; 17: 66.

[4] Apigian AK, Landry GJ. Basic data underlying decision making in nonatherosclerotic causes of intermittent claudication. Ann Vasc Surg. 2015; 29: 138–153.

[5] Perlowski AA, Jaff MR. Vascular disorders in athletes. Vasc Med. 2010; 15: 469–479.

[6] Slovut DP, Olin JW. Fibromuscular dysplasia. N Engl J Med. 2004; 350: 1862–1871.

[7] Okazaki J, Guntani A, Homma K, Kyuragi R, Kawakubo E, Maehara Y. Fibromuscular dysplasia of the lower extremities. Ann Vasc Dis. 2011; 4: 143–149.

[8] Plouin PF, Perdu J, La Batide-Alanore A, Boutouyrie P, Gimenez-Roqueplo AP, Jeunemaitre X. Fibromuscular dysplasia. Orphanet J Rare Dis. 2007; 2: 28.

[9] Pontes Tde C, Rufino GP, Gurgel MG, Medeiros AC, Freire EA. Fibromuscular dysplasia: a differential diagnosis of vasculitis. Rev Bras Rheumatol. 2012; 52: 70–74.

[10] França M, Pinto J, Machado R, Fernandez GC. Bilateral adventitial cystic disease of the popliteal artery. Radiology. 2010; 255: 655–660.

[11] Porras D, Stein DR, Ferguson MA, Chaudry G, Alomari A, Vakili K, Fishman SJ, Lock JE, Kim HB. Midaortic syndrome: 30 years of experience with medical, endovascular and surgical management. Pediatr Nephrol. 2013; 28: 2023–2033.

[12] Stanley JC, Criado E, Eliason JL, Upchurch GR Jr, Berguer R, Rectenwald JE. Abdominal aortic coarctation: surgical treatment of 53 patients with a thoracoabdominal bypass, patch aortoplasty, or interposition aortoaortic graft. J Vasc Surg. 2008; 48: 1073–1082.

[13] Kim HB, Vakili K, Modi BP, Ferguson MA, Guillot AP, Potanos KM, Prabhu SP, Fishman SJ. A novel treatment for the midaortic syndrome. N Engl J Med. 2012; 367: 2361–2362.

[14] Sumboonnanonda A, Robinson BL, Gedroyc WM, Saxton HM, Reidy JF, Haycock GB. Middle aortic syndrome: clinical and radiological findings. Arch Dis Child. 1992; 67: 501–505.

[15] Saif I, Seriki D, Moore R, Woywodt A. Midaortic syndrome in neurofibromatosis type 1 resulting in bilateral renal artery stenosis. Am J Kidney Dis. 2010; 56: 1197–1201.

[16] Peach G, Schep G, Palfreeman R, Beard JD, Thompson MM, Hinchliffe RJ. Endofibrosis and kinking of the iliac arteries in athletes: a systematic review. Eur J Vasc Endovasc Surg. 2012; 43: 208–217.

[17] Rousselet MC, Saint-Andre JP, L'Hoste P, Enon B, Megret A, Chevalier JM. Stenotic intimal thickening of the external iliac artery in competition cyclists. Hum Pathol. 1990; 21: 524–529.

[18] Radonić V, Koplić S, Giunio L, Bozić I, Masković J, Buća A. Tex Heart Inst J. 2000;27(1):3-13. Popliteal artery entrapment syndrome: diagnosis and management, with report of three cases. Tex Heart Ins J. 2000; 27: 3–13.

[19] Akkersdijk WL, de Ruyter JW, Lapham R, Mali W, Eikelboom BC. Colour duplex ultrasonographic imaging and provocation of popliteal artery compression. Eur J Vasc Endovasc Surg. 1995; 10: 342–345.

[20] Sapienza P, Tartaglia E, Venturini L, Gallo P, di Marzo L. Adductor canal compression syndrome: a forgotten disease. Ann Ital Chir. 2014; 85(ePub).

[21] Verta MJ Jr, Vitello J, Fuller J. Adductor canal compression syndrome. Arch Surg. 1984; 119: 345–346.

[22] Balaji MR, DeWeese JA. Adductor canal outlet syndrome. JAMA. 1981; 245: 167–170.

[23] Demir S, Akin S, Tercan F, Ariboğan A, Oğuzkurt L. Ergotamine-induced lower extremity arterial vasospasm presenting as acute limb ischemia. Diagn Interv Radiol. 2010; 16: 165–167.

[24] Kaneyama J, Kawarada O, Sakamoto S, Harada K, Ishihara M, Yasuda S, Ogawa H. Vasospastic limb ischemia presenting acute and chronic limb ischemia. Ann Vasc Dis. 2014; 7: 169–172.

[25] Berlit P, Kessler C, Reuther R, Krause KH. New aspects of thromboangiitis obliterans (von Winiwarter-Buerger's disease). Eur Neurol. 1984; 23: 394–399.

[26] Beschorner U, Goebel H, Rastan A, Sixt S, Zeller T. Histological diagnosis of atypical Takayasu arteritis using percutaneous transluminal atherectomy. J Endovasc Ther. 2008; 15: 241–243.

[27] Kawano H, Hanibuchi M, Yoshijima T, Toyoda Y, Kishi J, Tezuka T, Nishioka Y. A case of atypical Takayasu arteritis initially presenting with peripheral artery disease. Case Rep Clin Pathol. 2015; 2: 34–40.

[28] Finlayson R, Robinson JO. Giant-cell arteritis of the legs. Br Med J. 1955; 2: 1595–1597.

[29] Tatò F, Hoffmann U. Giant cell arteritis: a systemic vascular disease. Vasc Med. 2008; 13: 127–140.

[30] Cid MC, Prieto-González S, Arguis P, Espígol-Frigolé G, Butjosa M, Hernández-Rodríguez J, Segarra M, Lozano E, García-Martínez A. The spectrum of vascular involvement in giant-cell arteritis: clinical consequences of detrimental vascular remodelling at different sites. APMIS Suppl. 2009; 127: 10–20.

[31] Loo ZY, Thwaites S, Kyaw P. Giant cell arteritis presenting as critical lower limb ischemia. Vasc Endovascular Surg. 2013; 47: 660–662.

[32] Czihal M, Tato F, Rademacher A, Kuhlencordt P, Schulze-Koops H, Hoffmann U. Involvement of the femoropopliteal arteries in giant cell arteritis: clinical and color duplex sonography. J Rheumatol. 2012; 39: 314–321.

[33] Assie C, Janvresse A, Plissonnier D, Levesque H, Marie I. Long-term follow-up of upper and lower extremity vasculitis related to giant cell arteritis: a series of 36 patients. Medicine. 2011; 90: 40–51.

[34] Kermani TA, Matteson EL, Hunder GG, Warrington KJ. Symptomatic lower extremity vasculitis in giant cell arteritis: a case series. J Rheumatol. 2009; 36: 2277–2283.

[35] Schmidt WA, Natusch A, Möller DE, Vorpahl K, Gromnica-Ihle E. Involvement of peripheral arteries in giant cell arteritis: a color Doppler sonography study. Clin Exp Rheumatol. 2002; 20: 309–318.

[36] Merkel PA. Overview of vasculitis. Vascular Medicine: A Companion to Braunwald's Heart Disease. Elsevier 2013, 507–524.

[37] Sakane T, Takeno M, Suzuki N, Inaba G. Behcet's disease. N Engl J Med 1999; 341: 1284–1291.

[38] von Winiwarter F. Ueber eine eigenthumliche form von endarteriitis und endophlebitis mit gangran des fusses. Arch Klin Chir. 1879; 23: 202–226.

[39] Buerger L. Thrombo-angiitis obliterans: a study of the vascular lesions leading to presenile spontaneous gangrene. Am J Med Sci. 1908; 136: 567–580.

[40] Shionoya S. Diagnostic criteria of Buerger's disease. Int J Cardiol. 1998; 1: 243–245.

[41] Olin JW. Thromboangiitis obliterans (Buerger's disease). N Engl J Med. 2000; 343: 864–869.

[42] Del Conde I, Peña C. Buerger disease (thromboangiitis obliterans). Tech Vasc Interv Radiol. 2014; 17: 234–240.

[43] Edo N, Miyai K, Ogata S, Nakanishi K, Hiroi S, Tominaga S, Aiko S, Kawai T. Thromboangiitis obliterans with multiple large vessel involvement: Case report and analysis of immunophenotypes. Cardiovasc Pathol. 2010; 19: 59–62.

[44] Kawarada O, Ayabe S, Yotsukura H, Nakaya T, Kanayama J, Harada K, Ishihara M, Yasuda S, Ogawa H. Subintimal angioplasty of lengthy femorotibial total occlusion in Buerger's disease. J Endovasc Ther. 2013; 20: 578–581.

[45] McKusick VA, Harris WS, Ottesen OE, Goodman RM, Shelley WM, Bloodwell RD. Buerger's disease: a distinct clinical and pathologic entity. JAMA. 1962; 181: 5–12.

[46] Talwar S, Choudhary SK, Bhan A. Buerger's disease. Indian J Cardiol. 1998; 1: 31–34.

[47] Celecova Z, Krahulec B, Lizicarova D, Gaspar L. Vasculitides as a rare cause of intermittent claudication. Bratisl Lek Listy. 2013; 114: 353–356.

[48] Hammentgen R, Stojanova-Scholz M, Martin M, Gresshöner-Solf IM, Haupt H, Fiebach BJ, Magnus L, Trobisch H. Bilateral popliteal artery occlusion in systemic lupus erythematosus in a 15-year-old girl. Vasa. 1987; 16: 86–88.

[49] Gladstein GS, Rynes RI, Parhami N, Bartholomew LE. Gangrene of a foot secondary to systemic lupus erythematosus with large vessel vasculitis. J Rheumatol. 1979; 6: 549–553.

[50] Bakker FC, Rauwerda JA, Moens HJ, van den Broek TA. Intermittent claudication and limb-threatening ischemia in systemic lupus erythematosus and in SLE-like disease: a report of two cases and review of the literature. Surgery. 1989; 106: 21–25.

[51] Asherson RA, Derksen RH, Harris EN, Bingley PJ, Hoffbrand BI, Gharavi AE, Kater L, Hughes GR. Large vessel occlusion and gangrene in systemic lupus erythematosus and "lupus-like" disease. A report of six cases. J Rheumatol. 1986; 13: 740–747.

[52] Harmon SM, Oltmanns KL, Min KW. Large vessel occlusion with vasculitis in systemic lupus erythematosus. South Med J. 1991; 84: 1150–1154.

[53] Wheatley MJ, Hennein HA, Greenfield LJ. Lower extremity arterial disease in systemic lupus erythematosus. Arch Surg. 1991; 126: 109–110.

[54] Pyrpasopoulou A, Chatzimichailidou S, Aslanidis S. Vascular disease in systemic lupus erythematosus. Autoimmune Dis. 2012; 2012: 876456.

[55] Herrick AL, Oogarah PK, Freemont AJ, Marcuson R, Haeney M, Jayson MI. Vasculitis in patients with systemic sclerosis and severe digital ischaemia requiring amputation. Ann Rheum Dis. 1994; 53: 323–326.

[56] Schwarz-Eywill M, Rinaldi N, Barth T, Nüsslein HG. Rare manifestation of large vessel vasculitis in systemic lupus erythematosus. Z Rheumatol. 2000; 59: 330–333.

[57] Giannakakis S, Galyfos G, Stefanidis I, Kastrisios G, Maltezos C. Hybrid treatment of lower limb critical ischemia in a patient with systemic lupus erythematosus. Ann Vasc Surg. 2015; 29: 596. e1–5.

[58] Jeffery RC, Narshi CB, Isenberg DA. Prevalence, serological features, response to treatment and outcome of critical peripheral ischaemia in a cohort of lupus patients. Rheumatology (Oxford). 2008; 47: 1379–1383.

[59] da Rocha MC, Vilar MJ, Freire EA, Santiago MB. Arterial occlusion in systemic lupus erythematosus: a good prognostic sign? Clin Rheumatol. 2005; 24: 602–605.

[60] Stafford L, Englert H, Gover J, Bertouch J. Distribution of macrovascular disease in scleroderma. Ann Rheum Dis. 1998; 57: 476–479.

[61] Deguchi J, Shigematsu K, Ota S, Kimura H, Fukayama M, Miyata T. Surgical result of critical limb ischemia due to tibial arterial occlusion in patients with systemic scleroderma. J Vasc Surg. 2009; 49: 918–923.

[62] Struthers GR, Pugh MT, Woodward DA. Polyarteritis nodosa following angioplasty. Ann Rheum Dis. 1993; 52: 247.

[63] Takaoka H, Takano H, Nakagawa K, Kobayashi Y, Hiroshima K, Komuro I. Buerger's disease-like vasculitis associated with Kimura's disease. Int J Cardiol. 2010; 140: e23–6.

[64] Gleich GJ, Leiferman KM. The hypereosinophilic syndromes: current concepts and treatments. Br J Haematol. 2009; 145: 271–285.

[65] Kawata E, Kuroda J, Wada K, Yoshida M, Kamiuchi K, Nakayama-Harusato I, Kimura S, Maekawa T, Kitagawa Y. Hypereosinophilic syndrome accompanied by Buerger's disease-like femoral arterial occlusions. Intern Med. 2007; 46: 1919–1922.

[66] Suzuki K, Uemura T, Kikuchi M, Ishihara Y, Ichioka S. Acute limb-threatening ischemia associated with antiphospholipid syndrome: a report of two cases. J Foot Ankle Surg. 2016; 55: 1318–1322.

[67] Dupont P, Jackson J, Warrens A, Lightstone L. Life-threatening thrombosis 18 years after first presentation of primary antiphospholipid antibody syndrome. Nephrol Dial Transplant. 2001; 16: 843–845.

[68] Biernacka-Zielinska M, Lipinska J, Szymanska-Kaluza J, Stanczyk J, Smolewska E. Recurrent arterial and venous thrombosis in a 16-year-old boy in the course of primary antiphospholipid syndrome despite treatment with low-molecular-weight heparin: a case report. J Med Case Rep. 2013; 7: 221.

[69] Ziaee V, Yeganeh MH, Moradinejad MH. Peripheral gangrene: A rare presentation of systemic lupus erythematosus in a child. Am J Case Rep. 2013; 14: 337–340.

[70] Ascherson RA, Cervera R, Klumb E, Stojanovic L, Sarzi-Puttini P, Yinh J, Bucciarelli S, Espinosa G, Levy R, Shoenfeld Y. Amputation of digits or limbs in patients with antiphospholipid syndrome. Semin Arthritis Rhrum.2008; 38: 124–131.

[71] Pari VS, Lakshmi M, Kumar S, Sathyamurthy P, Sudhakar MK, Sundaram S. A young female with catastrophic antiphospholipid syndrome. Int J Case Rep Images. 2014; 5: 513–518.

[72] Montes de Oca MA, Babron MC, Blétry O, Broyer M, Courtecuisse V, Fontaine JL, Loirat C, Méry JP, Reinert P, Wechsler B, Levy M. Thrombosis in systemic lupus erythematosus: a French collaborative study. Arch Dis Child. 1991; 66: 713–717.

[73] Hughson MD, McCarty GA, Brumback RA. Spectrum of vascular pathology affecting patients with the antiphospholipid syndrome. Hum Pathol. 1995; 26: 716–724.

[74] Emmi G, Silvestri E, Squatrito D, Amedei A, Niccolai E, D'elios MM, Bella CD, Grassi A, Becatti M, Fiorillo C, Emmi L, Vaglio A, Prisco D. Thrombosis in vasculitis: from pathogenesis to treatment. Thromb J. 2015; 13: 15.

[75] Bastug DE, Dominic A, Ortiz O, DiBartolomeo AG, Kotzan JM, Abraham FM. Popliteal artery thrombosis in a patient with Cogan syndrome: treatment with thrombolysis and percutaneous transluminal angioplasty. Cardiovasc Intervent Radiol. 1997; 20: 57–59.

[76] Liu H, Al-Quran SZ, Lottenberg R. Thrombotic storm in Kimura disease. J Thromb Thrombolysis. 2010; 29: 354–357.

[77] Herrick AL, Oogarah PK, Freemont AJ, Marcuson R, Haeney M, Jayson MI. Vasculitis in patients with systemic sclerosis and severe digital ischaemia requiring amputation. Ann Rheum Dis. 1994; 53: 323–326.

[78] Shiba M, Ieko M, Kawarada O. Symmetric peripheral gangrene in antiphospholipid syndrome. Heart Asia 2016; 8: 8.

[79] Palatinus A, Adams M. Thrombosis in systemic lupus erythematosus. Semin Thromb Hemost. 2009; 35: 621–629.

[80] Asherson RA, Cervera R. Microvascular and microangiopathic antiphospholipid-associated syndromes ("MAPS"): semantic or antisemantic? Autoimmun Rev. 2008; 7: 164–167.

[81] Kitchens CS, Erkan D, Brandão LR, Hahn S, James AH, Kulkarni R, Pericak-Vance M, Vance J, Ortel TL. Thrombotic storm revisited: preliminary diagnostic criteria suggested by the thrombotic storm study group. Am J Med. 2011; 124: 290–296.

[82] Ortel TL, Erkan D, Kitchens CS. How I treat catastrophic thrombotic syndromes. Blood. 2015; 126: 1285–1293.

[83] Koyama T, Kawada T, Kitanaka Y, Katagiri K, Ohno M, Ikeshita M, Yamate N. Congenital anomaly of the external iliac artery: a case report. J Vasc Surg. 2003; 37: 683–685.

[84] Rob CG, Owen K. Congenital hypoplasia of the iliac arteries. Postgrad Med J. 1958; 34: 391–392.

[85] Tamisier D, Melki JP, Cormier JM. Congenital anomalies of the external iliac artery: Case report and review of the literature. Ann Vasc Surg. 1990; 4: 510–514.

[86] McLellan GL, Morettin LB. Persistent sciatic artery: Clinical, surgical, and angiographic aspects. Arch Surg. 1982; 117: 817–822.

[87] Imerci A, Ozaksar K, Gürbüz Y, Sügün TS, Canbek U, Savran A. Popliteal artery injury associated with blunt trauma to the knee without fracture or dislocation. West J Emerg Med. 2014; 15: 145–148.

[88] Flanigan DP, Keifer TJ, Schuler JJ, Ryan TJ, Castronuovo JJ. Experience with iatrogenic pediatric vascular injuries. Incidence, etiology, management, and results. Ann Surg. 1983; 198: 430–442.

[89] Bassett FH III, Lincoln CR, King TD, Canent RV Jr. Inequality in the size of the lower extremity following cardiac catheterization. South Med J. 1968; 61: 1013–1017.

[90] Bloom JD, Mozersky DJ, Buckley CJ, Hagood CO Jr. Defective limb growth as a complication of catheterization of the femoral artery. Surg Gynecol Obstet. 1974; 138: 524–526.

[91] Jacobsson B, Carlgren LE, Hedvall G, Sivertsson R. A review of children after arterial catheterization of the leg. Pediatr Radiol. 1973; 1: 96–99.

[92] Rosenthal A, Anderson M, Thompson SJ, Pappas AM, Fyler DC. Superficial femoral artery catheterization: effect on extremity length. Am J Dis Child. 1972; 124: 240–242.

[93] Currarino G, Eagle MA. The effects of ligation of the subclavian artery on the bones and soft tissues of the arms. J Pediatr. 1965; 67: 808–811.

Percutaneous Reconstruction Techniques: Popliteal Artery Approach for Chronic Total Occlusion of Superficial Femoral and Iliac Arteries

Omer Tanyeli

Abstract

Peripheral artery disease (PAD) is one of the most common diseases affecting quality of life. Claudication is the most frequent sign. If left untreated, PAD may cause serious daily life disturbances and may cause extremity losses, especially in elderly and diabetic patients. Restoration of blood flow from the aorta to the femoral arteries and from the femoral arteries to the popliteal arteries necessitates complex operational procedures. Most of these patients have concomitant coronary diseases. In such patients, open surgical repair with vascular grafts by the aid of general anesthesia increases both mortality and morbidity. Although femoral arteries are the most common site for PAD, iliac impairment is not so rare. In patients with combined iliac and femoral artery diseases, popliteal artery approach is a safe and effective technique for percutaneous revascularization. In this chapter, we share our experience with interventional percutaneous revascularization through popliteal approach, mainly using drug eluting balloons and stents, by the aid of mechanical thrombectomy devices with the highlights of current literature review.

Keywords: peripheral artery disease, popliteal artery approach, stenting, balloon angioplasty, mechanical atherectomy, total occlusion

1. Introduction

PAD is third most common cause of cardiovascular mortality and mortality worldwide, following coronary artery disease and stroke [1]. Although the exact number of patients suffering from PAD is unknown, it is commonly agreed that there is a global increase in the amount of patients mainly by increased age and life expectancy of the populations, mainly in underdeveloped countries. Fowkes et al. reported that there were 202 million people estimated to suffer from PAD, with a stronger change in the prevalence of low- and middle-income countries [1].

Elderly patients with diabetes mellitus and smoking habits are under great risk for PAD. Hyperlipidemia or hypertension is less likely to be the predisposing factors for the development of PAD.

Intermittent claudication (IC) is the most common symptom factor affecting quality of life. In order to improve walking distance, and prevent extremity losses, a wide variety of treatment strategies are offered including lifestyle changes, medical therapy, supervised exercise therapy, interventional procedures and surgical revascularization.

Ever since Seldinger discovered the needle-in, wire-in, needle-out, catheter in, interventional radiologists and cardiologists gained a favorable expertise not only in diagnosis of cardiovascular diseases, but also for treatment of vascular lesions. Over the past decade, with improvement of diagnostic procedures, catheter-based treatment strategies also increased and now almost became the first-line treatment strategy in almost all vascular diseases, mainly being performed by new generation qualified vascular surgeons and interventionists. Balloon angioplasty or stenting for a stenotic segment of the superficial femoral artery (SFA) became a routine process and endovascular procedures for complex chronic total occlusions (CTO) are more commonly being treated with interventional procedures using mechanical thrombectomy/atherectomy devices, which put the common surgical revascularization techniques in second order. In this chapter, we aimed to discuss the treatment of iliofemoral PAD, using combined endovascular treatment strategies, mainly focusing on the retrograde popliteal artery (PA) approach.

2. Peripheral artery disease

On the basis of anatomical and functional considerations, lower extremity occlusive PAD can be defined as atherosclerotic arterial disease and arterial narrowing, causing a mismatch between the blood supply and demand. Whatever is the cause, this mismatch results in symptoms including IC, exercise limitations, rest pain or tissue loss. These two definitions help divide the PAD patients into asymptomatic or symptomatic disease states [2]. About 10% of men at the age of 65 years are affected by atherosclerotic PAD. This ratio increases to 20% in men and women ≥75 years [3]. Besides its common nature, most of the patients remain asymptomatic and the disease is underdiagnosed. For every symptomatic patient with PAD, up to six patients are asymptomatic and miss the diagnosis. In a study of patients with PAD including 60-year-old men and women, Schroll et al. found that only 19% of patients were symptomatic [4].

2.1. The frequency of PAD location

Determining the location of PAD is crucial for decision-making and planning the treatment. The PAD may be classified according to the location of the involved arterial segment as aortoiliac, femoropopliteal and tibioperoneal segment. Location of PAD segment may vary

according to gender, associated disease, especially diabetes mellitus (DM) and the age group. Motsumi et al. reported that diabetic patients have severe occlusive disease involving the tibioperoneal segment [5]. Diabetic patients also have diffuse nature of PAD. Patients with DM, hypertension, dyslipidemia and smoking habits have significant occlusive disease of the femoropopliteal arterial segment. Smoking obviously increases the severity of arterial occlusive disease in the femoropopliteal segment or more proximal arterial segments. Diehm et al. reported that smoking had a higher relative risk ratio for severe involvement of the aortoiliac segment [6]. Interestingly, aortoiliac involvement in female diabetic patients was uncommon, irrespective of risk factor grouping and they had relative sparing of the arterial foot arch compared to their male counterparts [5].

When the frequency of the involved arterial segment in PAD was analyzed, researchers found that femoropopliteal location was the most common [6–8]. The involvement of femoropopliteal arterial segment varied between 47.3% and 77% in these studies. On the contrary, there are also a few studies reporting different results, mainly in the younger age groups. A study mainly focused on relatively younger age groups (<50 years) with early-onset PAD demonstrated that these patients had 65% aortoiliac disease [9]. In another study, common femoral arteries (CFA) were more commonly affected than the distal arterial segment (57.6% and 42.9%, respectively) [10]. In this study, older age, male sex, diabetes, heart failure and critical limb ischemia were more significantly associated with distal disease, whereas female sex, smoking, hypertension, dyslipidemia, coronary heart disease, cerebrovascular disease and chronic obstructive pulmonary disease were more significantly associated with proximal disease.

PAD resulting from atherosclerosis is a multisegmental disease in about two-thirds of symptomatic patients [11]. About 25–50% of patients have stenoses and/or occlusions in two or more segments [7, 12]. Knowing the fact that multisegmental disease affects about one in every 2–4 patients, determining the access site before any interventional procedure is very important.

2.2. Characteristics of Iliofemoral peripheral artery disease

Patients with PAD may have different symptoms depending on the anatomical location of the diseased arterial segments, onset of disease (acute or chronic) or presence/absence of the collateral circulation. Since the disease is progressive in nature, the patients may remain asymptomatic for years until the luminal obstruction is >50%. During this period, patients may have IC in strenuous exercise or may remain completely asymptomatic as stated earlier. As the disease progresses, and the luminal obstruction is >50%, patients may have progressively worsening IC, and the walking distance becomes to decrease. In following years, if the patient is left untreated symptoms intensify to rest pain, arterial ulceration, tissue loss or amputation.

There is a significant correlation between the severity of limb ischemia and the distribution of PAD. IC is usually associated with proximal lesions, and critical limb ischemia is associated with crural involvement. Proximal aortoiliac disease may cause thigh, hip, or buttock pain while walking and they are usually preceded by calf pain. Distal tibial or peroneal obstructions may result in ankle or foot pain while walking [13]. PAD patients with more severe and limb-threatening ischemia usually have multisegment involvement.

Patients with distal disease had poorer prognosis compared with patients without distal disease, independent of age, sex, comorbid conditions, medication (lipid-lowering and aspirin) use and resting ankle-brachial index (ABI), whereas patients with proximal disease showed no difference in prognosis after similar adjustment compared with patients without proximal disease. These findings suggest PAD is complex and heterogeneous and not a uniform entity [10].

The mortality for asymptomatic PAD is similar to that of mild to moderately symptomatic patients. Besides its beneficial effect on diagnosis of the disease, ankle-brachial index is also shown to correlate with the overall mortality of the disease [14]. The majority of these patients die of vascular causes such as cardiac, cerebrovascular, or other vascular diseases. The main reason for morbidity or mortality is either myocardial infarction or stroke. All-cause mortality is approximately 30% at 5 years, 50% at 10 years and 70% at 15 years [15]. In a population study, large-vessel involvement in PAD patients was significantly predictive of all-cause mortality in both genders with a relative risk of 4–5, independent of other cardiovascular risk factors. Isolated small-vessel PAD was unrelated to mortality. In that study, large-vessel PAD involved all arteries above the level of ankle [16]. Ogt et al. also found that the relative risk of mortality was elevated from 2- to 7-fold in men and women with multi- and unisegmental disease involving the aortoiliac and femoropopliteal segments. In the same study, the presence of tibioperoneal disease did not significantly increase mortality [8].

2.3. Diagnosis of iliofemoral peripheral artery disease

Depending on basic medical rules, the initial evaluation should include a careful history and physical examination. Knowing the fact that almost half of patients with PAD remain asymptomatic, suspicion of PAD for a clinician is very important. Shoes and socks should be removed for assessment of distal perfusion. Any signs of peripheral ischemia, peripheral pulses, skin color, toe nails, hair loss and trophic skin changes should be noted. Every sign of physical examination should be compared to the contralateral extremity. Abdomen should also be palpated for any potential abdominal aortic aneurysm. The blood pressure should be measured in both arms.

Upon suspicion and physical examination findings, referral to the vascular laboratory should be the initial step. The diagnostic tests should start by noninvasive methods. These noninvasive tests are also important for the follow-up of patients or disease progress.

The ABI is the single best initial screening test to perform in a patient suspected for PAD. A ratio of <0.90 is considered abnormal, with mild obstruction defined as a ratio of 0.71–0.90, moderate as 0.41–0.70 and severe when the ABI is <0.40. The higher arm blood pressure is used for the ABI ratio calculation [17]. The overall accuracy of the ABI to establish the diagnosis of lower extremity PAD has been validated with a sensitivity of 79–95% and a specificity of 96–100%, based on different studies [18, 19]. It is a reproducible technique, cheap and can also be used for screening and initial evaluation of target population, as well as assessment of disease progression. In patients with noncompressible arteries due to medial calcification such as elderly, diabetes and end-stage renal disease, toe-brachial index calculation may be helpful and values <0.7 are considered diagnostic for lower extremity PAD [20].

Treadmill exercise testing can be helpful, especially in patients with normal ABI during resting, such as in patients with isolated iliac artery stenosis. A decrease in ABI of 15–20% with exercise is considered diagnostic for PAD. Climbing stairs, walking in the highway or 6-min walking test can also be performed not only for differentiation of claudication from pseudo-claudication, but also objectively assess the limitations of the patients and help to prescribe patient specific exercise programs. They are also important for patient follow-ups and disease progress [21].

Pulse volume recordings and Doppler waveform techniques are other techniques that can provide accurate information even in patients with noncompressible vessels. The normal waveform is triphasic. Loss of triphasic pattern and analysis of the peak velocity can localize the area of stenosis. They may be used to establish the initial diagnosis, assess the location and severity of PAD as well as follow-up of patients after any revascularization procedures [17].

Although they are not the first diagnostic test of choice in diagnosis of PAD, computed tomography angiography (CTA), magnetic resonance angiography (MRA) and digital subtraction angiography (DSA) are the other techniques that allow direct visualization of the vasculature in PAD patients.

CTA may be used with either intra-venous or intra-arterial contrast agents. The sensitivities and specificities are >95% for identifying stenosis >50% and for correctly identifying occlusions [22]. CTA produces images of vascular structures in cross-sectional slices that can be reformatted into three-dimensional angiographic-like images. CTA not only shows the intra-luminal space, but also shows the surrounding tissue. For this reason, it visualizes calcification well, which is advantageous when considering revascularization strategies [23]. The main disadvantage is radiation exposure and the use of large volumes of iodinated contrast media, which limits its use in acute renal failure patients or patients with borderline renal function.

MRA is a useful diagnostic method in determining the location and stenosis severity in PAD patients. MRA may identify outflow vessels which may not be visualized by conventional angiography [24]. MRA has a high sensitivity and specificity for detecting acute occlusive disease when compared with DSA [25]. It is very useful for preoperative evaluation of the PAD patient in order to make a road-map, whether surgical or endovascular revascularization. **Figure 1** shows MRA of two different patients showing total occlusion of SFA.

MRA may also be used for postoperative follow-up of patients. A meta-analysis comparing MRA with catheter angiography demonstrated that sensitivity and specificity of MRA for detection of stenoses >50% were both in the range of 90–100% [26]. The main limitation of MRA is that it tends to overestimate the degree of stenosis because of turbulence; it cannot scan patients with pacemakers or defibrillators; metal stents or clips can obscure vascular flow; and use of gadolinium rarely may cause renal toxicity and nephrogenic systemic fibrosis in patients with elevated creatinine [17].

In our daily practice, there are some patients who are planned for endovascular interventions for critical stenoses, but not critically stenotic by DSA. Also, patients with previous stent in iliac/SFAs may also be misdiagnosed as occluded by MRA; that is why each patient needs a careful physical examination before MRA including comparative ABI. Duplex ultrasound scanning (DUS) may also give supportive data in these patients.

Contrast angiography provides detailed information about the vasculature, including minor collateral vessels, run-off and the flow speed, and is recommended as 'gold standard' method

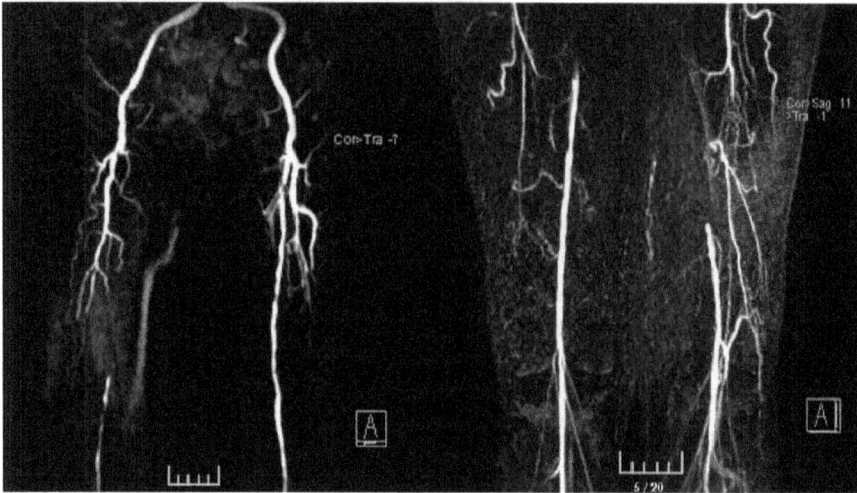

Figure 1. Contrast enhanced MR angiography, showing total occlusion of superficial femoral artery and well developed collateral circulation.

for evaluation of patients with PAD, especially when revascularization is considered. Image quality is enhanced by digital subtraction. The major advantage of DSA is the ability to selectively evaluate individual vessels, to obtain physiologic information such as pressure gradients and to serve as a platform for percutaneous intervention [23]. Angiography carries risk of any interventional procedure such as bleeding, infection, vascular damage, dissection, pseudoaneurysm formation and atheroembolism. Any of these factors can be reduced by experience of the interventionist [17]. As seen with other techniques, the use of contrast agent carries risk of contrast induced nephropathy, as well as anaphylactoid reactions. Angiography should not only be thought solely as a diagnostic method; at the same time, it also offers therapeutic options that are discussed later in this chapter.

Angiography, either noninvasive or invasive, should not be performed for the anatomic assessment of patients with PAD without leg symptoms because delineation of anatomy will not change treatment for this population.

3. Treatment options for iliofemoral peripheral artery disease

The management of lower extremity PAD is one of the most challenging problems for vascular surgeons/interventionists. As the population age increases and diagnostic tools improve, it is not surprising that the amount of patients seeking for treatment of PAD also increase day by day.

Treatment of any PAD, including iliofemoral PAD, can be classified into four categories including risk factor modification, exercise and cardiovascular rehabilitation, pharmacologic therapy, and invasive methods including surgery and interventional procedures [2]. Patients should not only be aware of their PAD, but also be informed and searched for other related diseases, including cerebrovascular and cardiovascular diseases. All the goals of these therapeutic options are to improve symptoms and quality of life, at the same time decrease cardiovascular event rates.

3.1. Risk factor modification

Since cardiovascular events are the major cause of death in patients with PAD, modification of atherosclerotic risk factors should be the mainstay of risk factor modification. Smoking cessation and aggressive glycemic control in diabetic patients, both represent the most dominant risk factors for PAD, are very important [17]. Smoking cessation among patients with symptomatic PAD does not improve walking capacity, but may reduce the severity of claudication and the risk of developing critical limb ischemia [27].

In addition to smoking cessation and glycemic control in PAD patients, hyperlipidemia should be treated to reduce the risk of cardiovascular events in patients with atherosclerosis. Statin treatment is shown to have beneficial effects in reducing pain-free walking distance in patients with PAD, so that there is a positive effect on IC [28].

Hypertension is associated with a two- to three-fold increased risk for PAD. Hypertension guidelines support the aggressive treatment of blood pressure in patients with atherosclerosis, indicating PAD. In this high-risk group the current recommendation is a goal of <140/90 mmHg and < 130/80 mmHg if the patient also has diabetes or renal insufficiency [29]. Regarding drug choice, all drugs that lower blood pressure are effective at reducing the risk of cardiovascular events. Most patients will require multiple agents to achieve desired blood pressure goals [21]. The angiotensin-converting enzyme (ACE) inhibitor drugs have also shown benefit in PAD, possibly beyond blood-pressure lowering in high-risk groups [30]. Beta-adrenergic blocking drugs have previously been discouraged in PAD because of the possibility of worsening IC symptoms. However, this concern has not been supported by randomized trials, especially for cardioselective beta-blockers; therefore, beta-adrenergic blocking drugs can be safely used in patients with claudication [31].

3.2. Exercise and cardiovascular rehabilitation

In patients with claudication, there is a considerable body of evidence to support the clinical benefits of a supervised exercise program in improving exercise performance and community-based walking ability [21]. Apart from medical therapy, exercise significantly improves walking time and overall walking ability in patients with IC and should be considered as a primary efficacious treatment in PAD. Several studies have suggested that some level of supervision is necessary to achieve optimal results (general, unstructured recommendations to exercise by the physician do not result in any clinical benefit). In prospective studies of supervised exercise conducted for 3 months or longer, there are clear increases in treadmill exercise performance and a lessening of claudication pain severity during exercise [32]. Current ACC/AHA guidelines recommend a supervised exercise therapy as a first-line treatment for IC, as it is equally effective as endovascular revascularization in the treatment of patients with IC [33]. Whether asymptomatic or symptomatic, any patients taking support for PAD (either medical or surgical/interventional), exercise therapy (namely structured exercise therapy) should be considered, not only to improve IC, but also for motivation and promote risk factor modification.

3.3. Pharmacologic therapy

Apart from medical therapies used to modify risk factors for PAD (antihypertensive, antidiabetic and antihyperlipidemic drugs), there are some drugs that are shown to improve IC or prevent occlusion-reocclusion after surgery/interventional procedures.

Based on the currently available literature, all patients with PAD should receive antiplatelet therapy to reduce cardiovascular risk with a slight preference for clopidogrel monotherapy. Antiplatelet therapy with aspirin alone (range 75–325 mg per day) or clopidogrel alone (75 mg per day) is recommended to reduce MI, stroke and vascular death in patients with symptomatic PAD [33]. The CAPRIE (clopidogrel versus aspirin in patients at risk of ischemic events) trial demonstrated a benefit of clopidogrel as compared with aspirin in cardiovascular risk reduction and bleeding events in a population of patients with symptomatic atherosclerotic vascular disease, including a subgroup of patients with symptomatic PAD [34]. However, there are two important subgroups that benefit from a different medical regime. Those receiving a venous bypass graft will have the most benefit when treated with a vitamin K antagonist and those receiving a below-knee prosthetic bypass graft will benefit the most when dual antiplatelet therapy (ASA and clopidogrel) [35].

Probably, the most effective pharmacologic treatment proven to be effective in relief of symptoms and improving IC in patients with PAD is cilostazol. ACC/AHA guideline strongly recommends the use of cilostazol in patients with PAD (class of recommendation IA) [33]. In a Cochrane review including 15 double-blind RCTs with a total of 3718 participants, cilostazol was associated with improvement in claudication symptoms but no changes in cardiovascular deaths or quality of life when compared with placebo [36]. The main limitation of the drug is congestive heart failure. Pentoxifylline is a xanthine and also acts as a nonselective inhibitor of phosphodiesterases, which causes an increase in intracellular cyclic AMP and decreased synthesis of tumor necrosis factor alpha and leukotrienes. It acts by improving red blood cell deformability, thus reducing blood viscosity as well as decreasing platelet aggregation and thrombus formation. By these properties, it was one of the agents used in PAD treatment. In a multicenter randomized control trial of pentoxifylline, cilostazol, or placebo for patients with moderate-to-severe claudication, there was no difference between pentoxifylline and placebo in the primary endpoint of maximal walking distance [37]. Therefore, pentoxifylline is not recommended as a treatment for claudication [33].

3.4. Invasive methods

An individualized approach to revascularization for claudication is recommended for each patient to optimize outcome. If a strategy of revascularization for claudication is undertaken, the revascularization strategy should be evidence based and can include endovascular revascularization, surgery, or both [33]. When deciding for an invasive method for treatment of PAD, patient's symptoms, localization of the affected arterial segment, patient specific factors including age, co-morbid diseases should be taken into consideration with a favorable risk–benefit ratio, with all combination therapies listed earlier.

In the last decade-or-two, endovascular procedures became one of the most popular concerns for treatment of PAD. There are numerous randomized clinical trials that compared endovascular procedures to various combinations of medical treatment with or without exercise programs.

When the aortoiliac disease is the concern, endovascular procedures are effective as a revascularization option for patients with lifestyle-limiting claudication and hemodynamically significant aortoiliac occlusive disease (class of recommendation IA) [33]. The CLEVER trial enrolled only patients with aortoiliac disease and compared endovascular therapy to supervised exercise therapy and to medications alone. At 6-month follow-up, both the endovascular therapy and supervised exercise groups had improved peak walking time compared with medication alone, with a greater improvement in the supervised exercise group [38]. The ERASE trial randomized patients with claudication and aortoiliac (as well as femoropopliteal) disease to endovascular revascularization plus supervised exercise or supervised exercise alone. After 1 year, patients in both groups had significant improvements in walking distances and health-related QoL, with greater improvements in the combined-therapy group [39].

When the femoropopliteal disease is the concern, endovascular procedures are reasonable as a revascularization option for patients with lifestyle-limiting claudication and hemodynamically significant femoropopliteal disease (class of recommendation IIa) [33]. There are a number of randomized clinical trials that showed short-term beneficial effects with endovascular treatment of femoropopliteal disease for claudication versus supervised exercise training or medical therapy, with benefit that diminishes by 1 year [40]. In a systematic review that included randomized clinical trials that enrolled patients with femoropopliteal disease, authors reported that endovascular treatment of claudication improved walking parameters and quality of life [41]. The durability of endovascular treatment for claudication is directly related to vessel patency. Long-term patency is greater in the iliac artery than in the femoropopliteal segment [33].

Since SFA and popliteal arteries are the most common sites of obstruction in PAD patients, when the surgery is the concern, femoropopliteal bypass is one of the most widely performed surgical processes in these patients with claudication. There is a clear and consistent primary patency benefit for autogenous vein versus to prosthetic grafts for popliteal artery bypass [42]. PTFE grafts should be preferred over Dacron grafts for femoropopliteal bypass when there is lack of autogenous grafts.

In this chapter, apart from the surgical revascularization, mainly endovascular treatment options for iliofemoral PAD and access sites will be discussed.

4. Endovascular management of iliofemoral lesions

Among those with appropriate indications for intervention, the procedure of choice, whether surgical or endovascular, depends on surgeon's/interventionist's experience, localization of the diseased arterial segment, anatomical suitability of disease and patient related factors, such as comorbid diseases. Most of the endovascular procedures are performed using local anesthesia on an outpatient manner.

Although the radiologists and cardiologists were the main pioneers of endovascular procedures, in the last decade, by the formation of hybrid operating rooms, vascular and cardiovascular surgeons became the leader of these interventional procedures. As a cardiovascular surgeon, in the last decade, we shared our patients with radiologists and cardiologists only for the reason that they had cath labs. The only way to re-face the patient was at the end of an unsuccessful attempt for percutaneous procedure, or a complication, such as rupture of the artery, pseudoaneurysm formation, bleeding, or emboli and so on. All the interventions can be of-course performed by different departments, but any department should be capable of fixing their own complications, related to their interventions. In this decade, probably one of the most important advancement in PAD diseases was involvement of vascular surgeons in the world of endovascular and hybrid procedures.

Given the widespread availability of percutaneous procedures, major vascular society guidelines recommend initial percutaneous revascularization. The endovascular techniques for the treatment of patients with lower extremity ischemia include balloon angioplasty, stents, stent-grafts and plaque debulking procedures. Although long segment stenosis/occlusions, multifocal stenoses, eccentric and calcified lesions are more prone to surgical revascularization, use of total occlusion catheters, rotational thrombectomy/atherectomy devices made these complex lesions also treatable with endovascular procedures.

In general, the outcomes of revascularization depend upon the extent of the disease in the subjacent arterial tree (inflow, outflow and the size and length of the diseased segment). IN TASC-II guideline, 'A' lesions represent those which yield excellent results from, and should be treated by, endovascular means; 'B' lesions offer sufficiently good results with endovascular methods that this approach is still preferred first, unless an open revascularization is required for other associated lesions in the same anatomic area; 'C' lesions produce superior enough long-term results with open revascularization that endovascular methods should be used only in patients at high risk for open repair; and 'D' lesions do not yield good enough results with endovascular methods to justify them as primary treatment [21]. For treatment of TASC A lesions, the choice of treatment is endovascular, whereas it is surgery for TASC D lesions. Endovascular treatment is the preferred treatment for type B lesions and surgery is the preferred treatment for good-risk patients with type C lesions, which should be decided on a patient basis. The same is also recommended for femoropopliteal lesions.

The technical and clinical success rate of percutaneous transluminal angioplasty (PTA) of femoropopliteal artery stenoses in all series exceeds 95% [43]. Device developments such as hydrophilic guide wires and technical developments, such as subintimal recanalization, provide high recanalization rates in total occlusions of more than 85% [44]. The technique of subintimal angioplasty is not as dependent on length, but rather on the presence of normal vessel above and below the occlusion to allow access [45]. There is general agreement that for acute failure of PTA of an SFA lesion, stent placement is indicated.

The mechanism of endovascular treatment using balloon angioplasty and stenting is based on plaque disruption and displacement within the arterial wall. By this way, the atheroma is not removed but pressed or crushed by the balloon and redistributed inside and along the arterial wall. Endovascular atherectomy may be performed under local anesthesia using standard caliber arterial sheaths, ranging from 4 to 8 Fr, and provides the theoretical advantage over balloon angioplasty that plaque is removed rather than pressed against the arterial wall, and subsequent balloon dilation is optional depending on the debulking effect. This contributes to substantial luminal gain with less barotrauma even if postdilation is performed, decreasing the risk of dissection and/or neointimal hyperplasia, while avoiding stent placement [46]. In order to improve patency, the combination of lesion debulking using percutaneous atherectomy and subsequent drug-coated balloon application has been implemented. Drug-coated balloons are proved to be an effective treatment option that does not require a permanent stent [47].

Atherosclerotic iliac artery disease is increasingly being treated with endovascular techniques. A number of new stent technologies can be utilized with high long-term patency, including self-expanding stents, balloon-expandable stents and covered stents, but comparative data on these stent types and in more complex lesions are lacking. Iliac stent choice can be largely categorized into choosing either a balloon-expandable or self-expanding stent based on lesion characteristics (i.e., calcified, fibrous, soft, eccentric, concentric, focal, diffuse, etc.), access site, introducer size, vessel tortuosity and lesion location [48].

For the last few years, our main strategy in treating iliac and femoropopliteal lesions are endo-first, if the lesion has suitable anatomy. For the patients with long segment stenosis and calcified lesions, we prefer rotational atherectomy for debulking of atherosclerotic plaque and then dilatation with drug-coated balloons. If there is a residual dissection, stenting is preferred. Mainly balloon inflatable stents are preferred for proximal iliac lesions, since the plaque over the iliac segments are generally stiff and prone to re-occlusion. For common and SFAs, our main preference is self-expanding nitinol stents, unless the problem is not solved by drug-coated balloons. As surgeons, we always should think of a possibility of reocclusion in these patients and that is why, stenting in the popliteal and distal CFAs should be avoided for alternative surgical sites.

4.1. Retrograde popliteal artery approach for femoral and iliac arterial lesions

To go inside a building, we should open the door first with the right key and in order to perform complex interventions, choosing the right access site is mandatory. There are several access sites described in the literature for endovascular procedures including ipsilateral retrograde common femoral access, ipsilateral antegrade common femoral access, superficial femoral access, contralateral common femoral access, retrograde popliteal access, pedal access, aortic access, radial access and so on. Whatever is the access site, the main goal is to approach stenotic/occluded arterial segments and perform endovascular interventions with success avoiding complications. Since PAD is not a uniform disease, and coexistence of femoral and iliac lesions are present in favorable amount of patients, retrograde contralateral common femoral access can result in procedural failure, especially in patients with unfavorable anatomy of the aortic bifurcation.

The SFA occlusions are generally managed by antegrade ipsilateral or retrograde contralateral femoral approach ending in intraluminal or subintimal recanalization of the vessel lumen [49]. In case of failure, a retrograde popliteal access is considered a valid alternative [50].

The retrograde popliteal approach is a type of subintimal arterial flossing with antegrade-retrograde intervention; it was first described by Tonnesen et al. in 1988 [51]. The main indications for this technique are a short SFA stump, flush occlusion or tandem common/SFA lesions and failure of antegrade approach. Also, coexistence of femoral and iliac lesions necessitates contralateral femoral approach; crossover in the abdominal aorta may complicate the procedure in patients with angled iliac arteries and aorta. Also, in chronic total occlusions (TASC D), it may be rather difficult to crossover the aorta by the atherectomy devices, even if the patient had normal anatomy in the aortic segment. In SFA lesions, the access over the inguinal region may rather be hard, especially in obese patients.

For the abovementioned patients, popliteal access is a useful method for interventional procedures. The procedure begins in prone position. Prone position has the advantage of contralateral popliteal artery use, either for proximal visualization of the totally occluded artery, or crossover if the retrograde access is not successful. Puncture of the artery and replacement of sheath should always be made by the aid of an ultrasonography, since the popliteal vein is in close proximity to the popliteal artery and sometimes lies over the artery. Visualization of the vein and artery avoids iatrogenic AV fistula formation (**Figure 2**). Since majority of the patients have absent/weak popliteal artery pulses, ultrasonography aided catheterization should always be part of routine practice. After placement of 6–8 Fr sheath, a hydrophilic 0.0035 wire is advanced, and supported either by a slightly angled diagnostic catheter or total occlusion catheter. In total occlusions, the lesion is usually crossed intimally/subintimally by the aid of 6 Fr total occlusion catheter. Confirming that the guidewire is in the patent true lumen proximally, verification is made by angiography. In total occlusion of femoral/iliac arteries, our strategy is to make debulking of atherosclerotic plaque with rotational atherectomy devices and then use drug-coated balloons, or stents according to type and localization of the lesions (**Figure 3**).

A good preoperative evaluation is important before the procedure. Minimum popliteal artery diameter should be at least 4 mm. Local anesthesia should not be made too much in amount

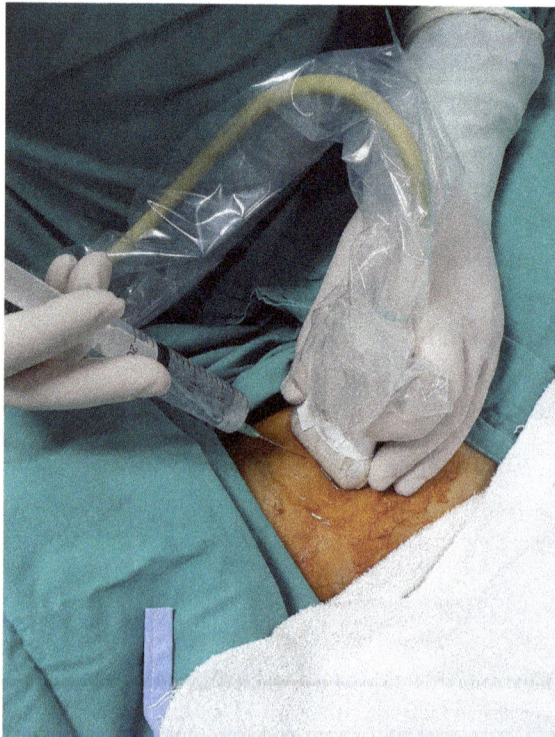

Figure 2. Popliteal artery access using ultrasonography probe after application of minimal local anesthesia.

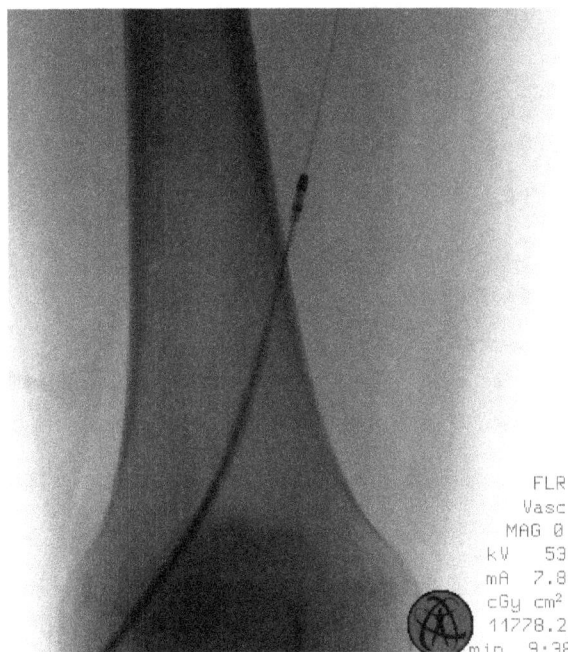

```
FLR
Vasc
MAG 0
kV    53
mA   7.8
cGy  cm²
11778.2
min  9.38
```

Figure 3. Rotational mechanical atherectomy catheter inserted through the 8F sheath over the popliteal artery in a retrograde fashion.

not to cause compression of the vasculature and obtain a clear image of ultrasound. Just a little amount of local anesthesia is usually enough; after insertion of the needle and guidewire, additional local anesthetic provides comfort of the patient.

Popliteal access is also advantageous in patients with occluded femoropopliteal artery bypass grafts. The atherectomy/thrombectomy can be made either from the native artery or the occluded graft, which usually results in high operational success in our cases. Videos (https://mts.intechopen.com/download/index/process/195/authkey/b9bb94b883d527ae-1b201a3ea2901c84) shows pre- and post-procedural angiograms showing total opening of SFA after rotational mechanical atherectomy and drug-coated balloons.

Subintimal guidewire extension and atherectomy usually results in residual dissection in the entry area; but since the direction of dissection is opposite to the direction of flow, in our opinion, this access becomes advantageous. As mentioned before, vascular surgeons should always leave a potential area for future surgical revascularization in the popliteal and common femoral arteries (CFA), after an eventful reocclusion of these segments.

The main disadvantage of this process is mainly based on the prone position of the patient. In complex cases, prolonged procedural times may disturb patients, especially if the patient has chronic obstructive pulmonary disease. Direct cannulation of the artery needs experience of ultrasonography and a learning curve in the very first few cases. Hematoma and post-procedural lack of compression may be overcome by routine use of vascular closure devices (**Figure 4**). Vascular closure devices are especially important when 6F or 8F sheaths are used for vascular access in the popliteal region; because, after the interventional procedure is completed, external compression may cause runoff failure, leading acute obstruction of the popliteal artery.

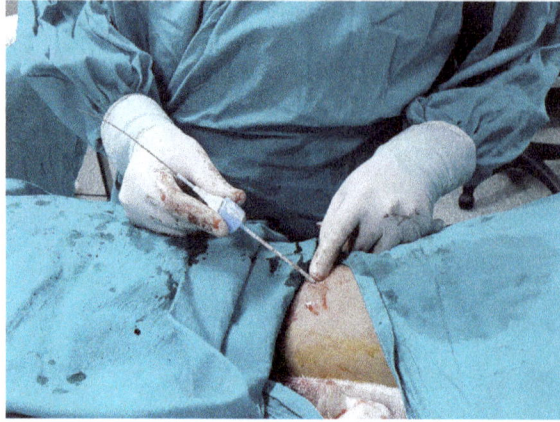

Figure 4. At the end of the endovascular procedure, popliteal artery is closed by vascular closure device to avoid compression.

Retrograde transpopliteal approach is an innovative technique that allows complex endovascular procedures, and should be a part of every vascular interventinal's skill set. Proper case selection, operator experience and appropriate technique are essential for clinical and procedural success.

5. Conclusions

PAD is one of the most common diseases affecting quality of life, especially in the elderly population. Since most of these patients are asymptomatic, a careful physician should always be suspicious about the diagnosis. Symptomatic patients should be encouraged to structured exercise therapy, in combination with risk factor modification, pharmacological treatment and invasive treatment strategies when needed.

Endovascular treatment options and the number of procedures dramatically increased in the last decade. A careful preoperative evaluation and plan should be made to achieve success in interventional procedures. Although femoral arteries are the most common site for PAD, iliac impairment is not so rare. In patients with combined iliac and femoral artery diseases, popliteal artery approach is a safe and effective technique for percutaneous revascularization. Interventionists should always have an alternative plan and access site in their reserve for the success of complex procedures.

Notes/Thanks/Other declarations

Thanks Prof. Dr. Niyazi Gormus, for his expert opinion, patience and excellent guidance in our practice.

Author details

Omer Tanyeli

Address all correspondence to: otanyeli@gmail.com

Department of Cardiovascular Surgery, Meram Medicine Faculty, Necmettin Erbakan University, Konya, Turkey

References

[1] Fowkes FG, Rudan D, Rudan I, Aboyans V, Denenberg JO, McDermott MM, et al. Comparison of global estimates of prevalence and risk factors for peripheral artery disease in 2000 and 2010: A systematic review and analysis. Lancet. 2013;382:1329-1340. DOI: 10.1016/S0140-6736(13)61249-0

[2] Dieter RS, Chu WW, Pacanowski JP, McBride PE, Tanke TE. The significance of lower extremity peripheral artery disease. Clinical Cardiology. 2002;25:3-10

[3] Criqui MH, Fronek A, Barrett-Connor E, Klauber MR, Gabriel S, Goodman D. The prevelance of peripheral arterial disease in a defined population. Circulation. 1985;71: 510-515

[4] Schroll M, Munck O. Estimation of peripheral arteriosclerotic disease by ankle blood pressure in a population study of 60-year-old men and women. Journal of Chronic Diseases. 1981;34:261-269

[5] Motsumi MJ, Naidoo NG. Pattern and distribution of peripheral arterial disease in diabetic patients with critical limb ischemia (Rutherford clinical category 4-6). South African Journal of Surgery. 2017;55:48-54

[6] Diehm N, Shang A, Silvestro A, Dick F, Schmidli J, Mahler F, et al. Association of cardiovascular risk factors with pattern of lower limb atherosclerosis in 2659 patients undergoing angioplasty. European Journal of Vascular and Endovascular Surgery. 2006;31:59-63

[7] Haltmayer M, Mueller T, Horvath W, Luft C, Poelz W, Haidinger D. Impact of atherosclerotic risk factors on the anatomical distribution of peripheral arterial disease. International Angiology. 2001;20:200-207

[8] Vogt MT, Wolfson SK, Kuller LH. Segmental arterial disease in the lower extremities: Correlates of disease and relationship to mortality. Journal of Clinical Epidemiology. 1993;46:1267-1276

[9] Barretto S, Ballman KV, Rooke TW, Kullo IJ. Early-onset peripheral arterial occlusive disease: Clinical features and determinants of disease severity and location. Vascular Medicine. 2003;8:95-100

[10] Chen Q, Smith CY, Bailey KR, Wennberg PW, Kullo IJ. Disease location is associated with survival in patients with peripheral artery disease. Journal of the American Heart Association. 2013;2:e000304

[11] Aboyans V, Desormais I, Lacroix P, Salazar J, Criqui MH, Laskar M. The general prognosis of patients with peripheral arterial disease differs according to the disease localization. Journal of the American College of Cardiology. 2010;**55**:898-903

[12] Weinberg I, Giri J, Calfon MA, Hawkins BM, Weinberg MD, Margey R, et al. Anatomic correlates of supra-normal ankle brachial indices. Catheterization and Cardiovascular Interventions. 2013;**81**:1025-1030

[13] Halperin JL. Evaluation of patients with peripheral vascular disease. Thrombosis Research. 2002;**106**:303-311

[14] Crique MH, Langer R, Fronek A, Feigelson H, Klauber M, McCann T, et al. Mortality over a period of 10 years in patients with peripheral artery disease. The New England Journal of Medicine. 1992;**326**(6):381

[15] TASC Working Group. Management of peripheral arterial disease. Journal of Vascular Surgery. 2000;**31**:1-296

[16] Criqui MH, Coughlin SS, Fronek A. Noninvasively diagnosed peripheral arterial disease as a predictor of mortality: Results from a prospective study. Circulation. 1985;**72**:768-773

[17] Kasapis C, Gurm HS. Current approach to the diagnosis and treatment of femoral-popliteal arterial disease. A systematic review. Current Cardiology Reviews. 2009;**5**:296-311

[18] Fowkes FG. The measurement of atherosclerotic peripheral arterial disease in epidemiological surveys. International Journal of Epidemiology. 1988;**17**:248-254

[19] Lijmer JG, Hunink MG, van den Dungen JJ, Loonstra J, Smit AJ. ROC analysis of noninvasive tests for peripheral artery disease. Ultrasound in Medicine & Biology. 1996;**22**:391-398

[20] Carter SA, Tate RB. Value of toe pulse waves in addition to systolic pressures in the assessment of the severity of peripheral arterial disease and critical limb ischemia. Journal of Vascular Surgery. 1996;**24**:258-265

[21] Norgren L, Hiatt WR, Dormandy JA, Nehler MR, Harris KA, Fowkes FG, et al. Inter-society concensus for the management of peripheral arterial disease (TASC II). European Journal of Vascular and Endovascular Surgery. 2007;**33**(Suppl 1):1-75

[22] Sun Z. Diagnostic accuracy of multislice CT angiography in peripheral artery disease. Journal of Vascular and Interventional Radiology. 2006;**17**:1915-1921

[23] Chen Q, Shi Y, Wang Y, Li X. Patterns of disease distribution of lower extremity peripheral artery disease. Angiology. 2015;**66**:211-218

[24] Carpenter JP, Baum RA, Holland GA, Barker CF. Peripheral vascular surgery with magnetic resonance angiography as the sole preoperative imaging modality. Journal of Vascular Surgery. 1994;**20**:861-869

[25] Huegli RW, Thalhammer C, Jacob AL, Jaeger K, Bilecen D. Intra-arterial MR-angiography on an open-bore MR-scanner compared to digital-subtraction angiography of the

infra-popliteal runoff in patients with peripheral arterial occlusive disease. European Journal of Radiology. 2008;**66**:519-525

[26] Nelemans PJ, Leiner T, de Vet HC, van Engelshoven JM. Peripheral arterial disease: Meta-analysis of the diagnostic performance of MR angiography. Radiology. 2000;**217**:105-114

[27] Girolami B, Bernardi E, Prins MH, Ten Cate JW, Hettiarachchi R, Prandoni P, et al. Treatment of intermittent claudication with physical training, smoking cessation, pentoxifylline, or nafronyl: A meta-analysis. Archives of Internal Medicine. 1999;**159**:337-345

[28] Baigent C, Keech A, Kearney PM, Blackwell L, Buck G, Pollicino C, et al. Efficacy and safety of cholesterol-lowering treatment: Prospective meta-analysis of data from 90056 participants in 14 randomised trials of statins. Lancet. 2005;**366**:1267-1278

[29] Chobanian AV, Bakris GL, Black HR, Cushman WC, Green LA, Izzo JL Jr, et al. Seventh report of the joint National Committee on prevention, detection, evaluation, and treatment of high blood pressure. Hypertension. 2003;**42**:1206-1252

[30] Yusuf S, Sleight P, Pogue J, Bosch J, Davies R, Dagenais G. Effects of an angiotensin-converting-enzyme inhibitor, ramipril, on cardiovascular events in high-risk patients. The heart outcomes prevention evaluation study investigators. The New England Journal of Medicine. 2000;**342**:145-153

[31] Radack K, Deck C. Beta-adrenergic blocker therapy does not worsen intermittent claudication in subjects with peripheral arterial disease. A meta-analysis of randomized controlled trials. Archives of Internal Medicine. 1991;**151**:1769-1776

[32] Hiatt W, Wolfel E, Meier R, Regensteiner J. Superiority of treadmill walking exercise vs. strength training for patients with peripheral arterial disease. Implications for the mechanism of the training response. Circulation. 1994;**90**:1866-1874

[33] Gerhard-Herman MD, Gornik HL, Barrett C, Barshes NR, Corriere MA, Drachman DE, et al. AHA/ACC guideline on the Management of Patients with Lower Extremity Peripheral Artery Disease: A report of the American College of Cardiology/American Heart Association task force on clinical practice guidelines. Journal of the American College of Cardiology. 2016, 2017;**69**:e71-e126

[34] CAPRIE Steering Committee. A randomised, blinded, trial of clopidogrel versus aspirin in patients at risk of ischaemic events (CAPRIE). Lancet. 1996;**348**:1329-1339

[35] Vos C, Vahl AC. Anticoagulation and antiplatelet therapy in patients with peripheral arterial disease of the femoropopliteal arteries. The Journal of Cardiovascular Surgery. 2018;**59**:164-171

[36] Bedenis R, Stewart M, Cleanthis M, Robless P, Mikhailidis DP, Stansby G. Cilostazol for intermittent claudication. Cochrane Database of Systematic Reviews. 2014:CD003748

[37] Dawson DL, Cutler BS, Hiatt WR, Hobson RW 2nd, Martin JD, Bortey EB, et al. A comparison of cilostazol and pentoxifylline for treating intermittent claudication. The American Journal of Medicine. 2000;**109**:523-530

[38] Murphy TP, Cutlip DE, Regensteiner JG, Mohler ER, Cohen DJ, Reynolds MR, et al. Supervised exercise, stent revascularization, or medical therapy for claudication due to aortoiliac peripheral artery disease: The CLEVER study. Journal of the American College of Cardiology. 2015;**65**:999-1009

[39] Fakhry F, Spronk S, van der Laan L, Wever JJ, Teijink JA, Hoffmann WH, et al. Endovascular revascularization and supervised exercise for peripheral artery disease and intermittent claudication: A randomized clinical trial. Journal of the American Medical Association. 2015;**314**:1936-1944

[40] Nordanstig J, Taft C, Hensäter M, Perlander A, Osterberg K, Jivegard L. Improved quality of life after 1 year with an invasive versus a noninvasive treatment strategy in claudicants: Oneyear results of the invasive revascularization or not in intermittent claudication (IRONIC) trial. Circulation. 2014;**130**:939-947

[41] Vemulapalli S, Dolor RJ, Hasselblad V, Subherwal S, Schmit KM, Heidenfelder BL, et al. Comparative effectiveness of medical therapy, supervised exercise, and revascularization for patients with intermittent claudication: A network meta-analysis. Clinical Cardiology. 2015;**38**:378-386

[42] Pereira CE, Albers M, Romiti M, Brochado-Neto FC, Pereira CA. Meta-analysis of femoropopliteal bypass grafts for lower extremity arterial insufficiency. Journal of Vascular Surgery. 2006;**44**:510-517

[43] Muradin G, Bosch J, Stijnen T, Hunink M. Balloon dilation and stent implantation for treatment of femoropopliteal arterial disease: Metaanalysis. Radiology. 2001;**221**:137-145

[44] London N, Srinivasan R, Naylor A, Hartshorne T, Ratliff D, Bell P, et al. Subintimal angioplasty of femoropopliteal artery occlusions: The long-term results. European Journal of Vascular Surgery. 1994;**8**:148-155

[45] Desgranges P, Boufi M, Lapeyre M, Tarquini G, van Laere O, Losy F, et al. Subintimal angioplasty: Feasible and durable. European Journal of Vascular and Endovascular Surgery. 2004;**28**:138-141

[46] Katsanos K, Spiliopoulos S, Reppas L, Karnabatidis D. Debulking atherectomy in the peripheral arteris: Is there a role and what is the evidence? Cardiovascular and Interventional Radiology. 2017;**40**:964-977

[47] Katsanos K, Spiliopoulos S, Karunanithy N, Krokidis M, Sabharwal T, Taylor P. Bayesian network meta-analysis of nitinol stents, covered stents, drug-eluting stents, and drug-coated balloons in the femoropopliteal artery. Journal of Vascular Surgery. 2014;**59**:1123-1133

[48] Aggarwall V, Waldo SW, Armstrong EJ. Endovascular revascularization for aortoiliac atherosclerotic disease. Vascular Health and Risk Management. 2016;**12**:117-127

[49] Dumantepe M. Retrograde popliteal access to percutaneous peripheral intervention for chronic total occlusion of superficial femoral arteries. Vascular and Endovascular Surgery. 2017;**51**:240-246

[50] Narins CR. Access strategies for peripheral arterial intervention. Cardiology Journal. 2009;**16**:88-97

[51] Tonnesen KH, Sager P, Karle A, Henriksen L, Jorgensen B. Percutaneous transluminal angioplasty of the superficial femoral artery by retrograde catheterization via the popliteal artery. Cardiovascular and Interventional Radiology. 1988;**11**:127-131

6

Angiography and Endovascular Therapy for Below-the-Knee Artery Disease

Akihiro Higashimori

Abstract

Critical limb ischemia (CLI) is growing in global prevalence and is associated with high rates of limb loss and mortality. "Endovascular-first" approach is considered to be the current standard care for symptomatic infrainguinal atherosclerotic disease. Given the facts that many CLI patients have severe comorbidities and endovascular-first approach is a common practice and may reduce the magnitude of the surgical trauma and systemic complications. In this chapter, updated angiographic approach for below-the-knee disease is described with endovascular technique.

Keywords: critical limb ischemia, below-the-knee disease, angiosome, indigo carmine

1. Introduction

Critical limb ischemia (CLI) is growing in global prevalence and is associated with high rates of limb loss and mortality. The "endovascular-first" approach is considered to be the current standard treatment for symptomatic infrainguinal atherosclerotic disease [1]. Given the fact that many CLI patients have severe comorbidities, the endovascular-first approach is most common since it reduces the magnitude of surgical trauma and systemic complications. In this chapter, an updated angiographic approach for below-the-knee artery disease is described with endovascular techniques.

2. Basic angiographic technique for below-the-knee artery

2.1. Vascular anatomy of the below the knee

Normally, from the direct continuation of the popliteal artery and past the branch of the anterior tibial artery (ATA) is the tibioperoneal trunk. This vascular segment splits into the posterior tibial artery (PTA) and the peroneal artery (**Figure 1**).

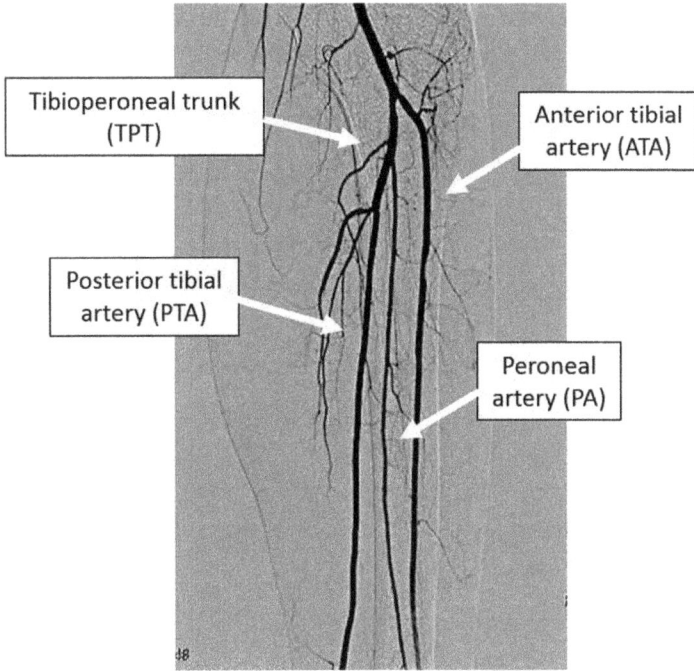

Figure 1. Anteroposterior view of the tibial trifurcation shows anterior tibial artery, tibioperoneal trunk, peroneal artery, and posterior tibial artery.

The distal peroneal artery splits into the anterior malleolar branch and the calcaneal branch (**Figure 2**).

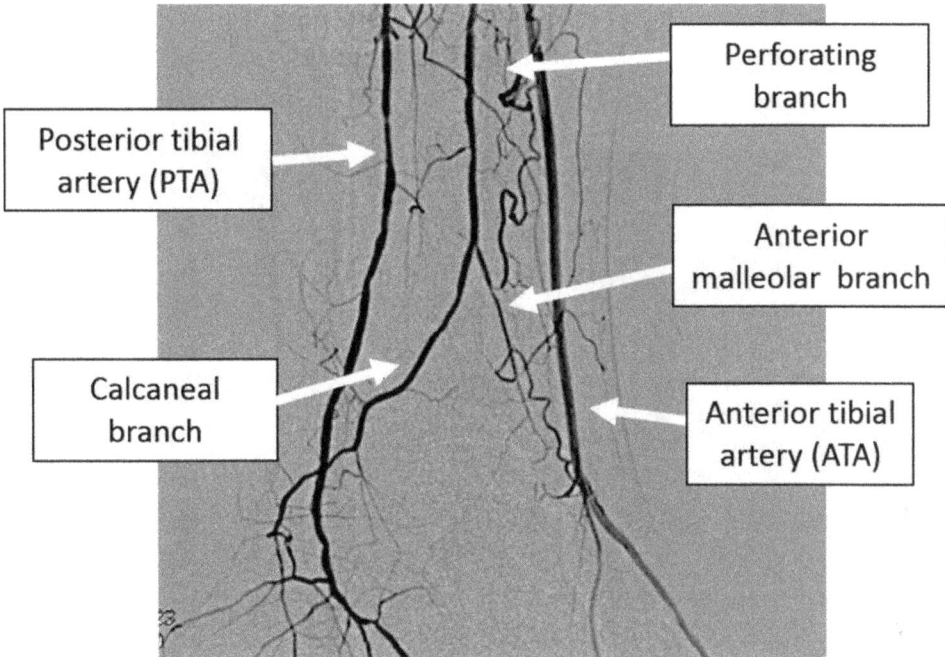

Figure 2. Lateral view at the distal leg shows the distal anterior and tibial arteries and peroneal artery. Distal peroneal artery splits into the anterior malleolar branch and calcaneal branch.

The dorsal pedis artery is a continuation of the ATA in the foot. The PTA bifurcates into the lateral plantar artery and medial plantar artery (**Figure 3**).

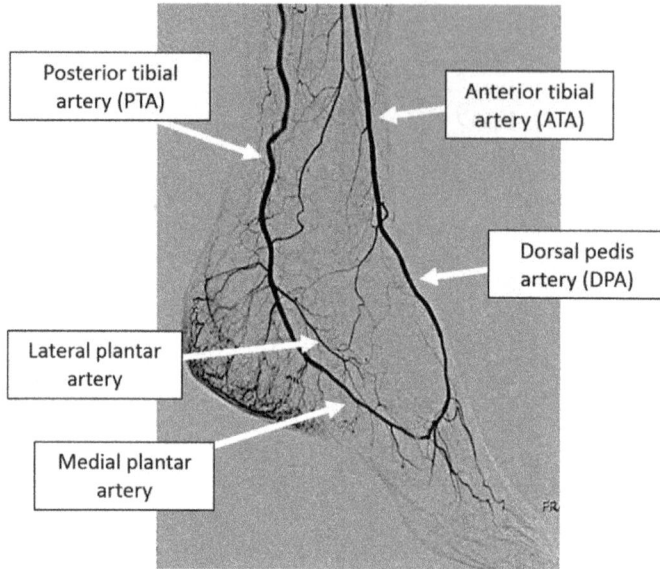

Figure 3. Lateral view of the ankle shows distal anterior tibial artery and posterior tibial artery. Dorsal pedis artery is a continuation of the anterior tibial artery in the foot. Posterior tibial artery bifurcates into the lateral plantar artery and medial plantar artery.

By definition, the popliteal artery ends at the origin of the first tibial artery, which typically is the ATA. In about 4% of cases, we find a so-called high origin of the ATA at the level of the knee joint or even some centimeters more proximal (**Figure 4**).

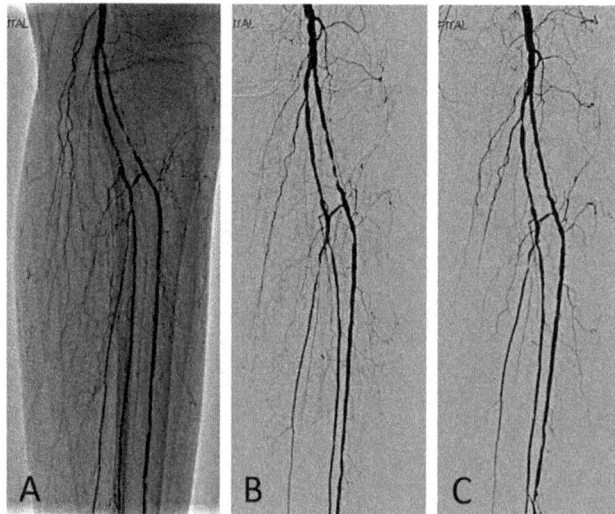

Figure 4. (A and B) High division of popliteal artery branching and anterior tibial artery at the knee joint. The anterior tibial artery was diseased. (C) Balloon angioplasty was performed in the anterior tibial artery.

Similarly, in just as small proportion of the population, a high origin of the PTA has been described. As a variation, a trifurcation of the popliteal artery into all three lower leg arteries at the same point has been observed in 0.4% of patients. The PTA may be missing completely in 1–5% of the normal adult population (**Figure 5**) [2].

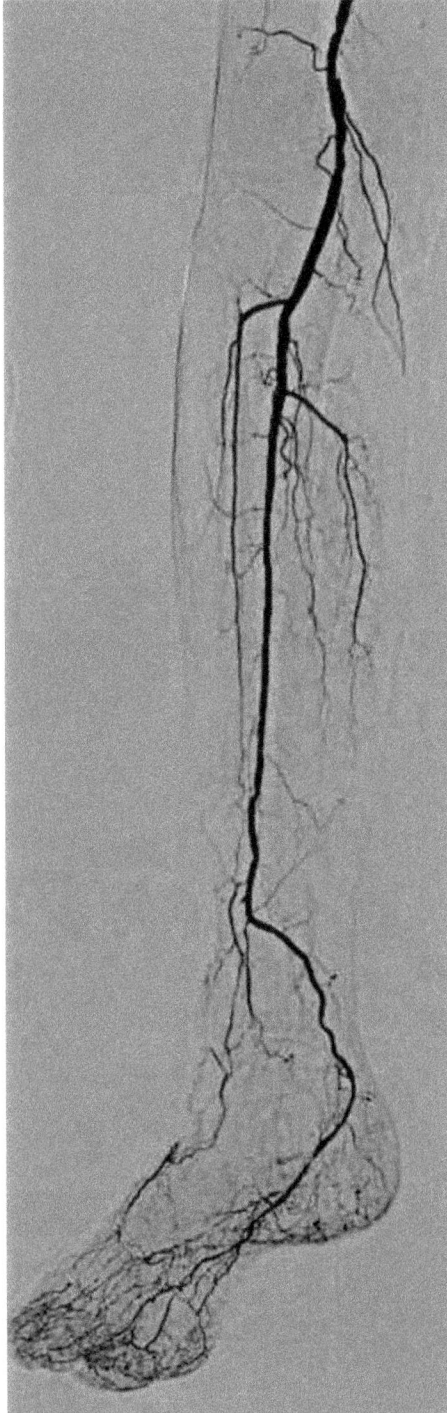

Figure 5. The posterior tibial artery is missing completely. Peroneal artery connects through the tibial arteries.

Branching variations of below-the-knee arteries are common. A practical triad classification of anatomical variations in the branching pattern has been reported [3], that is, Type 1, Type 1-B, Type 2-A, Type 3-A, and Type 3-B (**Figure 6**) [4].

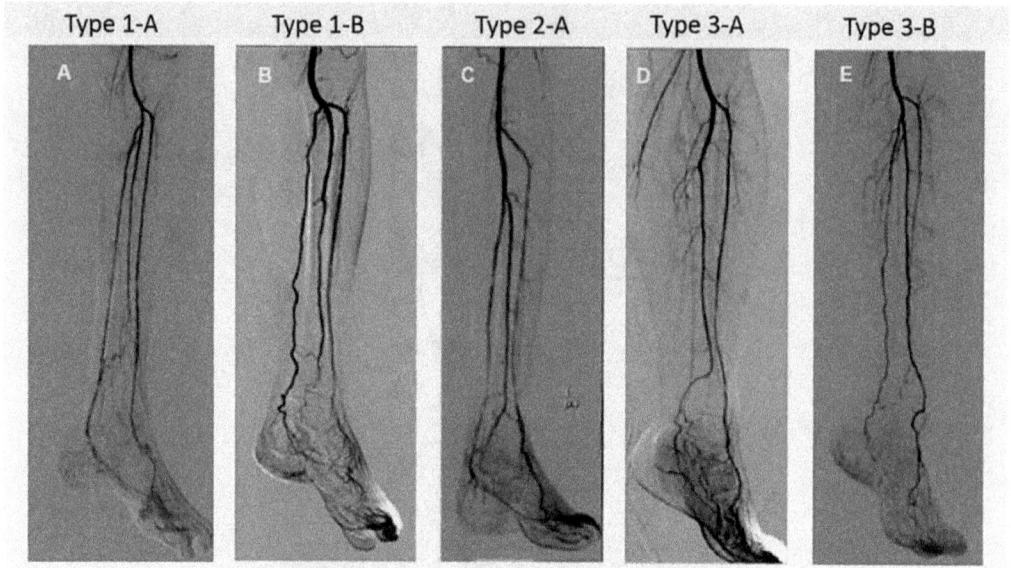

Figure 6. Anatomical variation of tibial arteries. (A) Type 1-A: normal level of arterial branching and most common pattern. The first branch is anterior tibial artery and peroneal trunk separates into peroneal and posterior tibial arteries. (B) Type 1-B: normal level of arterial branching. The three tibial arteries show trifurcation. (C) Type 2-A: high division of popliteal artery branching and the anterior tibial artery arises at the knee joint. (D) Type 3-A: hypoplastic posterior tibial artery and peroneal artery provide a distal supply to the plantar side of the foot. (E) Type 3-B: hypoplastic anterotibial artery and peroneal artery provide distal supply to the dorsal side of the foot.

There are many more anatomical variations and we have to keep in mind that these variant arteries are rather common (**Figures 7** and **8**).

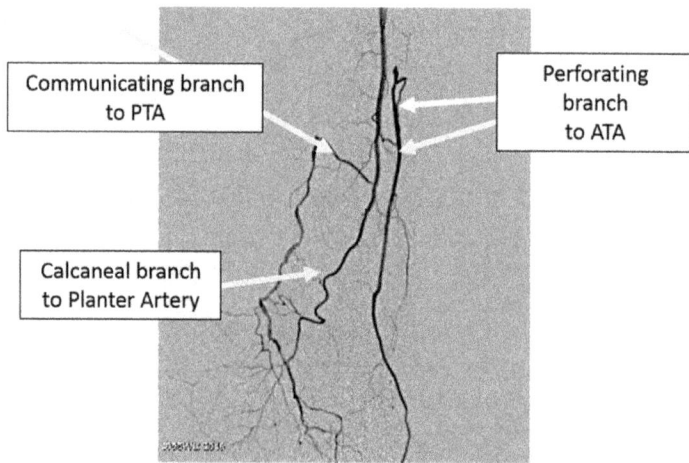

Figure 7. When ATA and PTA are occluded, the peroneal artery may function as the sole blood supply of the foot. Left ATA and PTA are occluded. Anterior terminal branch (perforating branch) of peroneal artery gives collateral to ATA. Similarly, posterior terminal branch (communicating branch) gives collateral to PTA.

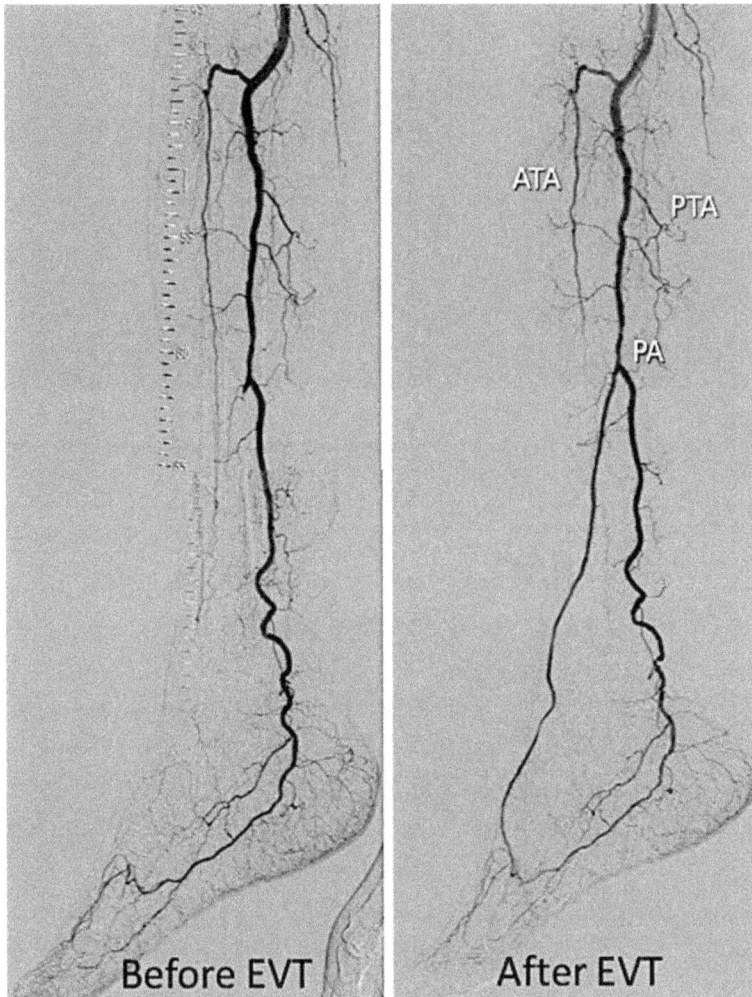

Figure 8. Based on pre-interventional below-the-knee angiography, it was assumed that anterior tibial artery is occluded. Post-interventional below-the-knee angiography showed that anterior tibial artery is hypoplastic. Peroneal artery continues to the dorsal pedis artery.

2.2. Angiography for below-the-knee arteries

Before intervention in below-the-knee vessels, the target vessel should be clearly identified. After confirming that no inflow disease is present, below-the-knee angiography is performed since the presence of inflow disease results in a less clear image [4]. **Figure 9** shows the basic image of below-the-knee angiography.

Only the AP view is insufficient to clearly visualize the below-the-knee anatomy and diseased segment. Four views are mandatory to see all below-the-knee arteries. There are two right anterior oblique (RAO) views and two left anterior oblique (LAO) views. In the upper RAO view, the proximal left ATA is well visualized and, in the lower RAO view, the three distal tibial arteries are well observed. In the upper LAO view, bifurcation of the peroneal artery and PTA is well visualized. In the lower LAO view, the ATA and peroneal artery overlap and these two vessels cannot be separated (**Figure 10**).

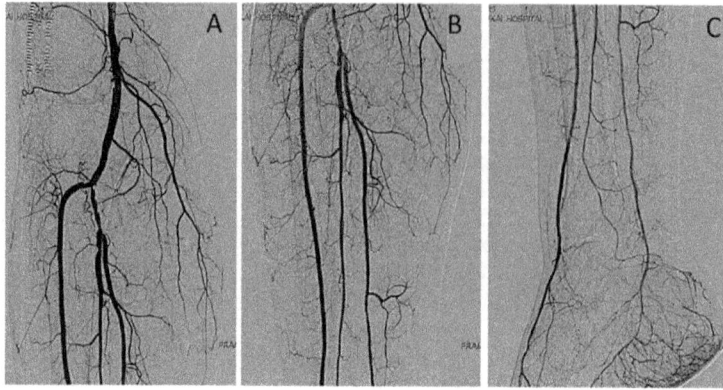

Figure 9. Basic below-the-knee angiography. Only AP view is insufficient to visualize the below-the-knee anatomy and diseased segment.

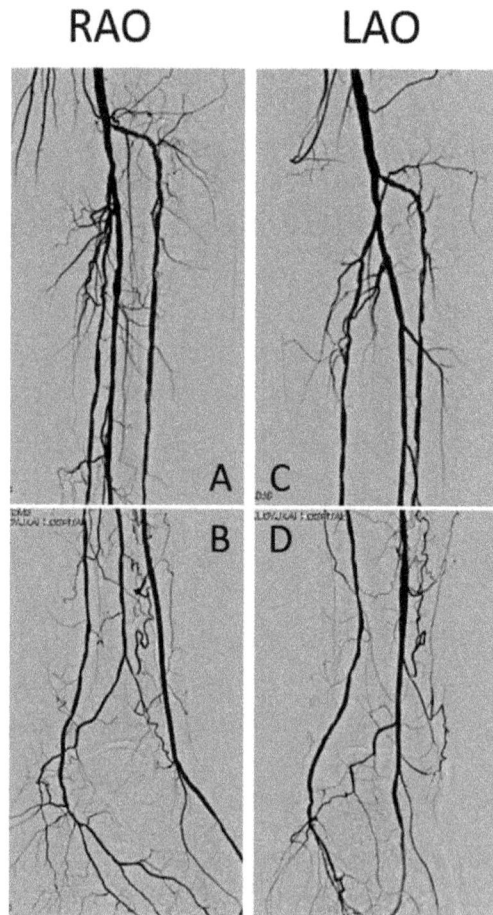

Figure 10. Basic below-the-knee angiography. (A) Upper right anterior oblique view. Proximal anterior tibial artery is well visualized, but peroneal artery and posterior tibial artery are overlapped. (B) Lower right anterior oblique view. In this view, distal three tibial arteries are separated. (C) Upper left anterior oblique view. Proximal peroneal artery and posterior tibial artery are well separated. (D) Lower left anterior oblique view. Distal posterior tibial artery is well visualized, but distal anterior tibial artery and peroneal artery are overlapped.

Figure 11 shows the basic angiographic steps. A femoropopliteal artery angiogram should be taken to rule out inflow disease (**Figure 11A**). After confirming that no inflow disease is present, below-the- knee angiography is performed through a catheter located at the distal popliteal artery (**Figure 11B**). Four views are taken before angioplasty (**Figure 11C**) and four more views after angioplasty (**Figure 11D**).

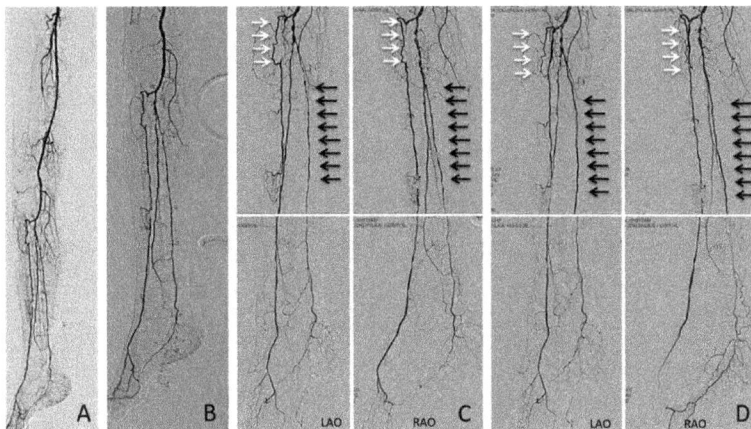

Figure 11. (A) Pre-interventional angiography for critical limb ischemia. Ipsilateral right femoropopliteal artery angiogram which can rule out inflow disease. (B) Below-the-knee angiography showed the entire three tibial arteries. (C) Pre-interventional below-the-knee angiography. This angiography showed the diseased proximal anterior tibial artery (white arrow) and mid-portion of the posterior tibial artery (black arrow). (D) Post-intervention below-the-knee angiography showed proximal anterior tibial artery and mid-posterior tibial artery successfully recanalized. Pre- and post-angiography were taken in the same angle and view.

If the patients have impaired renal function, four views are not mandatory. Moreover, pre- and post-interventional angiography should be taken in the same image size and angle (**Figures 12 and 13**).

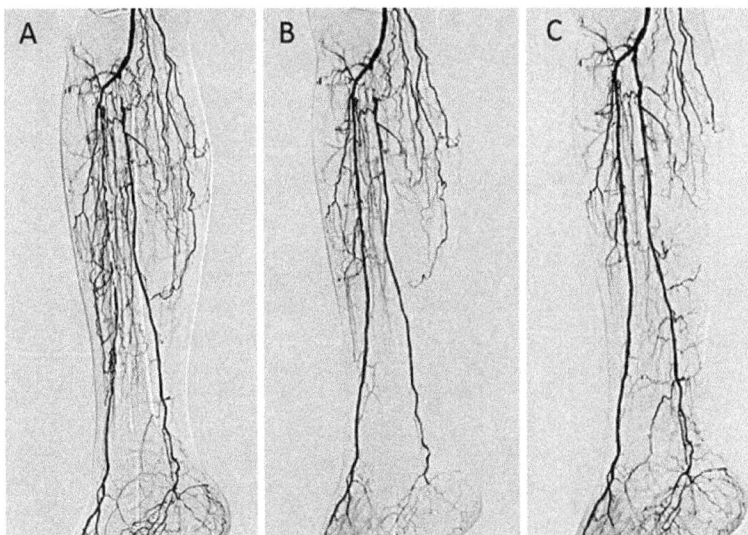

Figure 12. (A) Below-the-knee angiogram of pre-intervention. Right anterior tibial artery, peroneal artery, and posterior tibial artery were occluded. (B) Angiography of postanterior tibial artery intervention. (C) Angiography of postanterior and posterior tibial artery intervention. Peroneal artery was still occluded but sufficient blood flow seems to be obtained.

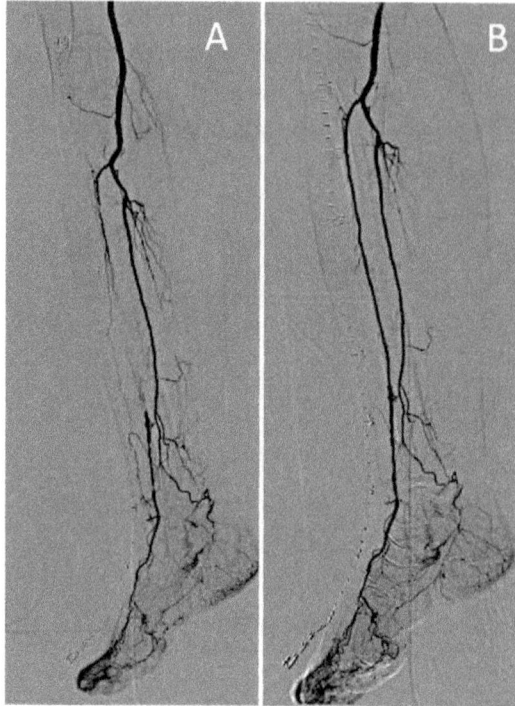

Figure 13:. Pre- (A) and post- (B) interventional angiography should be taken in the same image size and angle.

3. Basic angiographic technique for below-the-ankle arteries

3.1. Vascular anatomy of below-the-ankle arteries

The vascular anatomy of the foot is composed of the anterior and posterior circulation connected through the pedal arch. The anterior circulation consists of the dorsal pedis artery, lateral tarsal artery, and arcuate artery (**Figure 14**).

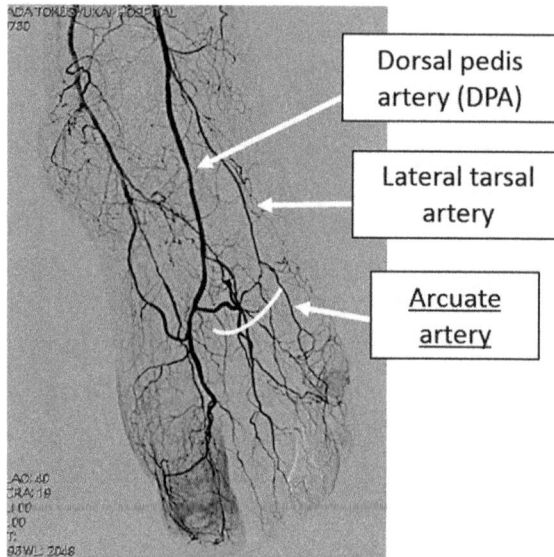

Figure 14. Anterior circulation consists of dorsal pedis artery, lateral tarsal artery, and arcuate artery.

The dorsalis pedis artery is a continuation of the anterior tibial artery distal to the ankle. The branches of the dorsalis pedis include the lateral and medial tarsal, first dorsal metatarsal, deep plantar, and arcuate arteries. The arcuate artery arises near the medial cuneiform, passing laterally over the metatarsal bases deep to the digital extensor tendons and gives rise to the second through fourth dorsal metatarsal arteries before anastomosing with the lateral tarsal artery. The arcuate artery is classically described as being the primary source of blood for the second, third, and fourth dorsal metatarsal arteries [5]; however, a combination of the arcuate, lateral tarsal, and proximal perforating arteries may be involved depending on an individual's vascular anatomy. The posterior circulation consists of the medial plantar artery and lateral plantar artery. These two arteries have an artery-to-artery connection which constitutes the deep plantar arterial arch. The first to fourth plantar metatarsal arteries are the branches of the deep plantar arterial arch (**Figures 15–17**).

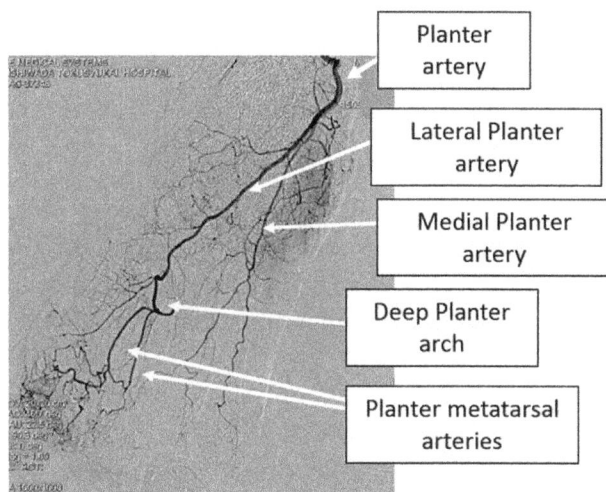

Figure 15. Posterior circulation consists of medial plantar artery and lateral plantar artery.

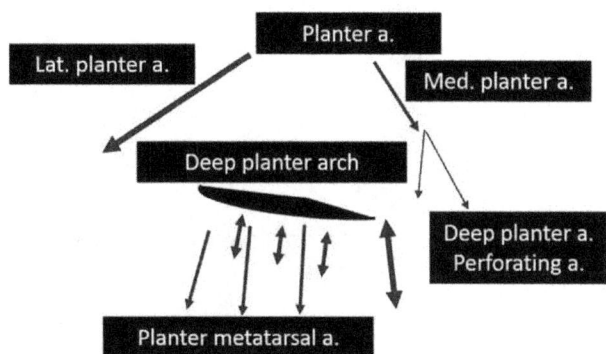

Figure 16. The digital branches originate from the anterior and posterior circulation. There are dorsal branches for each toe.

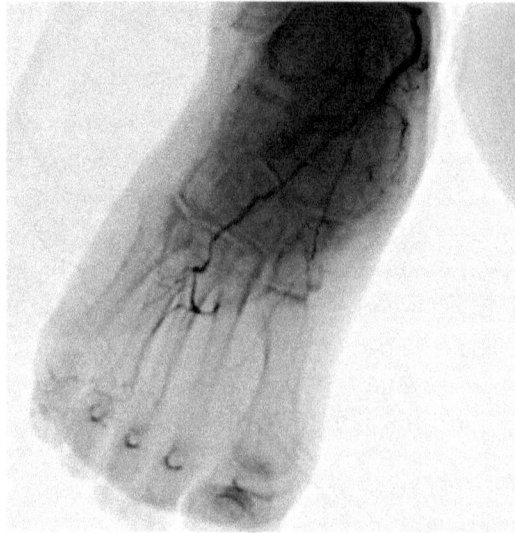

Figure 17. The digital branches originate from the anterior and posterior circulation. There are plantar branches for each toe.

Normally, the area between the anterior and posterior circulation forms the pedal arch. It primarily constitutes the deep perforating branches of the dorsal artery of the foot and the medial plantar artery. This arcade is the main supply for all distal forefoot circulation (**Figure 18**).

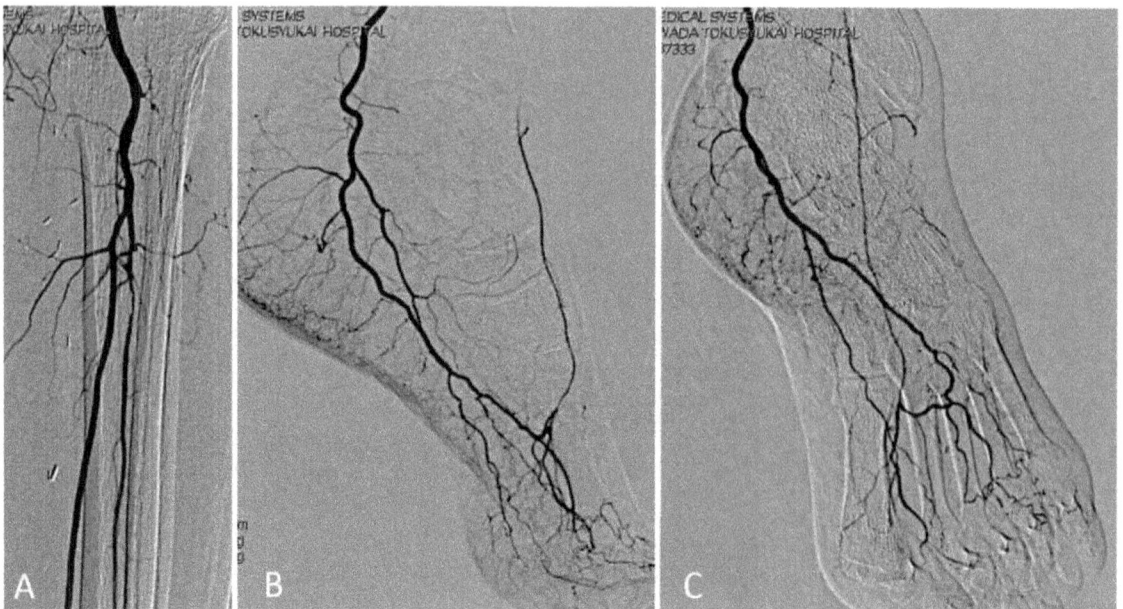

Figure 18. (A) Right anterotibial artery occluded at the proximal portion. (B) Lateral view of the right foot. Right dorsal pedis is retrograde visualized. (C) Dorsal pedis is visualized through the collateral via the deep plantar artery.

Moreover, we should keep in mind that anatomically variant arteries are quite common (**Figure 19**).

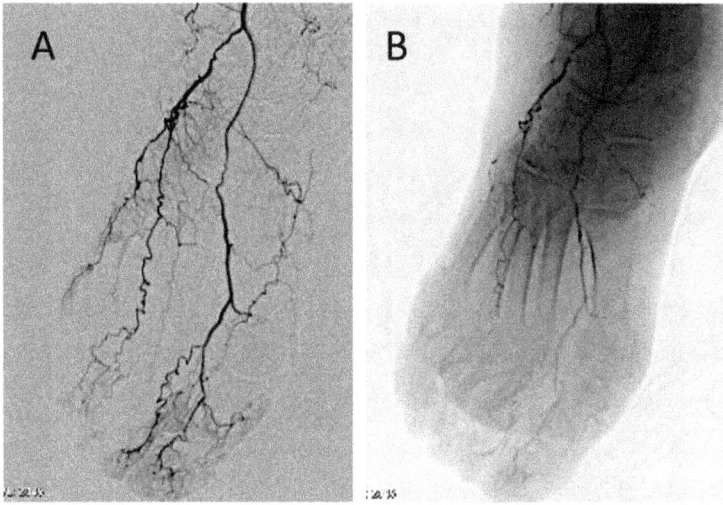

Figure 19. Angiography shows the absence of the arcuate artery and the anomalous origin of the dorsal metatarsal arteries (A) DSA image and (B) DA image.

The pedal arch at the completion of angiography has been classified as follows: Type 1, both dorsal pedis and plantar arteries are patent; Type 2A, only the dorsalis pedis artery is patent; Type 2B, only the plantar artery is patent; and Type 3, both the dorsalis pedis artery and plantar arteries are occlusive (**Figure 20**) [6].

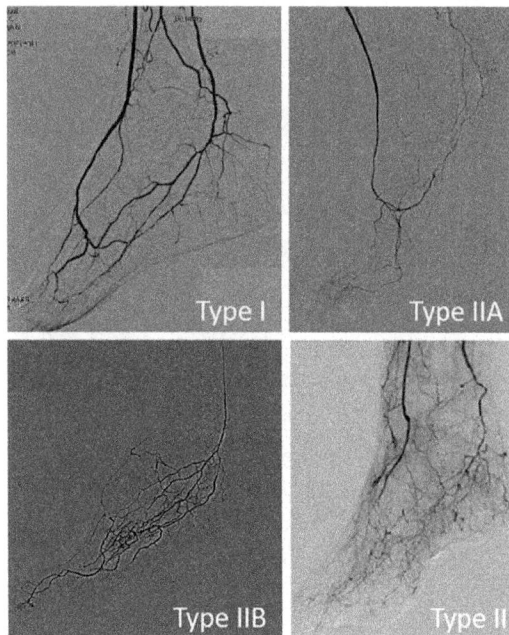

Figure 20. The pedal arch at the completion of angiography was classified into Types I, IIA, IIB, and III.

3.2. Angiography for below-the-ankle arteries

With severe ischemic limb, foot artery angiograms are hard to obtain due to patient leg movements. To minimize this problem, an injection of small amounts of contrast with inflow revascularization is essential. A typical below-the-ankle artery is shown in **Figure 21** [4].

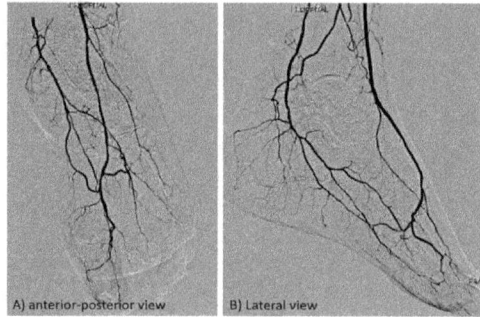

Figure 21. In the anterior view, plantaris medial and lateralis are well separated (A). In the lateral view, dorsal pedis artery is well seen but the lateral tarsal arteries are not well separated (B).

Basically, two views are sufficient: one is the anteroposterior view and the other a lateral view. In the lateral view, the dorsal pedis artery is well visualized but the lateral tarsal arteries are not well separated. In the anterior view, the medial and lateral plantar arteries are well separated. In the anterior view, the dorsalis pedis is well visualized and suited for retrograde dorsal pedis puncture (**Figures 22** and **23**).

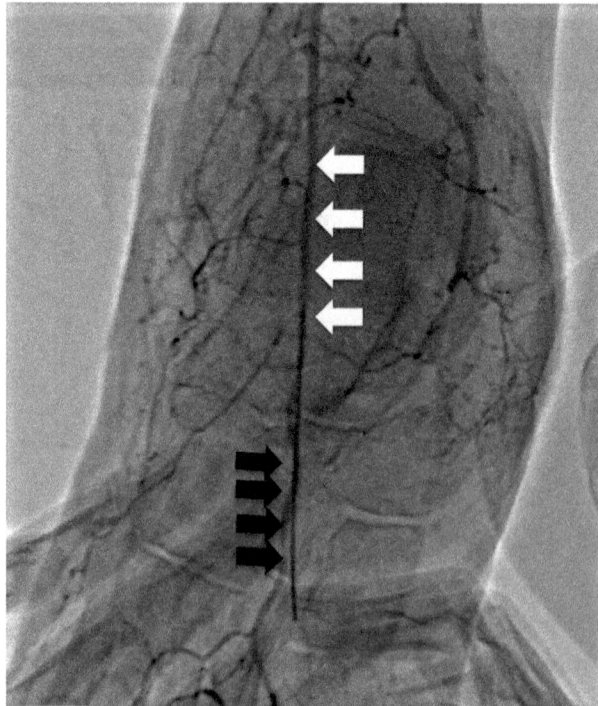

Figure 22. White arrow shows the dorsal pedis artery. Black arrow shows the puncture needle.

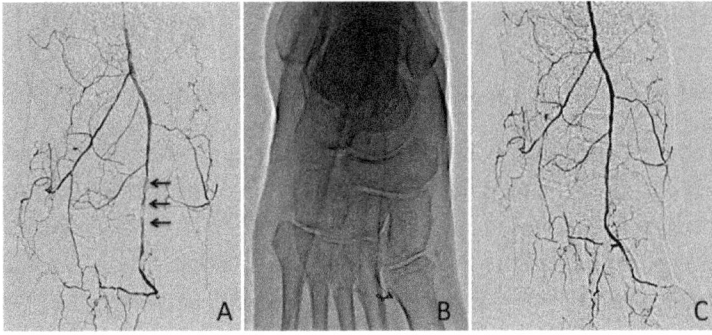

Figure 23. In anterior view, dorsal pedis artery is well visualized. Black arrow shows severe stenosis (A). This lesion was treated with 1.5 × 20-mm balloon (B). Post-angiography (C).

In the lateral view, the distal posterior tibial artery and proximal dorsalis pedis artery are well visualized and suitable for retrograde posterior tibial artery puncture (**Figures 24** and **25**).

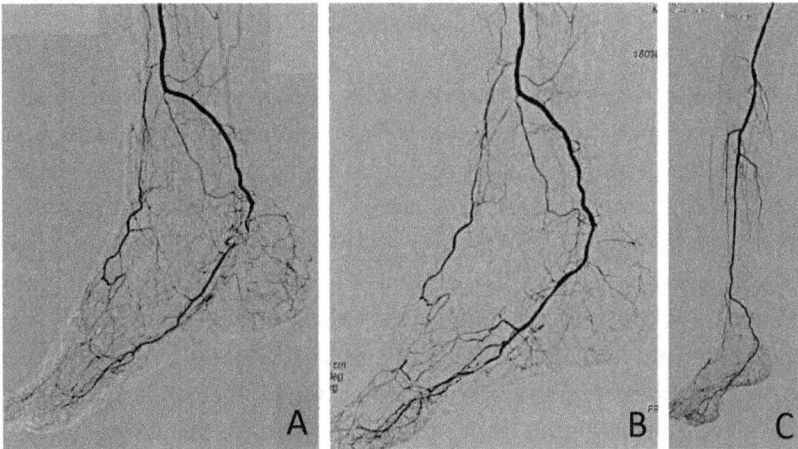

Figure 24. Balloon angioplasty to occluded plantar artery. Based on lateral angiogram, plantar artery was totally occluded (A). Using 2 × 40-mm balloon (B), the occluded vessel was recanalized (C).

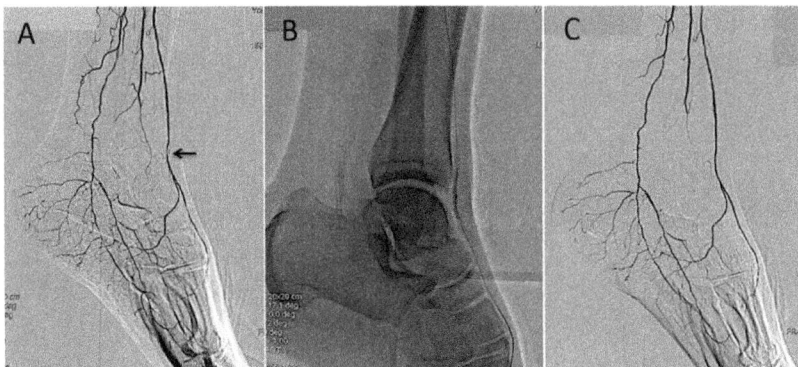

Figure 25. Based on lateral angiogram, proximal dorsal pedis artery disease is well visualized (black arrow) (A). This lesion was treated with 1.5 × 20-mm balloon (B). The stenosis lesion was recanalized (C).

4. Technical aspects of below-the-knee artery intervention

4.1. Endovascular therapy for below-the-knee artery disease

Endovascular therapy for the tibial vessels and foot arteries should be the first-line treatment in patients with CLI due to its good technical and clinical outcomes. Endovascular treatment is possible in most cases with a known low complication rate. The primary indications for tibial and foot artery intervention are limb salvage to avoid amputations. Patients with chronic leg ischemia face major future challenges and, in fact, the long-term survival rate with CLI is significantly lower than that of a matched population so that limb salvage is of major importance to such patients [2].

4.2. Access site

Antegrade access in the common femoral artery is, in our experience, the best approach to perform tibial and foot artery revascularization, with excellent guide ability of the wire and good pushability of the catheter balloons since this access site is closer to the lesions. Moreover, ultrasound-guided punctures may reduce radiation doses, screen time, and complications.

4.3. Guidewires

The tip load, tip stiffness, hydrophilic coat of the tip and body, guidewire flexibility, ability to shape, shaping memory, shaft support, torque transmission, trackability, and pushability are all critical components for a below-the-knee intervention guidewire [7]. Selection should be based on the specificities of the lesion such as localization, stenosis or chronic total occlusion (CTO), and lesion length. Non-hydrophilic guidewires allow a better tactile feel and a more controlled torque response when compared with hydrophilic wires. They are less likely to cause dissection of a vessel but have a higher resistance within the lesion, which decreases the chance of crossing, particularly "ronic total occlusions." But some guidewires, rather than increased sharpness, may have greater tip stiffness due to weight addition which increases their penetration ability. Hydrophilic wires typically advance with minimal resistance, providing good maneuverability in tortuous and long vessels but at a cost of reduced tactile feel [8]. In the field of coronary artery disease, we only use 0.014 inch wires, but in the field of peripheral artery disease, we use 0.014 inch and 0.018 inch wires. Our first wire is the 0.014 inch Runthrough peripheral (Terumo, Tokyo, Japan) and the second wires are the 0.014 inch Cruise (Asahi Intec, Nagoya, Japan) or 0.014 inch Command (Abott Vascular, Santa Clara, CA, USA). For chronic total occlusion lesions, we use 0.018 inch wires. **Table 1** shows the wires we use in our daily practice. These five wires cover almost all of our below-the-knee and below-the-ankle procedures.

0.014" guidewires	Hydrophilic	Tip load	Remarks
Runthrough peripheral (Terumo)	N	1 g	1st wire
Cruise (Asahi intecc)	Y	1 g	2nd wire
0.018" guidewires	Hydrophilic	Tip load	Remarks
Treasure (Asahi intecc)	N	12 g	CTO lesion
Astato (Asahi intecc)	N	30 g	CTO lesion

Table 1. Guidewires for below-the-knee artery intervention.

4.4. Balloon catheter

There are many low-profile balloons of various sizes and lengths for below-the-knee intervention. The balloon platforms are mostly dependent on either a 0.014-inch or 0.018-inch system. The main objective in below-the-knee intervention is to cross a total occlusion. For this purpose, we prefer a 0.018-inch lumen size for the over-the-wire angioplasty balloon (OTW) with increased shaft strength. These balloons give adequate pushability and wire support, particularly in complex chronic total occlusions when compared to the rapid exchange monorail technique. The over-the-wire balloon catheter system with the 0.018-inch platform allows good control of the wire without resistance and a smooth exchange to the 0.018 inch or 0.014 inch wire. They also allow wire exchange without sacrificing the progress made through the lesion. Additionally, their lumen can be used to inject contrast as well as verify position and distal outflow (**Figures 26** and **27**).

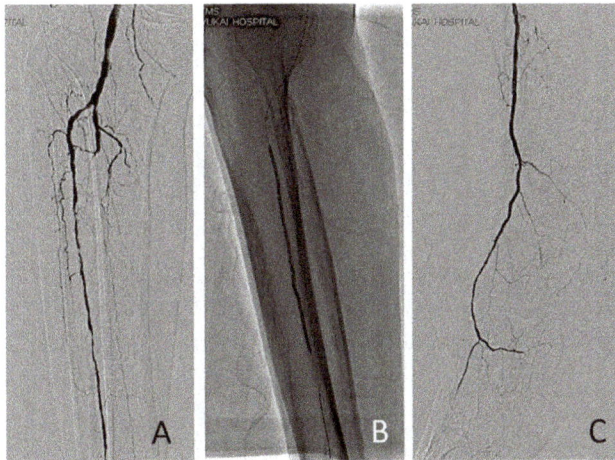

Figure 26. A 0.018-inch over-the-wire balloon catheter can be used to inject contrast, also verify position and distal outflow. (A) Pre angiography (B) Balloon delatation (C) Tip injection.

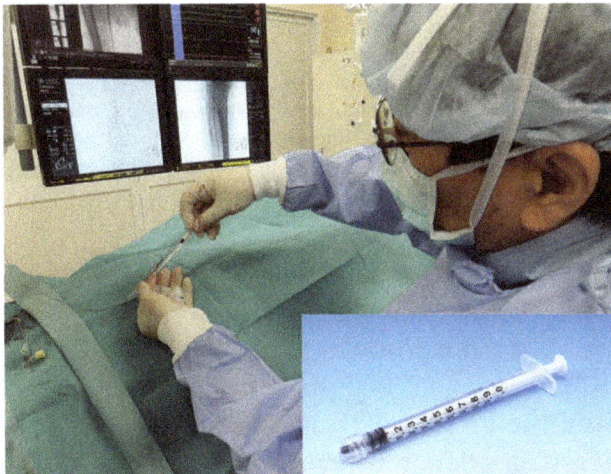

Figure 27. Injection of contrast through over-the-wire balloon. Contrast medium administered using a 1-ml Luer Lock syringe.

4.5. Transluminal recanalization for total occlusion

The first step in transluminal recanalization is to pass the proximal stenosis or negotiate the total occlusion by various wires until reaching the distal patent lumen. A drilling motion of the guidewire is used to properly penetrate and cross the lesion. As the initial wire, we prefer a 0.014-inch soft guidewire (**Table 1**) with an angulated tip since these very soft tips with coated wires have a higher chance of crossing the micro-channel without penetrating the subintimal space.

When we could not cross this soft 0.014 inch wire, it was exchanged with a 12-g 0.018-inch hard guidewire. The 0.018-inch wire has more controllability and penetration power compared to hard 0.014-inch wires. These wires are used with the OTW balloon catheter for wire support and exchange. In addition, the OTW balloon catheter can be used for tip injection to guide the wire and to understand what the problem is. However, in a 0.014-inch OTW balloon, there is a limitation for contrast injection (**Figure 28**).

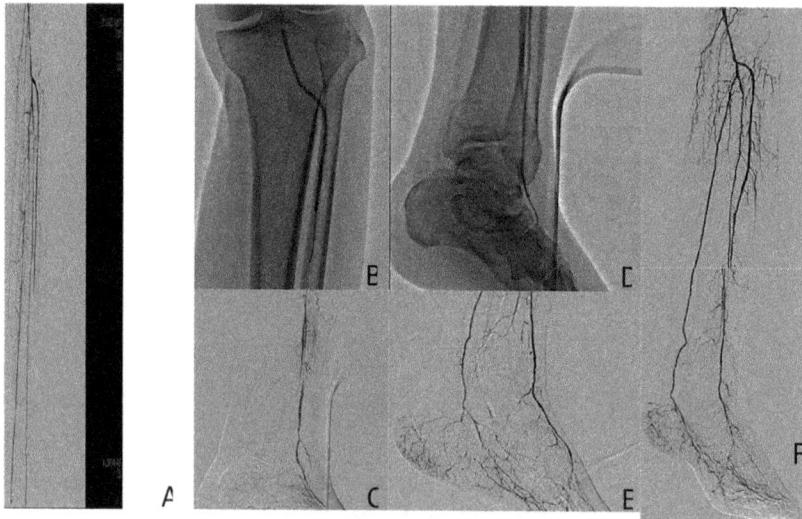

Figure 28. (A) Baseline angiography showed popliteal artery had severe stenosis and all below-the-knee vessels were occluded. (B) 0.014-inch soft guidewire was advanced into anterior tibial artery with 2.5 × 100-mm over-the-wire balloon catheter. The balloon was inflated at the distal popliteal artery and proximal anterior tibial artery. (C) Injection of contrast through over-the-wire balloon at proximal anterior tibial artery. Angiogram clarifies the position of the distal tip of the over-the-wire balloon and occluded segment. (D) 0.014-inch guidewire was changed to 0.018-inch hard guidewire which succeeded in crossing the occluded segment. A 2.0 × 100-mm balloon was inflated at the occluded segment. (E) Injection of contrast through over-the-wire balloon at the distal anterior tibial artery. Angiogram shows below-the-ankle vessels. (F) Final angiography shows complete revascularization was obtained.

4.6. Subintimal recanalization for total occlusion

A subintimal recanalization in below-the-knee arteries is one of the options after intraluminal attempts have failed and it was not possible to cross the lesion. Subintimal angioplasty was first described by Bolia [9], and since then there have been many publications to confirm its value and assess the clinical results of this technique to treat tibial vessels. We normally perform a subintimal recanalization in the crural arteries with a 0.018-inch J-tip guidewire (**Figure 29**) or 0.014-inch hydrophilic guidewire (Command, Abott Vascular). A balloon catheter is used to support the guidewire during subintimal progression.

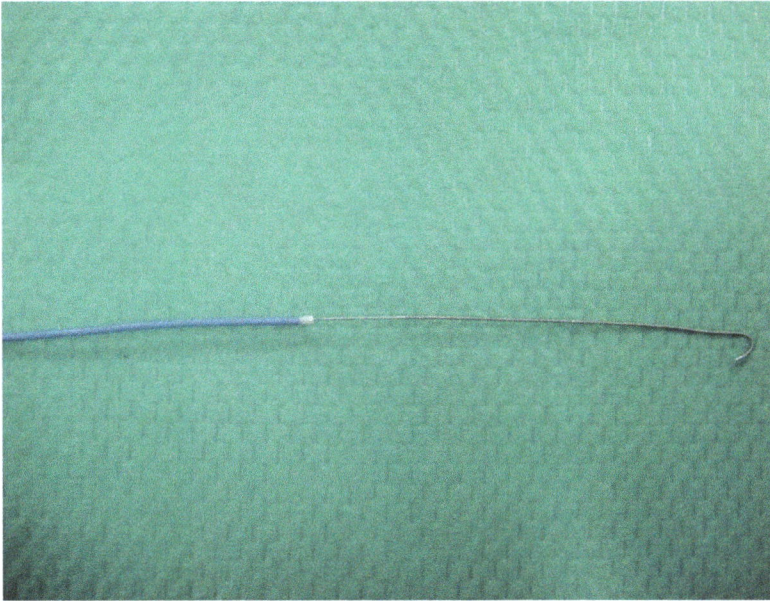

Figure 29. A 0.018-inch 1.5-mm J-tip wire (NEXUS NT 1.5J; Future Medical Design, Saitama, Japan).

4.7. Retrograde recanalization for total occlusion

When antegrade wiring cannot pass the lesion, such as the inability to reenter the patent distal true lumen after subintimal recanalization, a retrograde approach is the choice to cross the total occlusion. In these situations, the retrograde approach is an effective and safe technique for CTO interventions. Compared to other techniques such as the pedal plantar loop technique and/or collateral wiring, retrograde distal access is easier and less risky without damaging the collateral vessels. In our daily procedures, distal retrograde access is the best technical strategy for reentry or to resolve any problems.

4.8. Techniques for distal puncture

All tibial vessels, including the anterior tibial, posterior tibial, and peroneal arteries, can be accessed in retrograde fashion. Generally, the distal anterior tibial artery or posterior tibial artery is selected because these approaches are easier to establish hemostasis under external compression. The peroneal artery can be punctured but it is difficult to achieve hemostasis. The degree of vessel opacification can be enhanced using vasodilators through the femoral access site to maximize the caliber of the arterial target. Usually, nitroglycerin is administered from the distal tip of a catheter. Patient cooperation and proper use of sedation are of utmost importance for the success of this approach. Local anesthesia at the puncture site should be minimized to make the precise puncture into the 1–2-mm vessel. The position of the foot during the access procedure is also important. When puncturing the dorsal pedis or anterior tibial artery, the foot is placed in plantar flexion (**Figure 30**).

When accessing the posterior tibial artery, we place the foot in eversion and dorsal flexion (**Figure 31**).

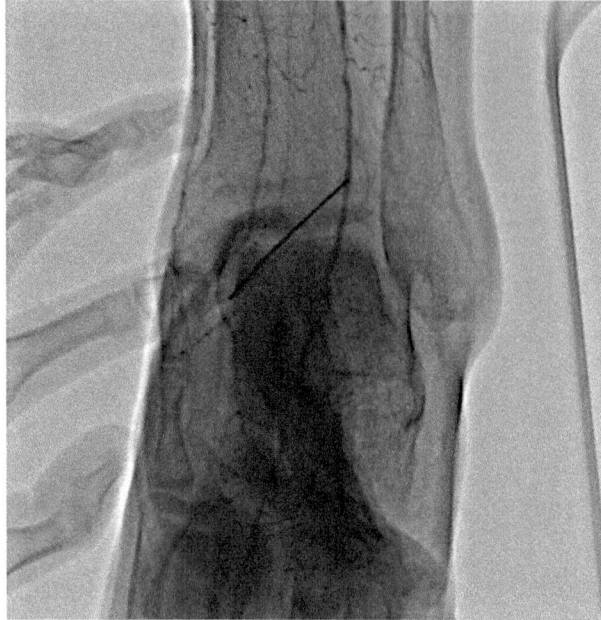

Figure 30. The dorsal pedis artery can be accessed percutaneously under fluoroscopic guidance with a micro-puncture. When accessing the dorsal pedis or anterior tibial artery, the foot is placed in plantar flexion.

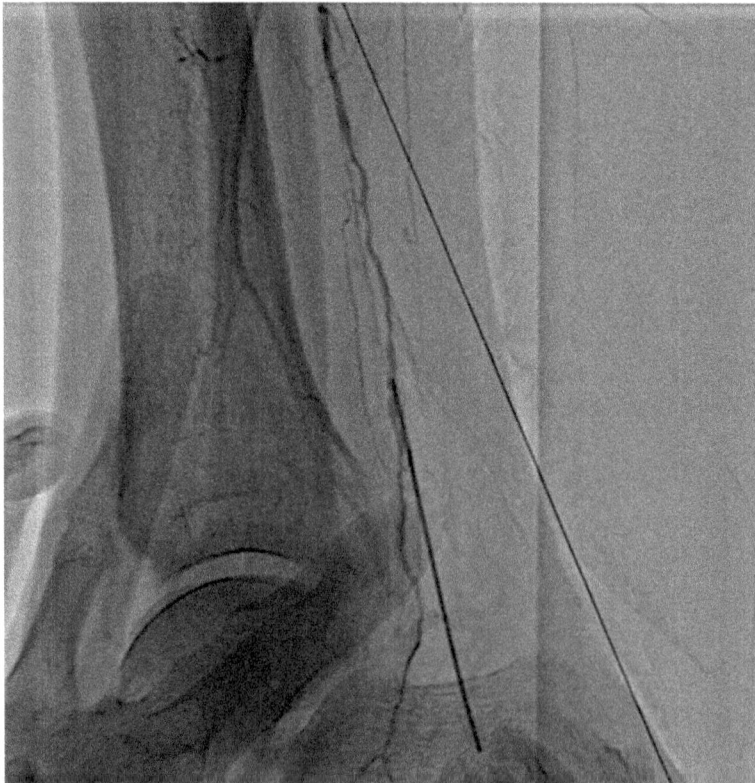

Figure 31. When accessing the posterior tibial artery, the foot is placed in eversion and dorsal flexion.

Selection of the puncture point is of vital importance in the cannulation of a 0.014-inch wire so that it is necessary to find a fairly normal vessel site. A micro-puncture needle (Cook Medical Inc., Bloomington, IN, USA) is best suited for this purpose. Under fluoroscopic guidance, a small amount of contrast is injected through a proximal vessel, most often the popliteal artery. After successful puncturing which is confirmed by back bleeding, the 0.014-inch hydrophilic wire (Cruise; Asahi Intec, Tokyo, Japan) is passed through the needle into the vessel under fluoroscopic guidance (**Figure 32**). The needle is then removed and inserted into a micro-catheter (Ichibanyari; Kaneka Medical Products, Osaka, Japan). This sheathless strategy can reduce the risk of disrupting the access vessel and is easier to achieve hemostasis (**Figure 32**).

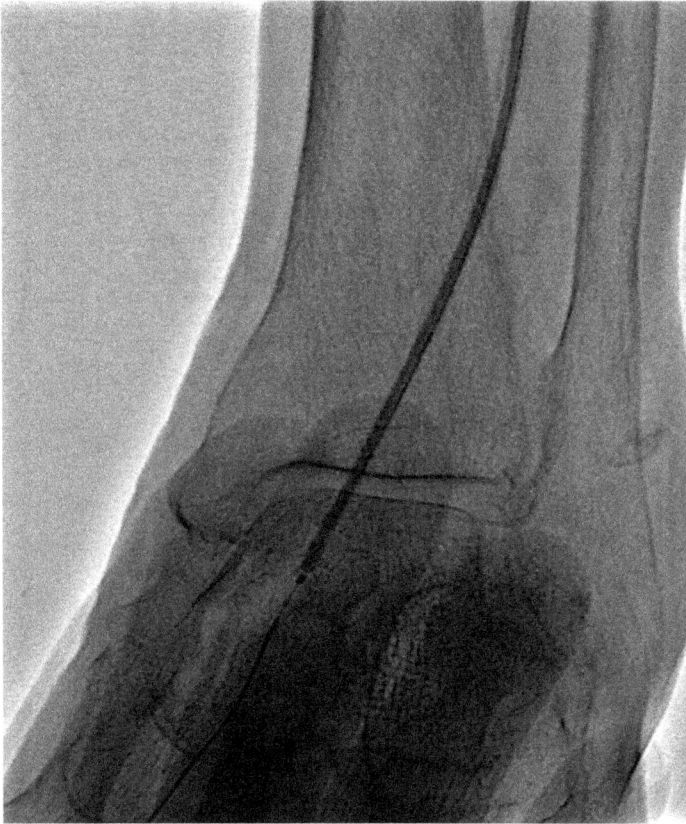

Figure 32. The retrograde micro-catheter is withdrawn and hemostasis is secured through digital compression and/or low-pressure balloon dilatation with appropriately sized balloons.

4.9. Complications

A vessel perforation by wiring could happen while attempting to cross a tibial chronic total occlusion. In most cases, bleeding due to wire perforation is of no clinical significance. However, the perforated site must be sealed. If the wire has crossed the lesion, balloon infla-tion is applied with low pressure and, in most cases, hemostasis can be established. However, when bleeding cannot be stopped or the wire did not cross the lesion, external compression guided by angiography or temporary balloon occlusion at the proximal to perforated site should be tried. In conjunction with proximal balloon occlusion, an external compression method should also be performed. The Tometa-Kun compression system (Zeon Medical, Tokyo, Japan) is generally used to achieve complete hemostasis at the radial artery. The Tometa-Kun compression system is easy to use and quite an effective method for external compression (**Figure 33**).

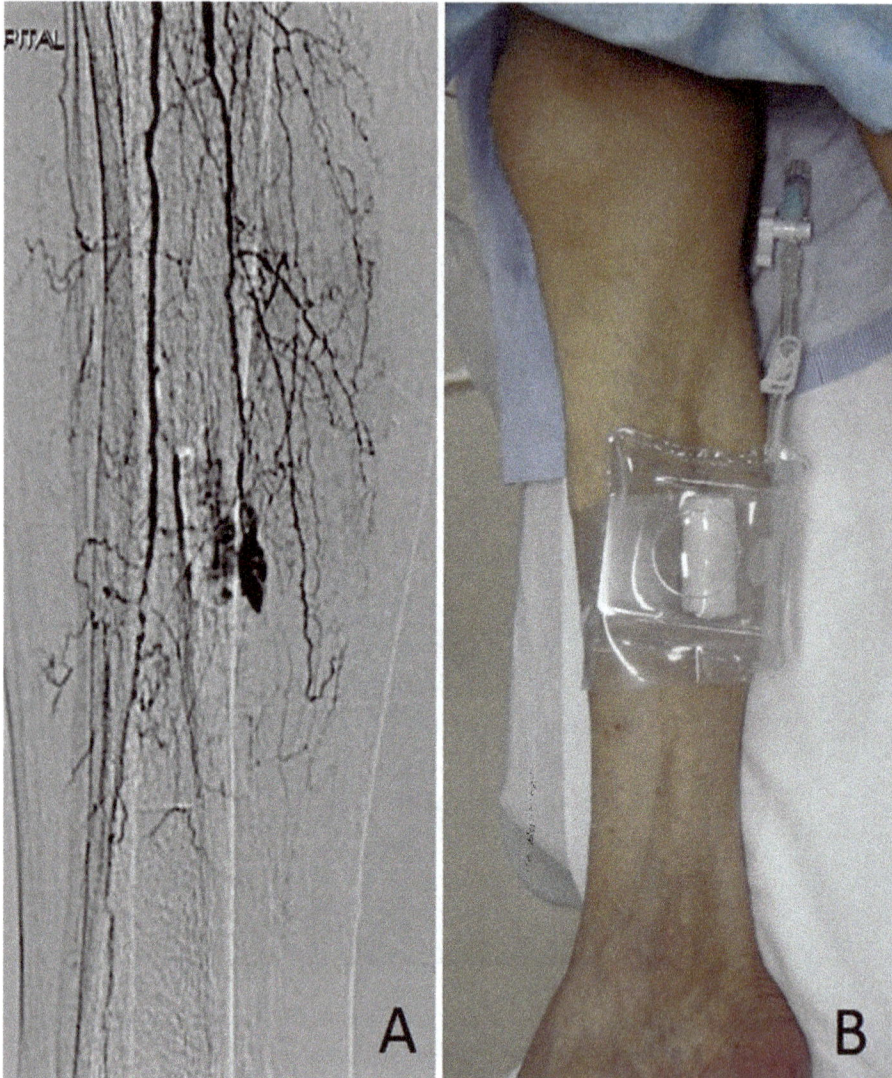

Figure 33. Perforation site is compressed with Tometa-Kun device which allows effective eternal compression.

5. Indigo carmine angiography

There are many issues regarding local perfusion problems of the foot. A non-healing ulce-ris often caused by macrovascular obstructions in combination with disease at the level of microcirculation in the foot. In addition to macrovascular ischemia, microcirculation, particularly in a diabetic foot, is often damaged. Endovascular revascularization of the macrovessels is the first-line treatment; however, there are no validated tests to predict the clinical outcome after successful revascularization and often ulcer healing is the hard end point.

5.1. Indigo carmine

In the field of oral surgery, the injection of indigo carmine to tumor-feeding arteries has been used to determine the main feeding artery to the tumor. After confirming the color change of indigo carmine, the super-selective administration of chemotherapy infusions is performed [10]. The application of indigo carmine in patients with CLI has previously been reported, providing visual information regarding foot perfusion at the microcirculation level (**Figure 34**) [11].

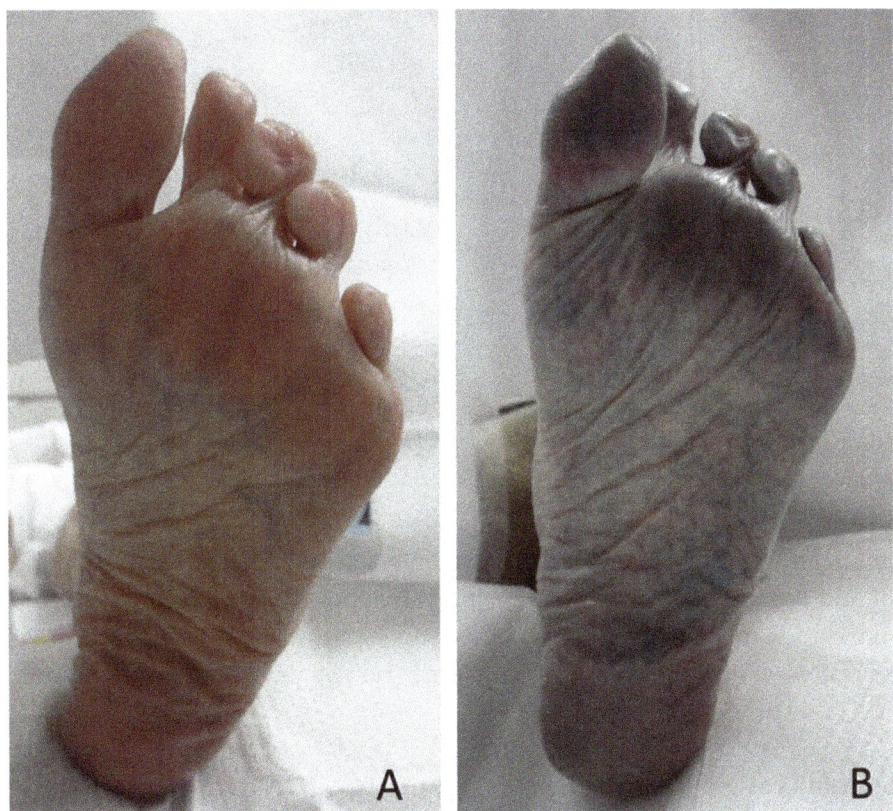

Figure 34. The application of indigo carmine in patients with CLI has been reported, providing visual information regarding foot perfusion at the microcirculation level.

5.2. The angiosome concept

The angiosome concept was introduced by Taylor and Palmer who showed the foot and ankle area to be composed of six distinct angiosomes supplied by the anterior tibial artery, posterior tibial artery, and peroneal artery [12, 13]. The ATA supplies the dorsal side of the foot and toes while the PTA supplies the plantar side of the foot, toes, interdigital web spaces, and inner side of the heel. The PA supplies the lateral ankle and lateral side of the heel (**Figure 35**) [8].

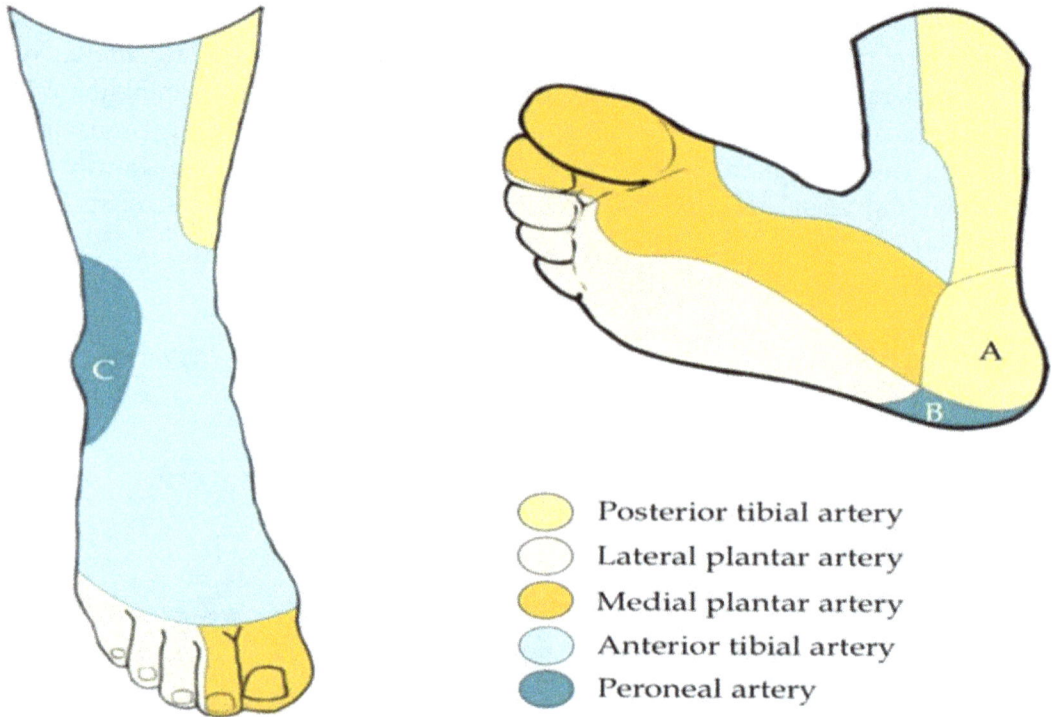

Posterior tibial artery
Lateral plantar artery
Medial plantar artery
Anterior tibial artery
Peroneal artery

Figure 35. Six distinct angiosomes supplied by the anterior tibial artery (ATA), posterior tibial artery (PTA), and peroneal artery (PA).

However, there are extensive connections between below-the-knee arteries coursing throughout the foot and the inter-angiosome connections by choke vessels could be more important for revascularization in ischemic foot. Whether angiosome-guided EVT is essential for revascularization is not yet well elucidated since there is no objective method to evaluate foot perfusion after successful revascularization.

5.3. Indigo carmine angiography

Indigo carmine angiography to provide visual information is not a difficult process. Generally, 5-ml indigo carmine is injected after endovascular therapy. If the indigo carmine is injected from the distal portion of the below-the-knee artery, indigo carmine angiography shows the territory of the vessel. If indigo carmine is injected from the distal popliteal artery, indigo carmine angiography shows all of the below-the-knee feeding territories (**Figure 36**).

Indigo carmine angiography depicts microcirculation clearly by making the circulated area visible with blue dye. If the ulcerated area remains undyed after the EVT procedure, we can speculate that sufficient blood flow was not established, informing us of the necessity for further revascularization with either distal bypass or EVT. Indigo carmine angiography is thus a completely new and effective method of evaluating distal microcirculation.

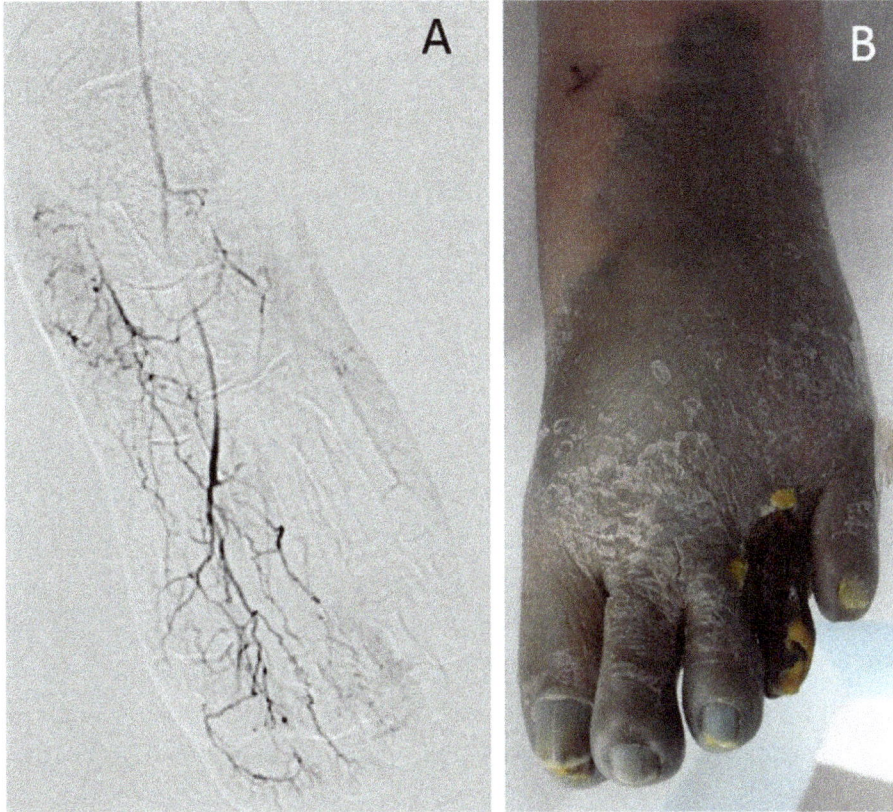

Figure 36. Indigo carmine angiography clearly depicts microcirculation by making the circulated area visible with blue dye.

Author details

Akihiro Higashimori

Address all correspondence to: akihiro.higashimori@gmail.com

Kishiwada Tokushukai Hospital, Osaka, Japan

References

[1] Garg K, Kaszubski PA, Moridzadeh R, Rockman CB, Adelman MA, Maldonado TS, Veith FJ, Mussa FF. Endovascular-first approach is not associated with worse amputation-free survival in appropriately selected patients with critical limb ischemia. J Vasc Surg. 2014;59(2):392–9.

[2]   Marco M, Luis MP, Giacomo C. Revascularization of tibial and foot arteries: below the knee angiography for limb salvage. Angioplasty, Various Techniques in Treatment of Congenital and Acquired Vascular Stenoses. ISBN 978-953-0084-3, InTech, 2012.

[3]   Kawarada O, Yokoi Y, Honda Y, Fitzgerald PJ. Awareness of anatomical variations for infrapopliteal intervention. Catheter Cardiovasc Interv. 2010;76(6):888–94.

[4]   Yoshiaki Y. Angiography for peripheral vascular intervention. Angioplasty, Various Techniques in Treatment of Congenital and Acquired Vascular Stenoses. ISBN 978-953-0084-3, InTech, 2012.

[5]   Standring S, Ellis H, Healy J, Johnson D, Williams A. Pelvic Girdle and Lower limb. In Sandring S, ed. Gray's Anatomy: The Anatomical Basic for Clinical Practice. 39th ed. Edinburgh: Elsevier, Churchill Livingstone, 2005. p. 1600.

[6]   Kawarada O, Fujihara M, Higashimori A, Yokoi Y, Honda Y, Fitzgerald PJ. Predictors of adverse clinical outcomes after successful infrapopliteal intervention. Catheter Cardiovasc Interv. 2012;80(5):861–71.

[7]   Godino C, Sharp AS, Carlino M, Colombo A. Crossing CTOs-the tips, tricks, and specialist kit that can mean the difference between success and failure. Catheter Cardiovasc Interv. 2009;74(7):1019–46.

[8]   Daniel B, Joana F, Armando M, Antonio GV. Below the knee technique: now and then. Angioplasty, Various Techniques and Challenges in Treatment of Congenital and Acquired Vascular Stenoses. ISBN 978-953-0084-3, InTech, 2012.

[9]   Bolia A, Miles KA, Brennan J, Bell PR. Percutaneous transluminal angioplasty of occlusions of the femoral and popliteal arteries by subintimal dissection. Cardiovasc Intervent Radiol. 1990;13:357–63.

[10] Korogi Y, Hirai T, Nishimura R, Hamatake S, Sakamoto Y, Murakami R, Baba Y, Arakawa A, Takahashi M, Uji Y. Superselective intraarterial infusion of cisplatin for squamous cell carcinoma of the mouth: preliminary clinical experience. AJR Am J Roentgenol. 1995;165(5):1269–72.

[11] Higashimori A, Yokoi Y. Use of indigo carmine angiography to qualitatively assess adequate distal perfusion after endovascular revascularization in critical limb ischemia. J Endovasc Ther. 2015;22(3):352–5.

[12] Taylor GI, Palmer JH. The vascular territories (angiosomes) of the body: experimental study and clinical applications. Br J Plast Surg. 1987;40(2):113–41.

[13] Taylor GI, Palmer JH. Angiosome theory. Br J Plast Surg. 1992;45(4):327–8.

7

Cardiovascular Risk Evaluation in Patients with Critical Leg Ischemia before Vascular Surgery

Mirela-Anca Stoia, Mihaela Mocan,
Cerasela Mihaela Goidescu,
Diana Larisa Hognogi Mocan and Roxana Chiorescu

Abstract

Assessment of the role and investigation particularities (comparative and complementary aspects, hierarchies, preferential indication) adapted to the context of a global cardiovascular (CV) evaluation, including clinical elements, non-invasive and invasive imagistic examination in order to estimate the cardiovascular risk (CVR) and to define the revascularization therapeutic strategy in patients with critical leg ischemia (CLI). Complete and accessible evaluation involves accessible means of investigation like clinical exam, electrocardiogram, cardiac biomarkers, arterial, cardiac, and carotid ultrasonography which could be affordable in all cardiovascular departments. Non-invasive stress tests, coronary and arterial cervical angiography imaging leads in selected cases and where is possible to the identification of significant coronary and/or carotid lesions potential responsible for cardiac and cerebrovascular events after vascular surgery. The evaluation algorithm allows better risk stratification of patients with CLI in high and intermediate CVR. The "poly-arterial" status in patients with CLI changes the intervention management with a more intensive pre-operative medical treatment, while the coronary and the carotid arteries revascularization might precedes the peripheral arterial revascularization procedures, in order to reduce the CV risk status.

Keywords: critical leg ischemia (CLI), cardiovascular risk (CVR), poly-arterial (multi-arterial sites lesions), perioperative evaluation, non-invasive stress tests, cardiac biomarkers

1. Introduction

Atherosclerosis (ATS) is a systemic pathological process that affects coronary, cerebral and peripheral arterial circulation. Peripheral arterial disease (PAD) is a distinct athero-thrombotic syndrome marked by stenosis and occlusion of arterial beds [1]. A large proportion of PAD patients are not diagnosed before having a major ischemic cardiovascular (CV) event (MACE), which limits the use of medical therapies with recognized evidence of cardiovascular risk (CVR) reduction [2]. Even if claudication can remain stable over 10 years in 70–80% of patients, the prevalence of myocardial infarction (MI), stroke and CV death is high. PAD patients triple their risk of mortality from any other cause and have a six fold higher risk of death by coronary artery disease (CAD) than those without this ATS lesions. All these problems lead to repeated hospitalizations, low quality of life for patients and increased CV morbidity [3].

2. Predictors of perioperative cardiovascular risk

2.1. The risk of PAD patients in noncardiac vascular surgery

It is estimated that more than 200 million patients suffer a surgery intervention every year worldwide, and the proportion might increase up to 300 million in time. Most of these patients are elderly men, 25% of them having a high or intermediate CVR. The rate of MACE ranges from 11% in patients with one CV risk factor (CVRF) up to 33% in patients with four CVRFs. Perioperative mortality ranges from 0.9% in patients with one CVRF to 11% in patients with four CVRFs. Approximately 60% of patients with PAD have coronary artery disease (CAD), up to 25% of PAD patients have carotid-cerebrovascular atherosclerotic lesions, and the rate of MACE (MI, stroke and CV death) reaches 7% per year. The main causes of mortality in patients with PAD are due to cardiac events, coronary MI (60%) first of all, followed by major or fatal stroke (35%) and only a small proportion (15%) of these patients dies due to complications of critical peripheral arterial ischemia (by gangrene, septicemia and multiorgan failure) [4]. Along with coronary and/or cerebrovascular disease, the type of surgery is an independent predictive risk factor for death of PAD patients with multisite arterial lesions [5, 6]. This is why, patients undergoing vascular surgery have a higher risk of MI (31%), CV death (5%) than general surgery patients (3%) [4, 7, 8]. A good diagnostic and management strategy for PAD patients reduces vital CVR in terms of short outcomes and identifies patients with coronary and/or cervical arterial lesions at risk for long-term CV events. noninvasive tests can provide both diagnostic information (by revealing coronary ischemic heart disease (IHD) or cervical arterial lesions) and CVR prognosis in patients who undergo noncardiac surgery [4, 9, 10].

2.2. Benefits and limits of perioperative risk stratification

Cardiac risk stratification separates patients for vascular surgery into high-risk, intermediate and low-risk categories, adapting the management of perioperative therapy to their needs. Low-risk patients will be further investigated by completing noninvasive and invasive tests, while for high-risk patients, perioperative management primordially changes.

The major objective of CVR stratification is the reduction of perioperative global morbidity and mortality. Clarifying the patient's risk status allows the clinician as well as the surgeon to consent to a better informed patient. From a socio-economic point of view, reducing postoperative complications allowed to reduce perioperative care and treatment costs. The main impediment of perioperative risk stratification procedure is the duration, the cost and the number of investigational tests, which implicitly leads to postponing the intervention moment [4, 7, 8, 10]. And that could be done in elective surgery, but it seems to be quite difficult to be done in emergencies interventions.

2.3. Clinical elements of perioperative cardiovascular risk

2.3.1. Overview

Retrospective clinical studies have shown that a history of coronary artery bypass surgery (CABG), percutaneous transluminal coronary angioplasty intervention (PCI) or coronary angiography without significant lesions indicates a low risk for perioperative cardiac events. The risk is similar to that of patients without clinical signs of significant CAD. The term "protection" given by the presence of a coronary graft cannot be specified. Many studies in large groups of patients have shown the independent predictors of perioperative CVR: the history of MI, angina pectoris (AP), and ischemic ST-T changes on the electrocardiogram (ECG/EKG), as well as the clinical symptoms of congestive heart failure (HF) [9–11].

2.3.2. Several clinical risk assessment scores for postoperative cardiac events

The revised cardiac risk index (RCRI) is used by anesthesiologists and surgeons to assess the perioperative CVR in patients who undergo noncardiac surgery. Parameters included in the evaluation are age over 70 years, estimated risk of surgery, history or presence of IHD (MI or history of AP), congestive heart failure (HF), HT with signs of left ventricular hypertrophy (LVH), presence of Q waves or ischemic ST changes on resting electrocardiogram (ECG) cerebrovascular disease (CVD), the presence of DM (treated with insulin, additional risk) and renal failure (e.g., **Table 1**) [4, 12, 13]. The presence of more than one of these six independent predictors of cardiac complications following surgery is mandatory for further investigation. Patients who do not have active cardiac conditions are stratified into three groups by the RCRI: low (0 risk factor), intermediate (1–2 risk factors) and high (≥3 risk factors) [14, 15]. In a meta-analysis of 24 studies that reported the association of the RCRI with MACE or death in the hospital or within 30 days of surgery, the RCRI discriminated moderately well between patients at low versus high risk for cardiac events after mixed noncardiac surgery.

However, its performance was considerably diminished when it was used in patients who underwent vascular surgery and emphasized the necessity of development and validation of a suitable CRI for use in vascular surgery patients [14, 16, 17]. The American College of Surgeons National Surgical Quality Improvement Program (ACS-NSQIP) database derived from general and other specialty surgery patients have allowed the development of another risk model, in which five risk factors (basically the same from RCRI) were determined to be associated with MI/cardiac arrest following an operation [13]. In the VSG-RCI assessment (published in 2010 by Vascular Study Group of New England (VSGNE), additional

Clinical risk factors	Clinical elements	Active cardiac condition	Clinical presentation
History of ischemic heart disease (IHD)	Previous MI Previous positive result on stress test Use of nitroglycerin Typical angina pectoris ECG Q waves Previous PCI or CABG	Unstable coronary syndromes	Unstable or severe angina (CCS class III–IV) Recent MI (7–30 days)
History of compensated previous congestive heart failure (HF)	Previous pulmonary edema Third heart sound Bilateral rales Evidence of heart failure on chest radiograph	De-compensated HF	NYHA functional class IV worsening or new-onset HF
History of cerebro-vascular disease (CVD)	Previous TIA disease Previous stroke	Significant arrhythmias	High-grade atrioventricular block Symptomatic ventricular arrhythmias Supraventricular arrhythmias (including atrial fibrillation) with uncontrolled ventricular rate (HR > 100 bpm at rest) Symptomatic bradycardia Newly recognized ventricular tachycardia
Diabetes mellitus (DM)	With or without preoperative insulin therapy	Severe valvular disease	Severe aortic stenosis (mean pressure gradient > 40 mm Hg, aortic valve area < 1.0 cm^2 or symptomatic) Symptomatic mitral stenosis (progressive dyspnea on exertion, exertional presyncope, or HF)
Renal failure	Creatinine level > 2 mg/dL		

Adapted from [4, 13]. CCS, Canadian Cardiovascular Society; MI, myocardial infarction; HF, heart failure; NYHA, New York Heart Association; HR, heart rate.

Table 1. Clinical risk factor to predict MACE and active cardiac conditions to be evaluated and to be treated before noncardiac surgery.

risk factors were introduced: CVRF (increasing age, DM insulin-dependent, HT, smoking), clinical features (presence of aortic aneurysm, peripheral arterial ischemic symptoms, CAD, congestive HF, chronic obstructive pulmonary disease, elevated creatinine, abnormal cardiac stress test), previous CV medication administered (β-blockers long-term therapy, antiplatelet, statins) and revascularization interventions (carotid endarterectomy, peripheral arterial bypass, endovascular/surgical interventions for aortic aneurysm). The RCRI predicted risk after carotid endarterectomy reasonably well, but substantially underestimated the other procedures for low- and higher-risk patients. VSG-CRI risk model predicted more accurately the risk of cardiac complications in vascular surgery patients than the RCRI, which underestimated in-hospital cardiac events in patients undergoing vascular surgery and that new VSGNE index was more accurate than the RCRI in predicting postoperative cardiac event. It should be noted that in this recent study only 45% of patients were evaluated by stress myocardial scintigraphy, the accessibility of the method still being limited [13, 18].

Generally, the type and the conditions of planned surgery cannot be fundamentally changed and can influence the postoperative CVR of patients. Urgent, prolonged (more than 5 h) and long hemodynamic stress (in major vascular interventions, intraabdominal and intrathoracic surgery) increase the risk of perioperative cardiac events. Peripheral vascular procedures present the highest risk (13%); the incidence of postoperative CV events could reach 10–15% [4, 7, 19].

2.4. Noninvasive cardiovascular parameters (biomarkers, coronary artery calcification)

Cardiac biomarkers have been studied for years in prediction of CV long-term outcomes, but less so for preoperative prediction. The most important and evaluated four biomarkers troponinI (TNI), N-terminal brain natriuretic peptide (NT-BNP), cystatin C, and C-reactive protein (CRP) significantly affected the prediction of death from CV causes. The statistical significance increased when the four biomarkers were incorporated into a model with established risk factors [20]. From six risk markers of interest (coronary artery calcium (CAC), carotid intima-media thickness (IMT), ankle-brachial index (ABI), brachial flow-mediated dilation (BFMD), CRP and family history of CAD, at a median follow up of 7.6 years, the CAC (had the highest predictive value), ABI, CRP and family history of CAD were independently associated with incident CAD [21, 22]. The addition of the degree of stenosis measured with computed tomography coronary angiography (CTCA), the presence of significant coronary artery stenosis (>50%) and/or multivessel CAD in completion with the CAC value and the RCRI significantly improved the predictive model for postoperative CV events [23]. Addition of CTCA determines a slight improvement in discrimination for CV death or MI. When added to the RCRI, information from CTCA is five times more likely to overestimate risk in low-risk individuals than to identify a previously misclassified high-risk individual. Thus, current data do not support CTCA as a first-line preoperative screening test for CAD in PAD patients (e.g., **Table 2**) [4, 24].

High CRP levels are positively associated with PAD, independent of smoking, and multiple other cofounders, demonstrating the important role of inflammation in ATS. High levels of inflammatory markers would identify vascular surgery patients at increased risk for adverse events (graft failure, MACE) after lower extremity bypass surgery. Among patients with an elevated CRP (>5 mg/L) before surgery, major postoperative MACE occurred in 60%, compared with a 32% rate in those with a baseline CRP < 5 mg/L (**Table 2**) [25].

High preoperative NT-BNP or CRP are independent predictors of perioperative MACE in noncardiac surgery; the addition of these two markers to the RCRI improves its predictive power for adverse events. There is a statistically significant association between an elevated preoperative NT-BNP level and various CV adverse outcomes within 30 days of surgery (composite of cardiac death, nonfatal MI and atrial fibrillation). NT-BNP concentrations of 99.5 pg./mL predicted cardiac events and 448 pg./mL predicted cardiac death (all-cause

Biomarker	Indication	Sensitivity	Specificity
NT-BNP	Obtain preoperatively in high surgical risk patients scheduled to undergo non-emergent vascular surgery	75–88%	62–100%
CRP		NA	NA
TnT		97%	54%
CAC	Evidence is currently lacking to recommend preoperative risk stratification with routine measurement	79%	61%

Adapted from [13].

Table 2. Indications and characteristics of various markers in preoperative cardiac risk stratification.

mortality in the short-, intermediate- and long-term postoperative periods). Over the threshold value of 448 pg./mL, NT-BNP had a positive predictive value of 100% and suggested that, if a preoperative NT-BNP level is in this vicinity, then it may be preferable to delay or cancel the procedure. Patients with high preintervention values of both CRP and NT-BNP are 10.6 times more likely to experience MACE than patients with normal CRP and NT-BNP values. Patients with a postoperative BNP ≥245 pg./ml or NT-proBNP ≥718 pg./ml had a significantly elevated risk for 30-day CV mortality, nonfatal MI, and cardiac failure. In addition, these postoperative elevations are able to predict long-term outcomes (i.e. ≥ 180 days after surgery) (e.g., **Table 2**) [26, 27].

Similar to postoperative troponin (Tn) levels, the current data for postoperative BNP suggest that it is the absolute postoperative threshold, rather than the increase in the BNP between the preoperative and postoperative period, that is associated with postoperative morbidity and mortality. Natriuretic peptides act as a cumulative marker of myocardial damage sustained during the perioperative period, possibly as a result of ischemic injury, volume overload or both. However, it remains unclear what the exact temporal relationship between postoperative BNP and Tn elevations is. In certain circumstances, it is possible that BNP elevation may precede Tn elevation, as may occur during fluid overload. In such cases, BNP elevations may identify patients at risk of subsequently developing myocardial injury and postoperative Tn elevation. Identification of patients at risk may provide a window for therapeutic intervention. It is likely that the more common scenario is postoperative BNP elevation that occurs together with, or shortly after, a postoperative Tn elevation. In these cases, elevated postoperative BNP may reflect the severity of myocardial injury and may prognosticate short- and long-term outcomes (e.g., **Table 2**) [26, 27].

In the perioperative period, it is clear that any Tn elevation is associated with an increased risk of death, even in the absence of a defining features (e.g., ischemic symptoms and ECG changes, evidence of MI on echocardiography) necessary for the diagnosis of MI. Owing to the effects of anesthesia, and widespread use of narcotics, the majority of perioperative ischemic events are clinically silent. In the Perioperative Ischemic Evaluation (POISE) trial, 65% of patients with a perioperative ischemic event did not experience ischemic symptoms [28]. The risk of death at 30 days was 9.7% in patients with a symptomatic MI and 12.5% in patients with an asymptomatic MI. Thus, the universal definition of MI may not be as sensitive in the perioperative period to detect ischemic events that are associated with poor, intermediate and long-term outcomes.

An isolated peak cardiac biomarker elevation (preferably Tn) with or without correlation with ischemia may be the most sensitive tool to detect perioperative ischemic events that are clinically important [29]. A peak postoperative TnT (>0.02 ng/ml) measured within the first 3 days after surgery is the strongest predictor of 30 days mortality and explained 41.8% of the deaths in population [30]. The current data suggest that the absolute postoperative threshold of Tn is a stronger independent predictor of postoperative MI and intermediate-term survival than the increase in the Tn level between the preoperative and postoperative period. Current data therefore suggest that a raised preoperative Tn level may identify patients who are at risk of increased short-term CV morbidity, mortality and long-term mortality (1 year after surgery, but no longer) due to his high sensitivity, but it may be an inappropriate additional test for improving preoperative risk stratification due to its poor specificity (**Table 2**) [26].

Preoperative cardiac biomarkers (especially BNP and Tn) evaluation adds incremental value to the risk stratification (by RCRI) for MACE (i.e. MI, pulmonary edema, CV death) and for in-hospital mortality [26]. While the body of evidence for the use of cardiac biomarkers for risk stratification is not extensive, the utility of assessing certain biomarkers in high-risk vascular surgical patients is suggested. A pharma-economic analysis of routine Tn surveillance in all patients who fulfilled the VISION study, based on a 25% relative risk reduction for vascular mortality and perioperative MI following the introduction of statin and aspirin therapy in high-risk patients who were Tn positive, found routine Tn surveillance to be cost-effective [30, 31].

2.5. Cardiac evaluation

2.5.1. Investigation of inducible myocardial ischemia

An ECG should be obtained in all moderate to high-risk vascular surgery patients and confers well-accepted prognostic information [11]. The two most common forms of stress testing are exercise ECG (not often feasible due to debility of many vascular surgery patients) and exercise or pharmacologic stress testing combined with imaging (e.g. dobutamine/dipyridamole stress echocardiography (DSE) and myocardial perfusion imaging scintigraphy (MPI)). There is an association between a positive test (ST depression) and the likelihood of postoperative cardiac complications [15]. Outpatient ECG monitoring is relatively affordable, but requires manual interpretation from the investigator, being time-consuming. The automatic or manual interpretation of the ischemic score depends on the correctness and the accuracy of the recorded ECG path. At a very variable percentage of patients (12–73%), recording irregularities are an obstacle to correct interpretation [32]. A study involving both noncardiac (general and vascular) surgery patients has not shown benefits in performing this type of ECG screening in preoperative monitoring [33]. Other studies focused only on patient groups in vascular surgery demonstrated both the positive and negative predictive value of the results of ECG monitoring of silent ischemia, but under the significance of the values provided by MPI. However, the combination of the two tests does not increase the predictive value [7, 28]. Ischemia and/or intra- and postintervention endocardial lesions (T-negative or ST-segment elevation) are more predictive for perioperative cardiac events (up to 85% of perioperative MI may also be preceded by episodes of ischemia-lesion on ECG), and the prognostic value increases if the cardiac Tn serum level reaction is associated [7].

2.5.2. Noninvasive clinical imaging tests for cardiac perioperative risk assessment

The American College of Cardiology (ACC) and the American Heart Association (AHA) as well as European Society of Cardiology (ESC) introduced guidelines to detect and manage perioperative cardiac risk and to prevent cardiac complications after vascular surgery [15, 19]. For preoperative noninvasive stress testing (NIST), the guidelines recommended that patients with active cardiac conditions should be evaluated and treated. NIST may be considered for patients with high or intermediate risk, if it will change management.

NIST include left ventricular (LV) function evaluation and inducible myocardial ischemia through ECG holter monitoring, ECG, echocardiography or scintigraphy coupled with exercise trial or pharmacological stress methods (**Table 3**). These noninvasive assessment tests should be able to detect cardiac abnormalities not revealed by clinical scores. The simple observation of some cardiac abnormalities does not necessarily means augmenting perioperative cardiac risk [32, 33].

NIST requires logistical and financial support. The PAD patients have less accessibility to MPI when compared to CAD patients. The interpretation of the investigation results in these studies is quite variable, which decreases the predictive accuracy. The explanations of these variable interpretations could be related to differences between the definition of fixed objectives, the follow-up strategies and the heterogeneity of the evaluated groups. Even though NIST are available and can be performed, they do not provide a "guarantee" for the perioperative period, as long as postoperative events have multifactorial causes that could not be accurately predicted [32, 33].

The perioperative period is characterized by myocardial ischemia due to hypercoagulability, increased consumption and oxygen demand, caused by catecholamine discharges, pain,

Tests	Prerequisites	Recommended indications
Electrocardiogram (ECG)	None in prior 3 months	CAD, PAD, CVD
	Perioperative risk death/MI >1%	Significant arrhythmia
		Structural heart disease
		Document baseline*
Echocardiogram	Potential to change management	HF with worsening symptoms
	Not for prognosis or as surrogate for exercise capacity	Dyspnea of unknown origin
		Clinical suspicion of structural heart disease
		HF or structural heart disease and no prior test within 1 year*
Non-invasive stress test (NIST)	Perioperative risk death/MI >1%	Unable to perform >4 METs based on subjective assessment or validated tool
	Elevated risk or known CAD	
	Potential to change management	

Adapted from [15].*Uncertain utility may be considered. CAD indicates coronary artery disease; CVD, cerebrovascular disease; HF, heart failure; MET, metabolic equivalents; PAD, peripheral arterial disease.

Table 3. Recommendations for preoperative cardiac investigations in vascular surgery.

anemia, anesthetic and surgical stress. Noninvasive clinical screening (via ECG, cardiac, carotid-vertebral and peripheral arterial ultrasound and where possible by NIST) coupled with cardiac Tn serum levels dosing increases the safety of postoperative evolution and improves the prognosis [34, 35].

Although available in many cardiology centers, stress tests could not be performed systematically in all presurgery intervention patients. Due to the pain caused by critical leg ischemia (CLI), 30–70% of PAD patients could not perform the exercise test; they are added to those who could not do it the same because of obesity, degenerative diseases of the hip and knee or postvascular sequelae. In this context, the results of the effort tests were inconclusive in several studies [7, 36]. For these patients, stress tests using pharmacological agents that increase consumption and demand for oxygen represent an alternative for detecting coronary ischemia. These stress tests are dipyridamole-coupled ECG, thallium myocardial scintigraphy and echocardiography coupled with dobutamine or dipyridamole. The presence of "reversible" segmental infiltration defects fixation, or alterations in segmental parietal kinetics has a predictive sensitivity with positive value greater than the presence of "fixed" defects (e.g., **Table 4**) [28].

Stress echocardiography with dobutamine (DSE) (or dipyridamole) has the theoretical advantage for evaluating both segmental ventricular parietal kinetics and altered LVF as determined by inducible myocardial ischemia. Most echocardiography stress studies conducted on vascular surgery patients suggested that DSE had a good negative predictive value, but the positive

Non-invasive stress tests	Advantages	Disadvantages
Stress ECG	Most affordable of the common testing modalities Widely available	Unable to use in many vascular surgery patients that suffer from claudication and poor functional capacity, as target heart rates cannot be achieved. No additional information about cardiac function that can be seen with cardiac imaging is provided
Stress echo-cardiography (dobutamine) DSE	If pharmacologic stress testing is necessary, may be preferred in patients with known bronchospastic lung disease or significant carotid stenosis. Preferable choice when any additional information about left ventricular function and/or valvular heart disease is desired. Shorter testing time with results available sooner. No ionizing radiation.	Dobutamine has the ability to induce arrhythmias and increases in blood pressure and/or myocardial contractility; avoid in patients with known arrhythmias and symptomatic or large aortic aneurysms
Myocardial perfusion imaging or scintigraphy (MPI with dipyridamole/ thallium)	If pharmacologic stress testing is necessary, may be preferred in patients with known arrhythmias and symptomatic or large aortic aneurysms. Preferable for the assessment of myocardial viability in patients with known left ventricular dysfunction, where the extent and severity of inducible ischemia is of importance.	Dipyridamole may induce bronchospasm or decreases in blood pressure; avoid in patients with bronchospastic lung disease or significant carotid stenosis. Longer testing time and delay for results to be available. Ionizing radiation. Failure to detect global ischemia

Adapted from [13].

Table 4. Comparison of noninvasive stress testing modalities.

predictive value was moderate. This does not increase the discriminatory value of the clinical criteria and does not change the appropriate risk group ranking after the RCRI score. In patients with one or two positive cardiac markers, the negative value of DSE was confirmed by the absence of postoperative cardiac events, while a positive result was followed by an incidence of up to 5% of cardiac events postoperative (MI, sudden death), so preoperative DSE offered no incremental value for determining postoperative adverse cardiac outcomes [7, 28, 37]. The second multicenter Dutch Echocardiographic Cardiac Risk Evaluation study showed no difference between the intermediate risk patients with positive NIST results group and negative results group in cardiac death or MI at 30 days after surgery (1.8 vs. 2.3%) (e.g., **Table 4**) [38].

Myocardial perfusion imaging (MPI) scintigraphy combined with pharmacokinetic stress test and EKG with dipyridamole are most used today in centers that benefit from this availability. Despite the initial expectations of better characterization and stratification of patients, especially from groups initially assessed as having intermediate or low risk for postoperative cardiac events, the results were not what they expected. Stress MPI has a relatively high sensitivity for the prediction of cardiac complications, but the specificity of this method is less satisfactory. Preoperative MPI has a high negative predictive value, but it has not proven to be sufficiently sensitive, and the benefit of MPI was unproven in low-risk patients and probably not cost-effective. There was no association between reversible defects on dipyridamole stress MPI and adverse cardiac events in moderate-risk patients undergoing elective vascular surgery. Based on the scintigraphy results, previously patients in the low-risk group switched to the intermediate risk group, but the rate of postsurgery intervention cardiac events do not change significantly, indicating the limited positive predictive value of these tests and proving no independent prognostic value superior to clinically stratified risk [7, 28]. Information about myocardial perfusion does not accurately predict adverse cardiac outcomes (e.g., as prolonged myocardial ischemia, MI, congestive HF and severe ventricular tachyarrhythmia) following univariate and multivariate analyses. The best correlates of cardiac complications were documented evidence of CAD and age greater than 65 years (e.g., **Table 4**) [12, 24, 39].

Two important questions remain unanswered related to the patient at risk: which stress test is best for which patient and what interventions outside of best medical management are of benefit to reducing perioperative ischemia events. No large head-to-head analyses of DSE versus MPI have been performed, although two well-known meta-analyses have compared the different modalities. DSE showed a positive trend toward better diagnostic performance than the other tests. Relative to MPI, DSE had a similar sensitivity, but significantly greater specificity (70% vs. 49%) (e.g., **Table 3**). Comparison with summary receiver operating characteristic analysis between all modalities revealed a trend toward better performance with DSE, but this was only significant when compared with MPI. DSE has better negative predictive value characteristics than MPI. In addition, a moderate-to-large perfusion defect by either DSE or MPI predicts postoperative MI and death, but DSE is slightly superior to MPI in predicting postoperative cardiac events [24, 39].

A typical pattern has emerged with stress testing for risk stratification prior to surgery; the positive predictive value is usually very low, and the negative predictive value is typically high. Routine preoperative NIST is not necessary in all patients undergoing revascularization for CLI, especially for patients in the low-risk group and for those undergoing endovascular treatment [40]. Widespread use of NIST in assessing the risk of perioperative CV complications remains controversial due to the low predictive value that affects the accuracy of the information. Therefore, the implications for CV risk stratification remain unclear. Even with the reported subtle differences between MPI and DSE, the fact remains that current guidelines do not distinguish between one or the other NIST for the preoperative workup of surgical patients. In line with current joint guidelines, we would recommend that surgeons take into account the availability and expertise in interpretation of the varying modalities and patients specifics at their respective institutions when deciding which test to obtain (e.g., **Figure 1**) [13]. A reversible defect on NIST is considered a predictor of postoperative MACE, and possible revascularization might be recommended. Some authors have suggested coronary angiography as a routine screening test, due to the significant prevalence of coronary involvement in vascular patients. Because coronary angiography is an invasive method with a risk of up to 0.05%, it was not used in studies as a routine examination in perioperative RCV assessment in noncardiac surgery patients. Last data suggested perioperative MI is quite common in

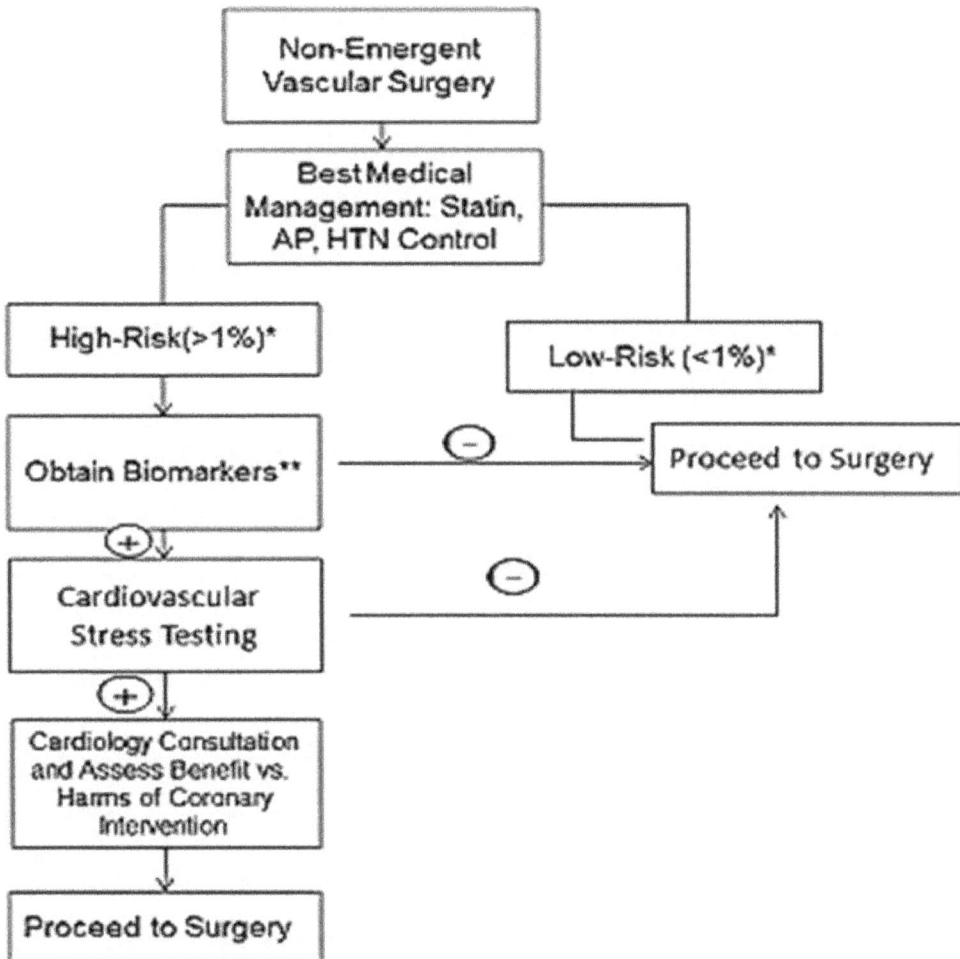

Figure 1. Suggested algorithm for preoperative optimization in vascular surgical patients. AP—Antiplatelet therapy; HTN—Hypertension. Adapted from [13].

nonvascular surgical patients, vascular patients being relatively protected by cardiovascular medication previously administered, and that postoperative events such as anemia play a major role in postoperative MI [41].

2.5.3. Cardiac ultrasound evaluation in perioperative assessment of PAD patients

With cardiac ultrasound (US) (or echocardiography), we can evaluate both the function and the morphology of the heart. The presence of LVH is associated with an increased risk of CV morbidity and all-cause mortality, which emphasizes the importance of diagnosis. The quantitative evaluation of the LV systolic function by LV ejection fraction (LVEF) is a simple and specific predictive index in relation to clinical utility [42]. End-systolic LV volume is an independent predictor of survival in CAD and LVEF has prognostic value for survival in post-MI patients. The presence of diastolic dysfunction represents an early indicator of LV function impairment. Although that high mortality of PAD patients was mainly attributable to coexisting coronary or cervical arteries disease, the prevalence of US abnormalities in patients with peripheral arterial ischemia was not systematically studied. Asymptomatic LV dysfunction is predictive for short- and long-term perioperative CV events in vascular surgery patients; therefore, the echocardiogram should be routinely performed in surgical patients for stratification of CV risk, even in the absence of HF symptoms [43].

The prevalence of CVRF (smoking, DM, dyslipidemia, HT) in PAD patients causes, in addition to peripheral arterial lesions, coronary arteries and myocardial involvement with ischemic, hypertensive and/or diabetic heart disease, aortic and mitral valve calcifications and sometimes myophatic evolution through dilated cardiac disease [44–46]. In PAD patients were found high prevalence of clinically significant cardiac US changes (61.6% vs. 35.3%), especially related to the LV dysfunction and the presence of aortic stenosis (AS) compared to patients without PAD. The presence of PAD is shown to be an independent predictor of LVEF <50%. In PAD patients, MI and HF are the main causes of mortality [47]. PAD patients develop a significantly higher degree of LVH compared with patients with the same means BP but with no PAD. By cardiac US examination, LVH was found in 75% of patients with HT, CAD and PAD and in 46% of patients with HT and CAD but without PAD, respectively. LVH was found in 93% of PAD patients, with ABI <0.6, and 62% of patients with ABI between 0.6 and 0.9 [43, 47–49]. PAD patients with CLI have higher CV morbidity than stable PAD patients. US evaluation is useful in defining the group of patients with low CV risk, in which can be performed with relative safety the revascularization of the limb by interventional/surgery procedures. In the case of the intermediate risk group, additional CV risk assessment tests are required [44–50].

2.6. Perioperative cardiac management strategies

2.6.1. The impact of perioperative risk stratification in the management of PAD patients

Approximately 10% of general surgery patients are included in the high-risk surgical perioperative group after the standard clinical and noninvasive assessment. But for vascular surgery patients, the percentage of high-risk patients may increase by 10–20%. From these, 5–10% may be eligible for myocardial revascularization (PCI or CABG) [7]. In vascular surgery patients in intermediate or low perioperative risk groups, it is advisable to perform NIST. It is possible, however, that NIST does not provide additional predictive perioperative risk elements. Also, these tests do not provide information about cerebrovascular ischemic risk, derived from cervical arterial lesions, almost equally founded as coronary involvement in vascular surgery patients [7, 29]. Clinical judgment is important in assessing the balance between the relative urgency of identified cardiac and noncardiac surgery problems. A relatively small proportion of surgical patients require urgent preoperative treatment of cardiac conditions: congestive HF, life-threatening arrhythmias or acute coronary syndrome (ACS) (recent MI with significant evidence of ischemic risk or unstable, severe AP). However, there are situations in which the surgical situation with an important vital risk imposes the operative decision, even under an incomplete cardiac evaluation [7, 29].

2.6.2. Impact of coronary revascularization decision on noncardiac surgery patients

Patients in noncardiac surgery are at risk of major perioperative cardiac events (sudden cardiac death, cardiorespiratory arrest, MI). In these patients, the in hospital mortality rate is among 15–25%. Patients who underwent a postsurgery intervention cardiac arrest have a mortality rate in the hospital up to 65% and represent a risk factor for cardiac death within the next 5 years postoperatively. Perioperative MI is an independent risk factor for the risk of CVD and the increase incidence of a new MI over the next 6 months postoperatively [7]. This is why the concern is both for the most discriminatory assessment of noncardiac surgery patients in different risk groups, as well as for finding the best prevention strategies (interventional, medical, etc.) for perioperative CV events. By preoperative coronary angiography, the prevalence of CAD ranged between 50 and 80% and is dependent on the specific distribution of the PAD. It is also clear that periprocedural myocardial ischemia, even non-ST segment MI and Tn leaks, confer a significant 26–55% decreased survival through 5 years, supporting the impetus for careful patient preparation [13].

In retrospective studies, for both vascular and nonvascular surgery patients, the "protective" effects of coronary revascularization in reducing perioperative MACE were controversial [7]. "Prophylactic" preoperative myocardial revascularization of significant lesions could reduce perioperative coronary complications in patients with unstable CAD (ACS) and high CVR. There is a significant difference in mortality among high CVR patients who underwent coronary revascularization prior to noncardiac surgery (0.9%) compared to high CVR patients who did not undergo coronary revascularization procedures (2.4%) [7]. Coronary revascularization performed prior to noncardiac surgery has as a primary objective the reduction of CV mortality in the long-term outcome and as a secondary objective, the reduction of CVR in patients with high coronary risk: unstable refractory AP, left main coronary artery stenosis, coronary multivessel significant lesions, including anterior descendent artery (ADA) and altered LV systolic function. Patients who underwent myocardial revascularization before noncardiac surgery had a lower rate of long-term postoperative cardiac events (up to 5 years after noncardiac surgery). The lowest incidence of CV events in long-term outcome after noncardiac vascular surgery was observed in the group of patients with PCI versus revascularized patients by CABG [50, 51].

The Coronary Artery Revascularization Prophylaxis (CARP) trial showed no difference in the rate of postoperative MI (defined by elevated Tn level) (12 vs. 14%) in 30-day mortality, and MACE and mortality at 2.7 years (22 vs. 23%) in patients scheduled for vascular surgery with coronary artery revascularization before surgery compared with patients with no revascularization before surgery, but there was a statistically significant survival benefit at 4 years (87% vs. 70%) that persisted up to 8 years. The CARP trial focused on patients who had stable CAD and those without left main coronary disease or significant valvular heart disease. Time to vascular surgery was significantly longer in the revascularization group [52, 53]. Although this evidence is encouraging, caution is warranted. Of note, excellent adherence with cardioprotective drugs was documented. At least one large database review of nonvascular surgical patients concluded opposite findings, suggesting a benefit of revascularization, so the controversy remains open [54].

A prospective study included patients evaluated before vascular surgery by MPI to complete the coronary angiography indication followed by myocardial revascularization by PCI and/ or CABG. The results of MPI have increased the rate of coronary revascularization from 4.1% to 14.7%, without significantly improving postoperative MACE (MI, sudden cardiac death in the first 30 days after surgery intervention). However, it should be noted that the patients included in the study had one or two coronary vessels significant lesions with preserved LV systolic function and with optimal medical therapy. Patients with CAD and with severe impairment of LV systolic function, unstable AP and AS were not included. In vascular surgery patients having three coronary vessels significant lesions, there was a slight decrease in the incidence of perioperative cardiac events in myocardial revascularized patients before vascular surgery (43%) versus those treated by standard medical therapy (33%) [7]. Therefore in the coronary revascularization decision made prior to noncardiac surgery, three elements should be considered: the coronary risk of the patient, the risk of bypass surgery and the risk of noncardiac surgery. These results do not suggest that there are benefits in prophylactic coronary revascularization in patients with stable CAD regarding the short-term evolution after vascular surgery intervention [50, 51].

One of the main objectives of preoperative cardiac evaluation should be the identification of patients with high-risk coronary anatomy, amenable to revascularization, by an appropriate and discriminatory noninvasive/invasive cardiac evaluation. Once identified, the next question that needs to be answered is what the best revascularization strategy would be, CABG or PCI? The indication and the accomplishment of PCI before noncardiac vascular surgery are directed toward patients with high coronary risk prior to noncardiac surgery. PCI has the advantage of a low periprocedural risk (0.01%) and avoids the stress of CABG. The disadvantage of the PCI is that some lesions could not be accessed by angioplasty and should be resolved later by CABG [7, 50, 51]. Long-term outcomes appear to be better in patients undergoing CABG when compared to PCI, but incomplete revascularization after PCI, impact of stent-related complications and progressive occlusive CAD should be considered while evaluating the disadvantages of PCI over CABG. The heightened thrombogenic potential of newly implanted stents and prothrombotic state induced by the surgical stress increase the risk of in stent thrombosis. Premature discontinuation of antiplatelet therapy in patients with bare metal stents (BMS) or drug eluting stent (DES) is associated with a high rate of stent thrombosis and perioperative mortality. Elective surgical procedures that carry a potential for increased perioperative bleeding should be postponed until a minimum course of dual antiplatelet therapy (DAPT) has been completed. In patients presenting for emergency noncardiac surgery after stenting, consideration should be given to the risk of interrupting thienopyridine antiplatelet therapy compared with the risk of bleeding from surgical proce-dures, to continuation of aspirin in the perioperative period and to restarting thienopyridine as soon as possible [4].

Coronary revascularization is not recommended before surgery for patients with stable CAD in both ACC/AHA and ESC guidelines for the management in patients undergoing noncardiac surgery and it is recommended only in circumstances where it would be indicated even in the nonoperative setting. In general, CABG is recommended for left main disease, triple-vessel disease, complex anatomy or high-risk comorbidities (e.g. diabetes). Given the uncertain ben-efits of preoperative PCI for improving outcome after noncardiac surgery, current guidelines suggest consideration of PCI only for patients with left main disease whose comorbidities preclude CABG and for patients with unstable CAD (e.g. ST-elevation MI, non-ST-elevation ACS) who are appropriate candidates for emergency or urgent revascularization. If revascu-larization by PCI is considered, BMS is preferred over DES for vascular surgery patients given the time pressure to proceed with vascular surgery [15, 19].

The additional risk of anesthesia and intervention stress in noncardiac surgery patients who also have simultaneous cardiac problems should be noted. Even under these conditions, the idea of "prophylactic" coronary revascularization, in all cases, could not be accredited to patients who undergo vascular surgery, on the premises that they have multisite arterial lesions and therefore they also have coronary ATS [36]. Probably only prophylactic coronary revascularization of significant lesions in confirmed CAD could prevent perioperative com-plications in noncardiac surgery patients [8].

In the Reduction of Atherothrombosis for Continued Health (REACH) Registry, more than 50% of PAD patients had a concomitant CAD [2]. This means that modification of ATS risk factors is important in the long term and perioperative CVR is high in the short term [55]. Patients with high CVR should benefit from a sustained medical treatment and control of CVRF, considering the context of a possible myocardial revascularization intervention by PCI or by CABG, as well as the perspective of a future vascular surgery. Patients at risk of having CAD (regardless of the risk group) should be given control of blood pressure, serum cholesterol (via statins), cardiac compensation (angiotensin converting enzyme inhibitors (ACEI), diuretics) and arrhythmia (β-blockers, amiodarone). Numerous scientific studies have demonstrated the beneficial role of β-blockers, antiplatelets, ACEI and statins in reduc-ing perioperative CV mortality in patients undergoing noncardiac vascular surgery. Statins and antiplatelet therapies are also involved in ATS plaque stabilization and improvement of endothelial dysfunction [56–58].

2.7. Cervical arterial ultrasound evaluation in perioperative assessment of PAD patients

With the increase in the use of cardiac and arterial ultrasound (US) in assessing the patient with suspected or known PAD, the diagnostic and prognostic accuracy of these explorations has increased, the sensitivity and specificity of US detection cervical arterial lesions may reach 95%. Noninvasive US methods can also be applied to a wide range of patients including those at high risk for myocardial stress testing. With respect to CVD, a history should ascertain any previous stroke or transient ischemic attack, as well as detail the associated presentation and deficits. It is important to document the etiology to distinguish ATS carotid stenosis from cardio-embolic disease [44].

Carotid intima media thickness (IMT) measured by US is a noninvasive predictive marker independent of the onset, progression and extension of ATS disease, demonstrated in numerous studies. The increase in carotid IMT is associated with a higher incidence of coronary events and multisite ATS lesions [59]. Increased IMT has common risk factors with the onset and progression of coronary and cerebrovascular ATS lesions (HT, DM, dyslipidemia, smoking) [60, 61]. Furthermore, increased IMT demonstrates good reproducibility for both the progression and regression of ATS disease and has been validated as a vascular marker of ATS evolution in numerous clinical trials. At the same time, invasive studies have shown that treating CVRF for CAD can also significantly reduce progression of IMT [62, 63]. Carotid and femoral IMT thickening are associated with the presence of CVRF; the occurrence of CV events is an indicator of the presence of PAD. It has been shown that these risk factors and CV events are significantly linked to increased carotid and femoral IMT. The treatment of CVRF is associated with a decrease in the progression of IMT thickening, parallel to the reduction of CV events and an improvement in the symptoms associated with PAD. This finding is particularly evident in the context of hypolipemiant therapy. IMT, as an additional predictor of CVR, may influence the decision of therapeutic intervention by medication [59–63].

Significantly elevated IMT values were seen in PAD patients at femoral artery, simultaneous with carotid artery, which allowed the conclusion that the presence of PAD is associated with morphological alterations and dynamic variations of both the femoral and the carotid artery walls. DM patients with PAD had a significantly higher IMT at the carotid bifurcation and at the distal common carotid artery, relative to those without PAD. Thus, carotid IMT may be a marker of ATS with different localizations in patients with type 2 DM and reflects morphological and hemodynamic similarities between arterial beds [64]. Today, IMT is one of the most commonly used parameters of noninvasive assessment of CV-ATS risk. In the initial stages, clinical latency of ATS, the increase of carotid IMT over normal value, often is an indicator of the asymptomatic arterial ATS lesions as well as an accompanied predictor for the increased risk of future CV events in already symptomatic arterial ATS territories [1, 65]. The amount of carotid IMT in PAD patients is correlated with body mass index (BMI), ABI, serum LDL-cholesterol and the number of arterial cervical ATS plaques. These results support the hypothesis that ATS is a systemic, generalized disease, leading to functional and structural changes in each of the segments of the arterial system, as confirmed by many other studies that described the concomitant occurrence of carotid, coronary and peripheral arterial ATS disease. Up to 81% of PAD patients with increased IMT had angiographic coronary artery lesions, while 57% had carotid ATS plaques. Therefore, there is a statistically significant correlation between increased carotid IMT and the severity of CAD and also the presence of carotid ATS plaques and PAD clinically manifested which are positive predictive factors for the presence of CAD [1, 65].

PAD patients had advanced cervical arterial ATS lesions expressed both by a higher IMT and an increased prevalence of ATS plaques. Stenotic and occlusive ATS is a systemic phenomenon commonly coexisting in several arterial territories (coronary, carotid, peripheral arteries), often symptomatic in one of the arterial areas and asymptomatic in other affected arterial areas [44–46]. There are fewer studies that investigated the lesions in the cervical arterial system in patients with PAD, compared to the large number of studies investigating the coronary-carotid relationship [65]. Noninvasive vascular imaging, especially CV ultrasound, plays a particularly important role in the carotid evaluation system, and in some aspects (the morphological characterization of the ATS lesion and the possibility of analysis in multiple "nonstandardized" incidences) is superior to conventional angiography allowing accurate measurement of the functional diameter and the lumen area of the vessel, precise localization and dimension (thickness/length/extension and volume) of the ATS plaque, the ecostructure and the surface characterization of the ATS plaque and defining the type of vascular remodeling. Thickness, ecogenicity and endoluminal surface of the ATS plaque are the first features related to a possible instability characterized by the US assessment of vascular lesions [67, 68].

There are studies that argue that US technique overestimates the severity of carotid stenosis compared to angiographic assessment, but these results depend on the US way of quantifying stenosis. The two-dimensional US combined with color and pulse doppler modules generally leads to superimposable results with angiographic quantification [68–71]. Carotid angiography is indicated in selected cases and, particularly in cases where US is difficult to perform and poses diagnosis problems, shows particular aspects or atypical pathological pathways. Angiography visualizes intracranial circulation, not quite accessible to extracranial US (even transcranial doppler), which delivers indirect and segmental information related to cerebral circulation, which may present morphological and trajectory abnormalities. Information on the patency of intracranial collateral supply is important in the prognosis of carotid occlusion. Carotid angiography, in this case, helps to diagnose a possible subocclusive carotid stenosis, which would make the patient a candidate for a probably invasive solution [44–46, 66–71].

3. Conclusions

Patients with PAD undergoing elective vascular surgery have a high prevalence of coronary and cerebrovascular ATS with associated comorbidities (DM, renal failure, anemia) and are at an increased risk of perioperative death and MACE (MI or stroke). The management of patients with PAD refered to high-risk vascular surgical procedure for intermittent claudication, CLI or expanding abdominal aortic aneurysm requires risk stratification, optimization of medical therapies and limited use of cardiac imaging prior to surgery. Preventive coronary revascularization in patients with stable CAD, prior to the vascular operation, with the sole intention of mitigating the risk of CV complications in the perioperative period, is not effective and may be associated with significant bleeding and thrombotic risks, in particular, if stents are used. The patient, surgeon and anesthesiologist can be initially informed about the risk of surgery using modern preoperative risk indices (RCRI, NSQIP, VSG-CRI calculator). Modern biomarkers, such as BNP and high-sensitivity Tn assays, are likely to play a more substantial role in preoperative assessment in the future, but for now they are indicated for high-risk patients. A strategy of universal use of cardiac Tn in the perioperative period for active surveillance of myocardial ischemia may be more reasonable and cost-effective than the current standard of care and widespread use of cardiac imaging prior to high-risk surgery. An elevated cardiac Tn after vascular surgery is recommended and predictive to detect perioperative ischemic events associated with a long-term mortality risk. If the cardiac biomarkers are negative and medical therapy is thought optimized, proceeding with the surgery seems safe. If the cardiac biomarkers are positive, NIST with either DSE or MPI is recommend (particular attention to whether it has potential to change management), taking into account specific patient characteristics that would afford benefit from one modality when compared to another. If the NIST is positive, then a cardiology consultation should be obtained with the appropriate preoperative steps and interventions taken to optimize the patient for their procedure. In general, preoperative coronary revascularization has a limited role, being reserved for the same indications as in routine circumstances. For the most part, chronic CV medications, such as aspirin, ACEI, ARBs and β-blockers, should be continued, but the decision should be individualized to each patient's circumstances. Ideally, thienopyridine antiplatelets therapy should be held before surgery, aside from cases of recent coronary stenting, where expert opinion should be sought. Using clinical risk assessment with biomarkers may decrease further expensive testing and might clarify, optimize risk stratification and indicate whether abnormal cardiac biomarker therapies will change outcomes [71, 72].

Author details

Mirela-Anca Stoia*, Mihaela Mocan, Cerasela Mihaela Goidescu,
Diana Larisa Hognogi Mocan and Roxana Chiorescu

*Address all correspondence to: mirelastoia@yahoo.com

Department of Cardiology, County Clinical Emergency Hospital, University of Medicine and Pharmacy "Iuliu Hatieganu", Cluj-Napoca, Romania

References

[1] Stoia M, Farcas A, et al. The complete arterial screening of patients with peripheral artery disease frequently reveals the polyarterial status with particular implications in the therapeutic strategy. Clujul Medical. 2005;**LXXVIII**(3):583-591

[2] Suarez C et al. Influence of polyvascular disease on cardiovascular event rates. Insights from REACH registry. Vascular Medicine. 2015;**15**(4):259-265. DOI: 10.1177/1358863X 10373299

[3] Jeffrey WO, Brett AS. Peripheral artery disease: Current insight into the disease and its diagnosis and management. Mayo Clinic Proceedings. 2010;**85**(7):678-692. DOI: 10.1177/ 1358863X10373299

[4] Arora V, Velanovich V, Alarcom W, et al. Preoperative assessement of cardiac risk and perioperative cardiac management in noncardiac surgery. International Journal of Surgery. 2011;**9**:23-28. DOI: 10.1016/j.ijsu.2010.09.010

[5]   Stoia M. Arterial Pathology in Vida-Simiti LA. Cluj-Napoca: Cardiologia, Ed. Medicala Universitara "Iuliu Hatieganu; 2013. pp. 448-463

[6]   Olinic D, Stoia M, et al. Doppler ultrasound evaluation of the topographic features of arterial lesions associated with chronic lower limb ischemia. Clujul Medical, 1999; **LXXII**(4):476-483

[7]   Poldermans D, Hoeks SE, Feringa HH. Preoperative risk assessement and risk reduction before surgery. Journal of the American College of Cardiology. 2008;**51**(20):1913-1924. DOI: 10.1016/j.jacc.2008.03.005

[8]   Eagle KA, Vaishnava P, Froehlich JB. Perioperative cardiovasculare care for patients undergoing noncardial surgical intervention. JAMA Internal Medicine. 2015;**175**(5):835-839. DOI: 10.1001/jamainternmed.2015.0150

[9]   Di Minno G, Spadarella G, Cafaro G, et al. Systematic reviews and meta-analyses for more profitable strategies in peripheral arteries disease. Clinical perspectives and PAD research. Annals of Medicine. 2014;**46**(7):475-489. DOI: 10.3109/07853890.2014.932618

[10] Ford MK, Beattie S, Wijeysundera DN. Systematic review: Prediction of perioperative cardiac complications and mortality by the revised cardiac risk index. Annals of Internal Medicine. 2010;**152**(1):26-35. DOI: 10.7326/0003-4819-152-1-201001050-00007

[11] Tsialtas D, Bolognesi MG, Tecchio T, Azzarone M, Quaini F, Bolognesi R. Clinical, electrocardiografic and echografic features in patients with major arterial vascular disease assigned to surgical revascularization. VASA. 2014;**43**(6):443-449. DOI: 10.1024/0301-1526/a000391

[12] Moran PJ, Ghidella T, Power G, et al. The use of lee and co-workers index to assist a risk adjusted of perioperativecardiac outcome. Anaesthesia and Intensive Care. 2008; **36**(2):167-173. (PMID:18361006)

[13] Zarinsefat A, Henke P. Update in preoperative risk assessment in vascular surgery patients. Journal of Vascular Surgery. 2015;**62**:499-509. DOI: 10.1016/j.jvs.2015.05.031

[14] Ford MK, Beattie WS, Wijeysundera DN. Systematic review: Prediction of perioperative cardiac complications and mortality by the revised cardiac risk index. Annals of Internal Medicine. 2010;**152**:26-35. DOI: 10.7326/0003-4819-152-1-201001050-00007

[15] Fleischer LA et al. ACC/AHA guideline on perioperative cardiovascular evaluation and management of patients undergoing noncardiac surgery. Journal of the American College of Cardiology. 2014;**64**(22):e77-e137. DOI: 10.1016 /j.jacc.201 4.07.944

[16] Moodley Y, Naidoo P, Biccard BM. The South African Vascular Surgical Cardiac Risk Index (SAVS-CRI): A prospective observational study. South African Medical Journal. 2013;**103**(10):746-750. DOI: 10.7196/SAMJ.6967

[17] de Hert SP, de Rango P. The concept of risk assessment and being unfit for surgery. European Journal of Vascular and Endovascular Surgery. 2016;**51**:857-866. DOI: 10.1016/j.ejvs.2016.02.00

[18] Bertges DJ, Goodney PP, et al. The Vascular Study Group of New England Cardiac Risk Index (VSG-CRI) predicts cardiac complications more accurately than the revised cardiac index in vascular surgery patients. Journal of Vascular Surgery. 2010;**52**:674-683. DOI: 10.1016/j.jvs.2010.03.031

[19] Kristensen SD, Knuuti J, et al. 2014 ESC/ESA guidelines on non-cardiac surgery: Cardiovascular assessment and management. European Heart Journal. 2014;**35**:2383-2431. DOI: 10.1093/eurheartj/ehu282

[20] Zethelius B, Berglund L, Sundstrom J, et al. Use of multiple biomarkers to improve the prediction of death from cardiovascular causes. The New England Journal of Medicine. 2008;**358**:2107-2116. DOI: 10.1056/NEJMoa0707064

[21] Yeboah J, McClelland RL, Polonsky TS, et al. Comparison of novel risk markers for improvement in cardiovascular risk assessment in intermediate-risk individuals. JAMA. 2012;**308**:788-795. DOI: 10.1001/jama.2012.9624

[22] Kavousi M, Elias-Smale S, Rutten JH, et al. Evaluation of newer risk markers for coronary heart disease risk classification: A cohort study. Annals of Internal Medicine. 2012;**156**:438-444. DOI: 10.7326/0003-4819-156-6-201203200-00006

[23] Ahn JH, Park JR, Min JH, et al. Risk stratification using computed tomography coronary angiography in patients undergoing intermediate-risk noncardiac surgery. Journal of the American College of Cardiology. 2013;**61**:661-668. DOI: 10.1016/j.jacc.2012.09.060

[24] Sheth T, Chan M, Butler C, et al. Prognostic capabilities of coronary computed tomographic angiography before non-cardiac surgery: Prospective cohort study. BMJ. 2015;**350**:h1907. DOI: 10.1136/bmj.h1907

[25] Owens CD, Ridker PM, Belkin M, et al. Elevated C-reactive protein levels are associated with postoperative events in patients undergoing lower extremity vein bypass surgery. Journal of Vascular Surgery. 2007;**45**:2-9. DOI: 10.1016/j.jvs.2006.08.048

[26] Biccard BM, Devereaux PJ, Rodseth RN. Cardiac biomarkers in the prediction of risk in the non-cardiac surgery setting. Anaesthesia. 2014;**69**:484-493. DOI: 10.1111/anae.12635

[27] Rodseth RN, Biccard BM, Le Manach Y, et al. The prognostic value of pre - operative and postoperative B-type natriuretic peptides in patients undergoing noncardiac surgery: B-type natriuretic peptide and N-terminal fragment of pro-B-type natriuretic peptide: A systematic review and individual patient data meta-analysis. Journal of the American College of Cardiology. 2014;**63**:170-180. DOI: 10.1016/j.jacc.2013.08.1630

[28] Devereaux PJ, Xavier D, Pogue J, et al. Characteristics and short-term prognosis of perioperative myocardial infarction in patients undergoing noncardiac surgery: A cohort study. Annals of Internal Medicine. 2011;**154**:523-528. DOI: 10.7326/0003-4819-154-8-201104190-00003

[29] Garcia S, McFalls E. Perioperative clinical variables and long-term survival following vascular surgery. World Journal of Cardiology. 2014;**6**(10):1100-1107. DOI: 10.4330/wjc.v6.i10.1100. ISSN 1949-8462 (online)

[30] Devereaux PJ, Chan MT, Alonso-Coello P, et al. Association between postoperative troponin levels and 30-day mortality among patients undergoing noncardiac surgery. JAMA. 2012;**307**:2295-2304. DOI: 10.1001/jama.2012.5502

[31] Moodley Y, Naidoo P, Biccard BM. The south African vascular surgical cardiac risk index (SAVS-CRI): A prospective observational study. South African Medical Journal. 2013;**103**(10):746-750. DOI: 10.7196/SAMJ.6967

[32] Koizumi M, Sata N, Yasuda Y, et al. Preoperative cardiac evaluation: When should the surgeon consult the cardiologist? Surgery Today. 2006;**36**(5):425-435. DOI: 10.1007/s00595-005-3169-2

[33] Wright DE, Hunt DP. Perioperative surveillance for adverse myocardial events. Southern Medical Journal. 2008;**101**(1):52-58. DOI: 10.1097/SMJ.0b013e31815d3d19

[34] Flu WJ, Schouten O, Kuijk JP, Poldermans D. Perioperative cardiac damage in vascular surgery. European Journal of Vascular and Endovascular Surgery. 2010;**40**:1-8. DOI: 10.1016/j.ejvs.2010.03.014

[35] Subherval S et al. Polyvascular disease and long term cardiovascular outcomes in older patients with non-ST segment elevation myocardial infarction. Circulation. Cardiovascular Quality and Outcomes. 2012;**5**(4):541-549. DOI: 10.1161/CIRCOUTCOMES.111.964379

[36] Cove C, Hamburg N, et al. The association of diagnostic criteria for myocardial infarction and perioperative cardiac risk factors in vascular surgery patients. Epidemiology and Prevention of CV Disease: Physiology, Pharmacology and Lifestyle; session title: Markers for prognosis in CVD. 2013;**2**:e000136

[37] Karagiannis SE, Feringa HH, et al. Value of myocardial viability estimation using dobutamine stress echocardiography in assessing risk ppreoperative before noncardiac vascular surgery in patients with left ventricular ejection fraction<35%. The American Journal of Cardiology. 2007;**99**(11):1555-1559. DOI: 10.1016/j.amjcard.2007.01.033

[38] Poldermans D, Bax JJ, Schouten O, et al. Should major vascular surgery be delayed because of preoperative cardiac testing in intermediate-risk patients receiving beta-blocker therapy with tight heart rate control? Journal of the American College of Cardiology. 2006;**48**:964-969. DOI: 10.1016/j.jacc.2006.03.059

[39] Weinstein H, Steingart R. Myocardial perfusion imaging for preoperative risk stratification. Journal of Nuclear Medicine. 2011;**52**:750-760. DOI: 10.2967/jnumed.110.076158

[40] Kim TY, Yun WS, Park K. Cardiac risk factors of revascularization in chronic atherosclerotic lower extremity ischemia. Journal of the Korean Surgical Society. 2013;**84**:178-184. DOI: 10.4174/jkss.2013.84.3.178

[41] Henke PK, Zamora-Berridi G, Englesbe MJ, et al. A case-cohort study of postoperative myocardial infarction. Surgery. 2014;**156**(4):pp.1018-1026, 1029. DOI: 10.1016/j.surg.2014.06.055

[42] Tsao C et al. Subclinical and clinical correlate of left ventricular wall motion abnormalities in the community. The American Journal of Cardiology. 2011;**107**(6):949-955. DOI: 10.1016/j.amjcard.2010.11.014

[43] Flu WJ, van Kujik JP, Hoeks SE, Poldermans D. Prognostic implications of asymptomatic
      left ventricular dysfunction in patients undergoing vascular surgery. Anesthesiology.
      2010;**112**:1316-1324. DOI: 10.1097/ALN.0b013e3181da89ca

[44] Stoia MA. Arterial and cardiac ultrasonography contribution in evaluation and establish-
      ing therapeutic strategy in patients with peripheral artery disease [thesis]. Cluj-Napoca:
      Editura Medicală Universitară "Iuliu Hațieganu"; 2015

[45] Stoia MA, Farcas AD, et al. Comparative analysis of cardiovascular risk profile, cardiac
      and cervical arterial ultrasound in patients with chronic coronary and peripheral arterial
      ischemia. In: Vlad S., Roman N editors. International Conference on Advancements of
      Medicine and Health Care through Technology, 2016. Cluj-Napoca, Romania: IFMBE
      Proceedings, Springer; 2017;**59**:p.53-56. DOI: 10.1007/978-3-319-52875-5_13

[46] Farcas AD, Stoia MA, et al. Cardiovascular risk profile, cardiac and cervical artery
      ultrasound in patients with peripheral artery disease. In: Vlad S, Roman N, editors.
      International Conference on Advancements of Medicine and Health Care through
      Technology; 2016. Cluj-Napoca, Romania: IFMBE Proceedings, Springer; 2017;**59**:
      pp. 57-60. DOI: 10.1007/978-3-319-52875-5_13

[47] Ward RP, Min JK, McDonough KM, Lang RM. High prevalence of important cardiac find-
      ings in patients with peripheral arterial disease referred for echocardiography. Journal of the
      American Society of Echocardiography. 2005;**18**(8):844-849. DOI: 10.1016/j.echo.2005.01.004

[48] Shigematsu H, Nishibe T, et al. Three year cardiovascular events and disease progres-
      sion in patients with peripheral arterial disease: Results from the Japan medication
      therapy for peripheral arterial disease (J-METHOD). International Angiology. 2010;(2
      suppl):2-13 PMID:20357743

[49] Van Kujik JP, Flu WJ, Valentijn TM, et al. Influence of left ventricular dysfunction (dia-
      stolic versus systolic) on long term prognosis in patients with or without diabetes mel-
      litus having elective peripheral arterial surgery. The American Journal of Cardiology.
      2010;**106**(6):860-864. DOI: 10.1016/j.amjcard.2010.05.010

[50] Cassar A, Poldermans D, Rihal CS, Gersh B. The management of combined coronary
      artery disease and peripheral vascular disease. European Heart Journal. 2010;**31**:
      1565-1572. DOI: 10.1093/eurheartj/ehq186

[51] Freeman WK, Gibbons RJ. Perioperative cardiovascular assessment of patients
      undergoing noncardiac surgery. Mayo Clinic Proceedings. 2009;**84**(1):79-90. PMCID:
      PMC2664575, PMID: 19121258

[52] McFalls EO, Ward HB, Moritz TE, et al. Coronary-artery revascularization before elec-
      tive major vascular surgery. The New England Journal of Medicine. 2004;**351**:2795-2804.
      DOI: 10.1056/NEJMoa041905

[53] Duncan D, Wijeysundera DM. Preoperative cardiac evaluation and management of
      the patient undergoing major vascular surgery. International Anesthesiology Clinics.
      2016;**54**(2):1-32. DOI: 10.1097/AIA.0000000000000091

[54] Livhits M, Gibbons MM, de Virgilio C, et al. Coronary revascularization after myocardial infarction can reduce risks of noncardiac surgery. Journal of the American College of Surgeons. 2011;**212**:1018-1026. DOI: 10.1016/j.jamcollsurg.2011.02.018

[55] Bhatt LD, (REACH Registry Investigators). Comparative determinants of 4-year cardiovascular events rates in stable outpatients at risk of or with atherotrombosis. JAMA, 2010;**304**(12):1350-1357. DOI: 10.1001/ jama.2010.1322

[56] Poredos P, Jezovnik M, Kalodiki E, et al. Medical management of patients with peripheral arterial disease. International Angiology. 2015;**34**(1):75-93 PMID:24916346

[57] Hammill BG, Curtis LH, Bennett-Guerrero E, et al. Impact of heart failure on patients undergoing major noncardiac surgery. Anesthesiology. 2008;**108**(4):559-567. DOI: 10.1097/ALN.0b013e31816725ef

[58] Stoia M, Lupu A, Farcaș A, Catalano M. Diffuse and extensive changes of the carotid and abdominal arteries distensibility and arterial resistivity in patient with diabetic mellitus. Romanian Journal of Angiology and Vascular Surgery. 2006;**3-4**:86-91

[59] Bots ML, Sutton-Tyrrell K. Lessons from the past and promises for the future for carotid intima-media thickness. JAMA. 2012;**60**(17):1599-1604. DOI: 10.1016/j.jacc.2011.12.061

[60] Baldassarre D, Hamsten A, et al. Measurement of carotid-media thickness and of interadventitia common carotid diameter improve prediction of cardiovascular events (results of the IMPROVE-carotid intima media thickness[IMT] and IMT-progression as predictors of vascular events in high risk European population) study. Journal of the American College of Cardiology. 2012;**60**(16):1489-1499. DOI: 10.1016/j.jacc.2012.06.034

[61] Ruijter HM, Peters SAE, et al. Common carotid intima-media thickness measurements in cardiovascular risk prediction-a meta-analysis. JAMA. 2012;**308**(8):796-803. DOI: 10.1001/jama.2012.9630

[62] Chironi G, Simon A. The prognostic of intima-media thickness revisited. Archives of Cardiovascular Diseases. 2013;**106**:1-3. DOI: 10.1016/j.acvd.2013.01.001

[63] Bots ML, den Ruijter HM. Variability in the intima-media thickness measurement as marker for cardiovascular risk? Not quite settled yet. Cardiovascular Diagnosis and Therapy. 2012;**2**(1):3-5. DOI: 10.3978/ j.issn.2223-3652.2012.01.06

[64] Peters SAE, den Ruijter M, Bots L, Moons KGM. Improvements in risk stratification for the occurrence of cardiovascular disease by imaging subclinical atherosclerosis: A systematic review. Heart. 2012;**98**:177-184. DOI: 10.1136/heartjnl-2011-300747

[65] Nicolaides A, Kakkos S, et al. Asymptomatic internal carotid stenosis and cerebrovascular risk stratification. Journal of Vascular Surgery. 2010;**52**(1):1486-1496. DOI: 10.1016/j.jvs.2010.07.021

[66] Olinic D, Stoia M, et al. Doppler ultrasound examination in the quantification and characterization of the carotid stenosis ecostructure. International Angiology. 1997;**16**(1-3): 1615-5939. ISSN: 1061-1711 (Print)

[67] Olinic D, Stoia M, et al. Carotid plaque echostructure: Relation to carotid stenosis severity and symptomatology. Romanian Journal of Angiology and Vascular Surgery. 2000;**2**(2):77-81

[68] Bekelis K, Labropoulos N, Pappas P, Gasparis A. B-mode estimate of carotid stenosis: Planimetric measurements complement the velocity estimate of internal carotid stenosis. International Angiology. 2013;**32**(5):506-511 PMID:23903310

[69] Beach KW, Bergelin RO, Leotta DF, Primozich JF, Sevareid PM, Stutzman ET, Zierler RE. Standardized ultrasound evaluation of carotid stenosis for clinical trials: University of Washington Ultrasound reading center. Cardiovascular Ultrasound. 2010;**8**(44):1-15. DOI: 10.1002/ajum.12080

[70] Byrnes KR, Ross CB. The current role of duplex ultrasonography in the management of carotid atherosclerosis: Foundations and advances. International Journal of Vascular Medicine. 2012:1-10. DOI: 10.1155/2012/187872

[71] AbuRahma AF, Srivastava M, et al. Critical appraisal of the carotid duplex consensus criteria in the diagnosis of carotid artery stenosis. Journal of Vascular Surgery. 2011;**53**: 53-56. DOI: 10.1016/j.jvs.2010.07.045

[72] Norgren L, Hiatt WR, Dormandy JA, Hirsch AT, Jaff MR, Diehm C, Baumgartner I, Belch JJF. The next 10 years in the management of peripheral artery disease: Perspectives from the 'PAD 2009' conference. European Journal of Vascular and Endovascular Surgery. 2010;**40**:375-380. DOI: 10.1016/j.ejvs.2010.05.005

8

Angiography and Endovascular Therapy for Femoropopliteal Artery Disease

Masahiko Fujihara

Abstract

Femoropopliteal artery disease accounts for a significant proportion of endovascular interventions (EVTs) for peripheral artery disease (PAD) in patients with disabling claudication or chronic limb ischemia. The femoropopliteal artery starts from the common femoral artery (CFA) to the superficial femoral artery (SFA) and ends at the popliteal artery. The SFA is the longest vessel, and it is hard to visualize the entire vessel in one image. However, it is the main target for endovascular works. Before EVT procedure, full evaluation by the angiography is needed. These include anatomical variation, lesion length, lesion characteristics, calcification, and stent restenosis pattern. Endovascular approach is based on these information. The benefit of revascularization is considered to correspond to the severity of ischemia. Their assessment led to optimal endovascular strategy for femoropopliteal occlusive disease. However, to keep the patency after procedure by current endovascular approach still remains unsolved.

Keywords: femoropopliteal artery, superficial femoral artery, popliteal artery, angiography, endovascular therapy

1. Introduction

Femoropopliteal artery disease accounts for a significant proportion of endovascular interventions (EVTs) for peripheral artery disease (PAD) in patients with disabling claudication or chronic limb ischemia. PAD is commonly classified into either the Fontaine stages or Rutherford classifications [1, 2]. The femoropopliteal artery is the longest vessel and crosses two joint structures, i.e., the hip and knee joints. This vessel courses through the muscular adductor canal in the thigh, which places the artery at increased mechanical stress; specifically on the distal superficial femoral artery (SFA) and proximal popliteal artery (PPA), which are the most common anatomic locations of lower extremity atherosclerosis.

There has been a marked increase in the use of endovascular interventions in the treatment of peripheral arterial disease, with femoropopliteal interventions accounting for more than 55% of cases [3]. Stents in the femoropopliteal system have historically been associated with increased rates of stent fracture, which is related to high rates of restenosis [4]. This vascular segment has limited long-term patency rates so that the clinical value of EVT requires more investigation. Even though new technology has been introduced to femoropopliteal artery disease, it is still challenging to treat and interventions are often limited by its unique anatomic, hemodynamic, and mechanical constraints. Contrast angiography provides detailed information on the arterial anatomy and is recommended as the "gold standard" method for evaluation of patients with lower extremity PAD, especially when revascularization is contemplated. In this chapter, a basic angiographic technique for femoropopliteal artery disease is presented along with various angiographic images of pre- and postangioplasty.

2. Basic angiography for the femoropopliteal artery

The femoropopliteal artery starts from the common femoral artery (CFA) to the superficial femoral artery (SFA) and ends at the popliteal artery. The first branch is the profunda femoral artery (PFA). The SFA is the longest vessel, and it is difficult to visualize the entire vessel in one image; however, it is the main target for endovascular works.

2.1. Bifurcation angiography

In the antero-posterior (AP) view, the profunda femoris (PFA) overrides the SFA (**Figure 1**).

In the proximal SFA, the initial angiography should be taken by an ipsilateral view (**Figure 2**).

In this angled view, the clear separation between the left SFA and left PFA was made by the left anterior oblique (LAO) view. In **Figures 1** and **2**, the same two images are shown. In the digital subtraction image (DSA), the background is not clearly visible so that the bifurcation point is difficult to identify. In contrast, digital angiography (DA) shows the background so that we could understand where the bifurcation point starts at the common femoral head. This angled view is of particular importance in visualizing a diseased proximal femoral artery or diseased deep femoral artery (DFA) (**Figure 3**).

2.2. Anatomy of the CFA in relation to the femoral head

In this angled view, we could locate the level of the bifurcation point at the common femoral head. In this angiography, whether the DFA shows high or low take-off needs to be evaluated. In **Figure 4A** and **B**, the DFA arises from the middle femoral head. In these cases, careful attention is mandatory before a puncture to the CFA by either a retrograde or antegrade approach.

According to a report by Ho-Young Ahn et al. [5] (**Figure 5**), the proportion of cases in which the location of femoral artery bifurcation was above the center of the femoral head was 4.59%, and the proportion of cases in which the location of femoral artery bifurcation was in zone 3 was 10.1%, zone 4 was 36.7%, and zone 5 in which bifurcation is below the femoral head was 48.6% (**Figure 6**).

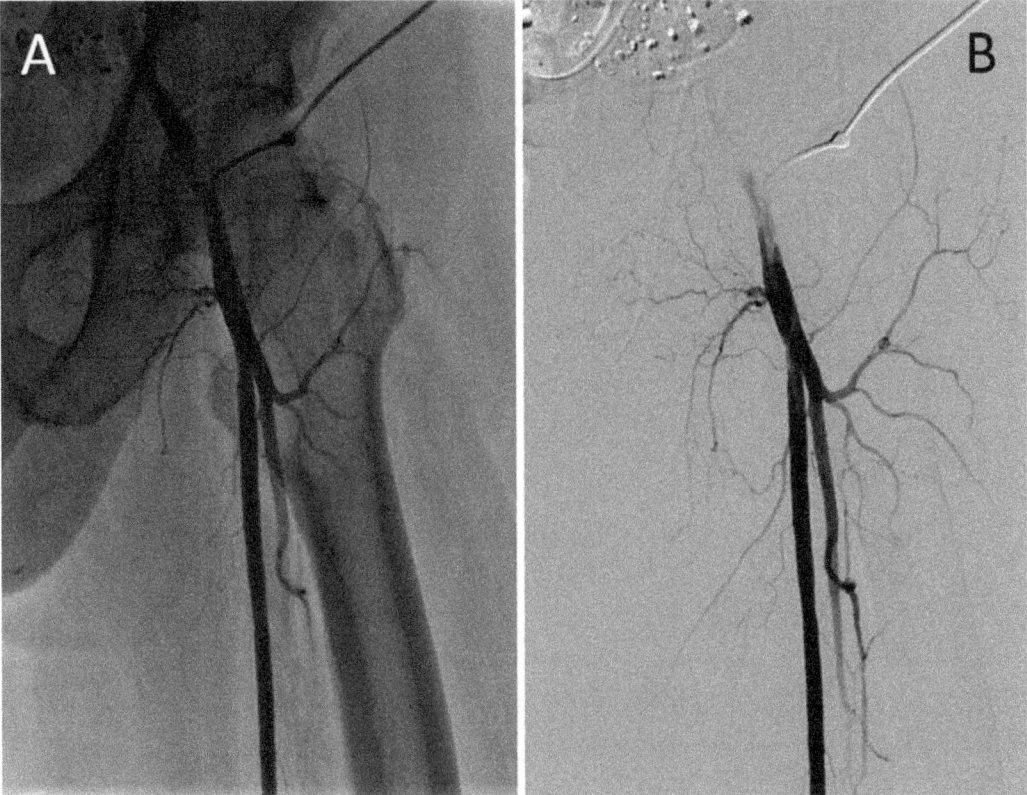

Figure 1. Anteroposterior view of proximal left femoral artery by (A) DA image; (B) DSA.

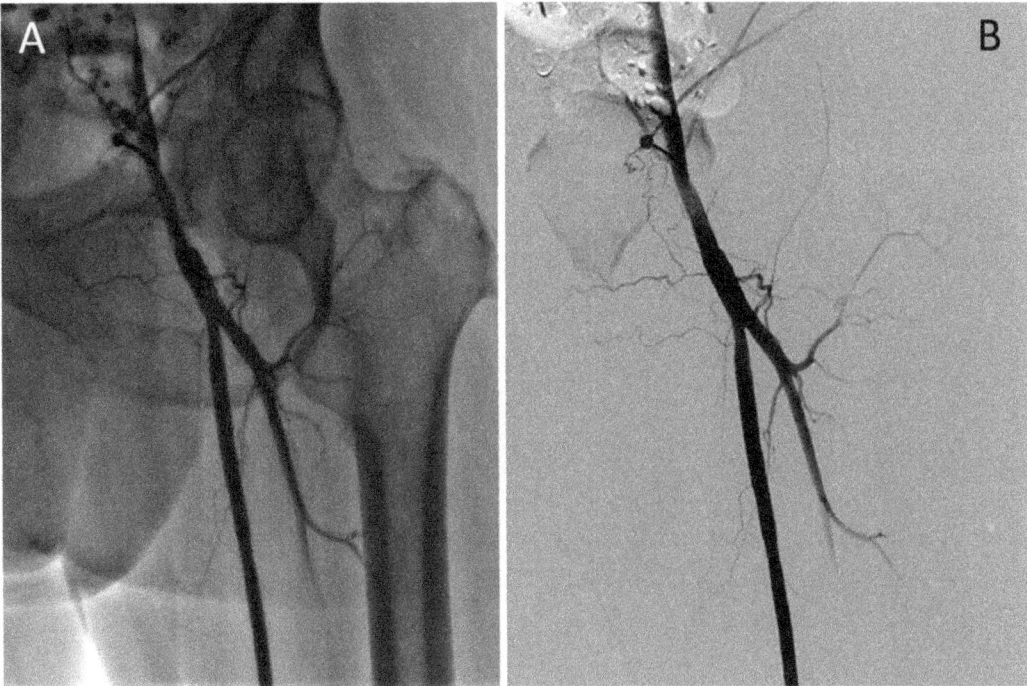

Figure 2. Left anterior oblique view of proximal left femoral artery by (A) DA image; (B) DSA.

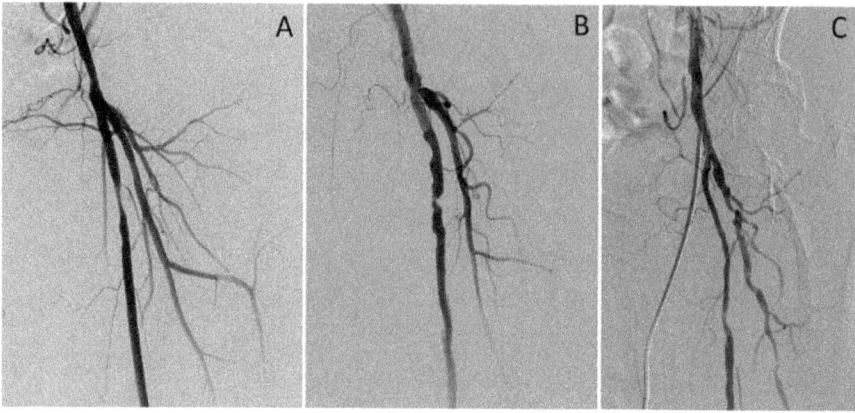

Figure 3. Left anterior oblique view for proximal left femoral diseased artery. (A) Proximal focal SFA stenosis is well visualized. (B) Complex SFA disease and ostial stenosis PFA are well visualized. (C) Both SFA and PFA are diffusely diseased.

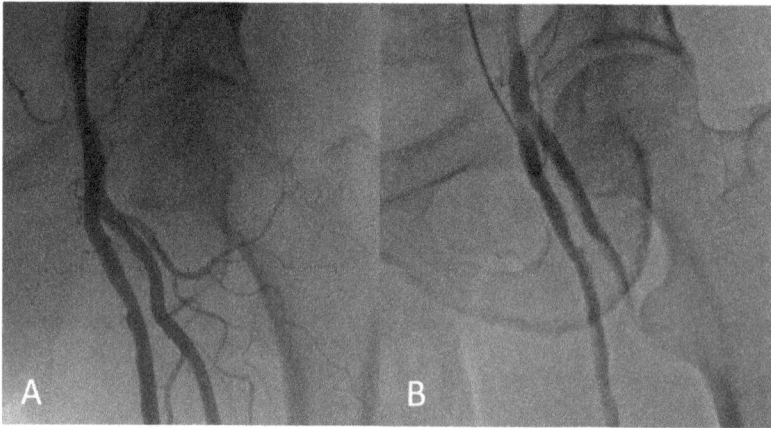

Figure 4. High take-off of profunda artery. (A) Located in zone 3. (B) Located in zone 4.

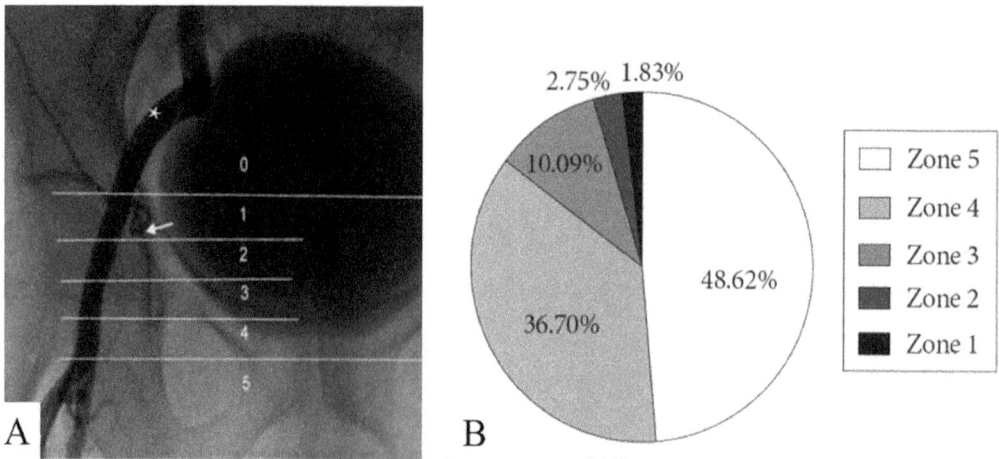

Figure 5. Angiographic anatomical study of the common femoral artery from Korea. (A) the definition of location for femoral artery bifurcation (B) the proportion of femoral artery bifurcation location, zone 5 in which bifurcation is below the femoral head was 48.6%.

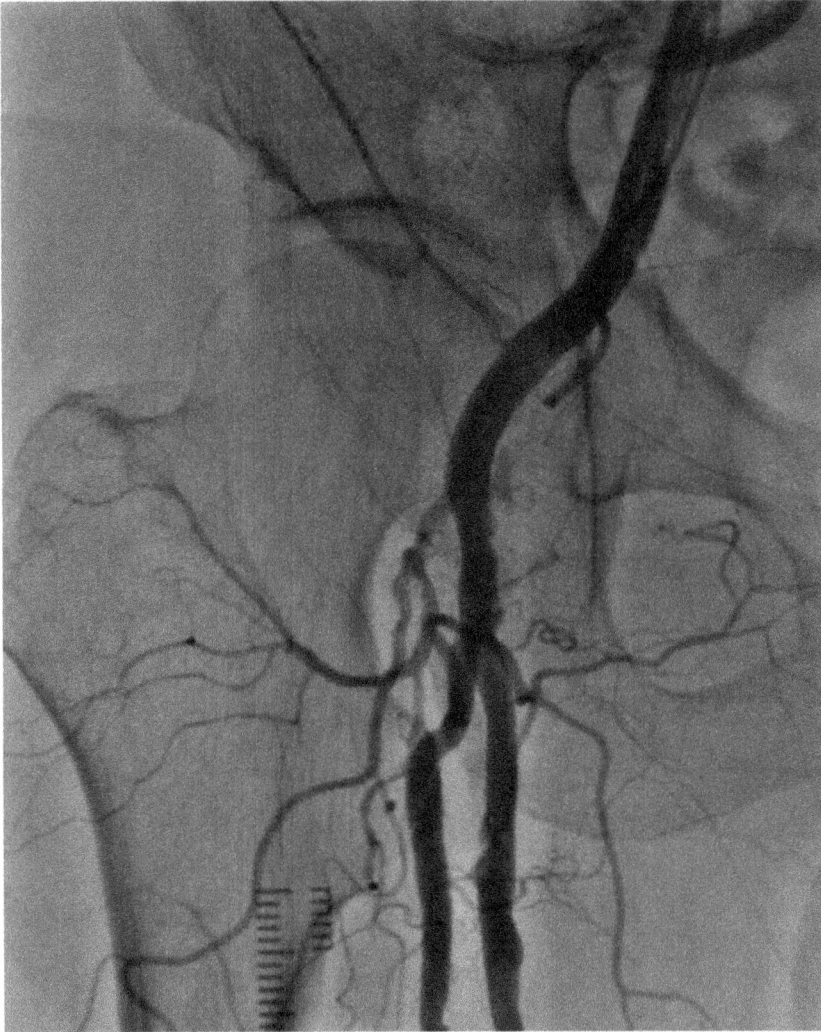

Figure 6. Low take-off of profunda artery.

To reduce vascular complications, the bifurcation point needs to be assessed to determine the optimal puncture location. The second point is the direction of the PFA. In most cases, the PFA is directed outward, but in some cases, the PFA goes inward then turns outward. This is an anomaly of the deep femoral artery bifurcation (**Figure 7**). Accurate knowledge of such anatomical variations regarding the origin of the PFA and femoral circumflex arteries is essential for clinicians. Information on the precise anatomy of the PFA will provide the foundation for assessments to minimize puncture-related complications.

2.3. Middle to distal SFA

From the mid to distal SFA portion, the angiographic view is the antero-posterior (AP) view (**Figure 8**).

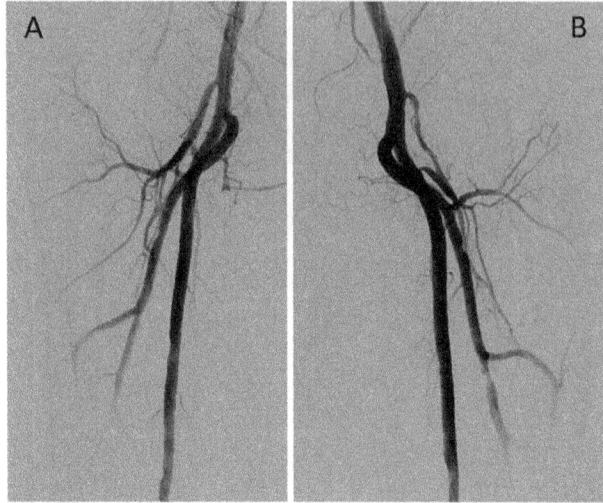

Figure 7. Variations of the profunda femoral artery. Both right (A) and left (B) deep femoral artery directed medially with separate origin of lateral circumflex artery.

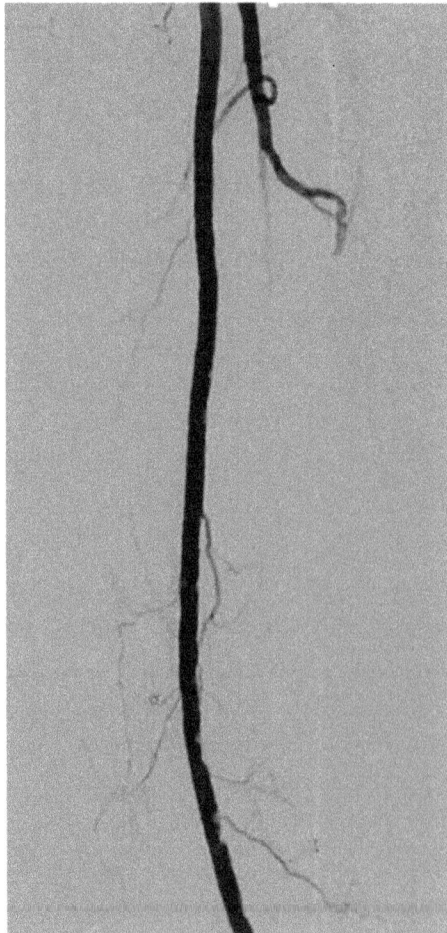

Figure 8. Anteroposterior view for middle SFA with a DSA image.

Distal SFA and popliteal artery angiography may require an angled view (**Figure 9**) since it runs posterior to the knee joint (**Figure 10**). Bolus chasing (running table) is a commonly employed method to visualize a long segment of the femoropopliteal to below the knee artery. In some angiographic systems, this angiography can be performed by digital subtraction with a small amount of contrast.

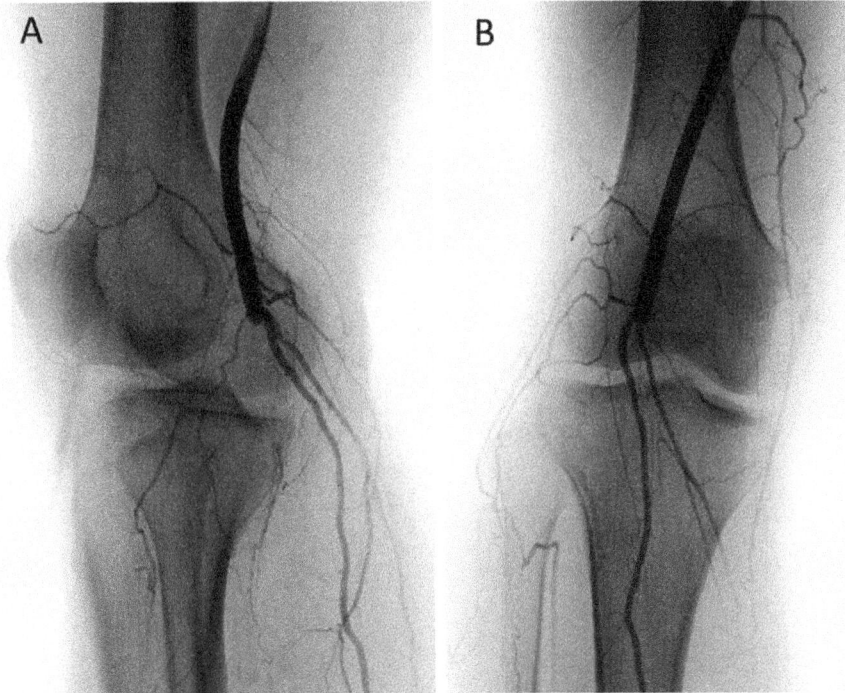

Figure 9. (A) Left anterior oblique view for distal to popliteal disease. (B) Anteroposterior view.

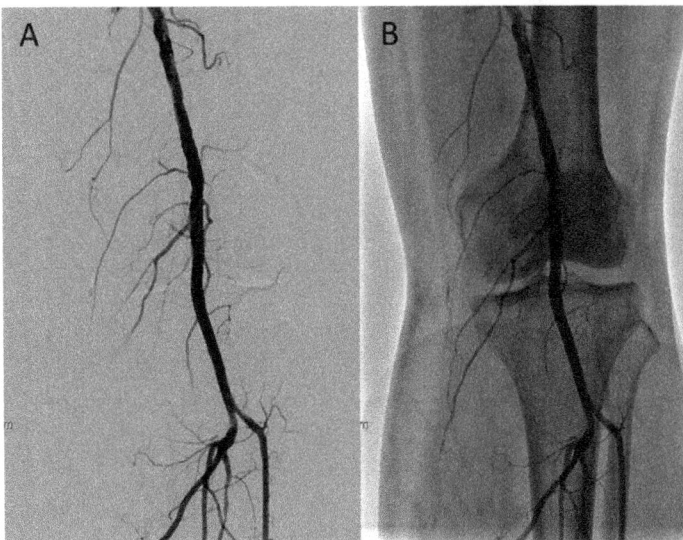

Figure 10. Anteroposterior view of left popliteal artery. (A) Left popliteal artery clearly shown by DSA image. (B) Due to boney structure overriding the popliteal artery, DA image has limitations in visualizing arterial edge and other branches.

We usually inject 4 cc/second for a total 16 cc of contrast to enhance visualization from the common femoral to the distal tibial artery (**Figure 11**).

2.4. Popliteal artery

The popliteal artery is a continuation of the distal SFA and courses through the popliteal fossa. It is located in the knee and back of the leg. Due to the bony structure of the knee joint, the popliteal artery is well visualized by DSA. In **Figure 12**, the DA image does not reveal any branches.

The popliteal artery segments are defined as follows: P1 segment, from the intercondylar fossa to proximal edge of the patella; P2 segment, from the proximal part of the patella to the center of the knee joint space; and P3 segment (below knee popliteal artery), from the center of the knee joint space to the origin of the anterior tibial artery (**Figure 13**) [6]. In the DSA image, the right superior lateral genicular artery and inferior lateral genicular artery are well visualized.

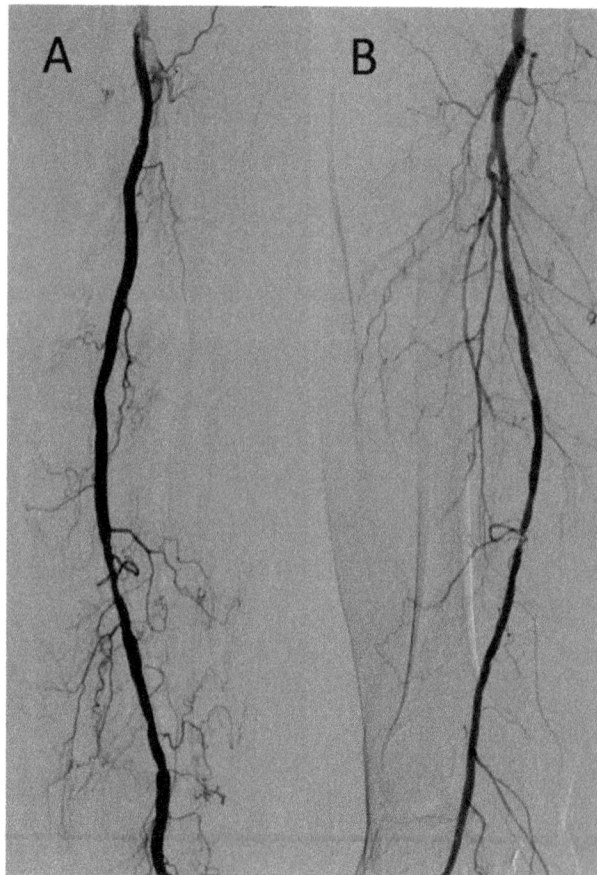

Figure 11. Bolus chase limb vessel angiography in DSA image. To see the whole femoropopliteal artery, bolus chasing is a very useful method. Angiogram can be obtained by digital subtraction with small amount of dye.

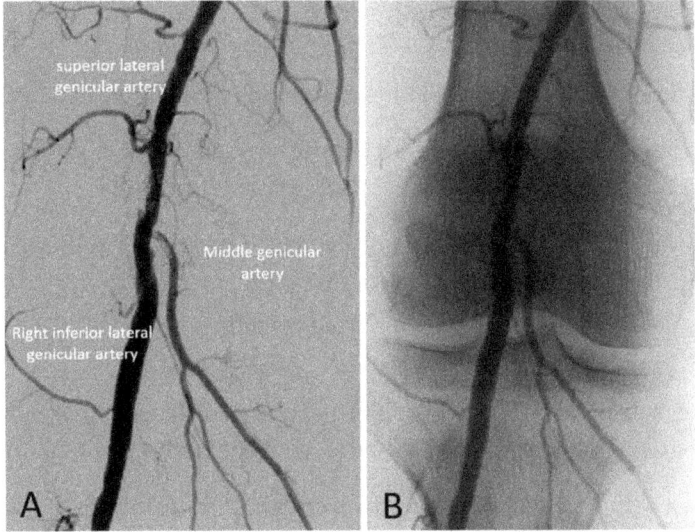

Figure 12. Anatomy of popliteal artery by (A) DSA image and (B) DA image.

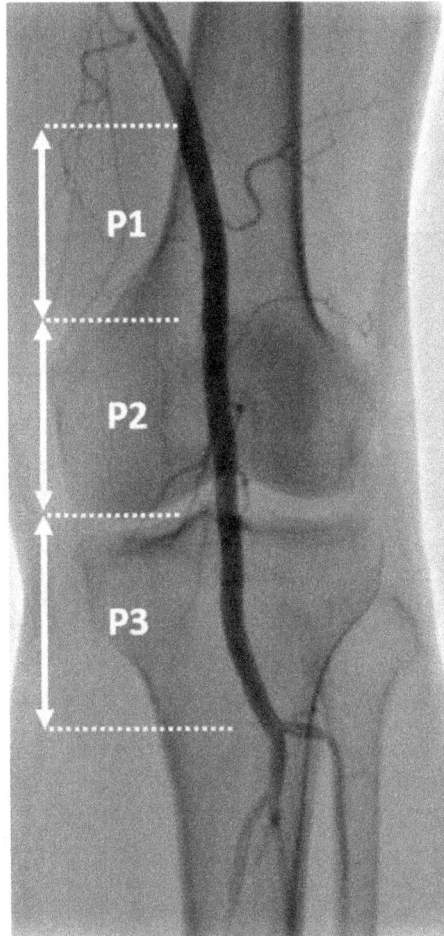

Figure 13. Definition of popliteal artery segments.

3. Common femoral artery disease

Most CFA diseases are localized short lesions and have coral-like calcifications (**Figure 14**).

The ideal angiographic image is provided by an ipsilateral view. This image shows the circumflex iliac artery and deep femoral artery bifurcation (**Figure 15**).

The CFA is the so-called nonstenting zone and stent implantation should be avoided due to issues regarding long-term durability and stent fracture. There are some cases in which acceptable results with long-term patency could be obtained by balloon procedure alone (**Figure 16**).

However, in most cases, ballooning is insufficient in retaining patency. Standard revascularization in CFA disease should be treated by endarterectomy (**Figure 17**).

Endarterectomy is a surgical cut-down and removal of the plaque. This so-called femoral endarterectomy with or without patch angioplasty has long been the favored approach for the treatment of patients with symptomatic common femoral artery disease. On the other hand, the endovascular approach is regarded as a less effective treatment strategy for CFA stenosis/occlusion. The plaque in the CFA is often bulky, eccentric, and heavily calcified and may not respond well to balloon dilation. Thus, stent implantation is contraindicated in the CFA.

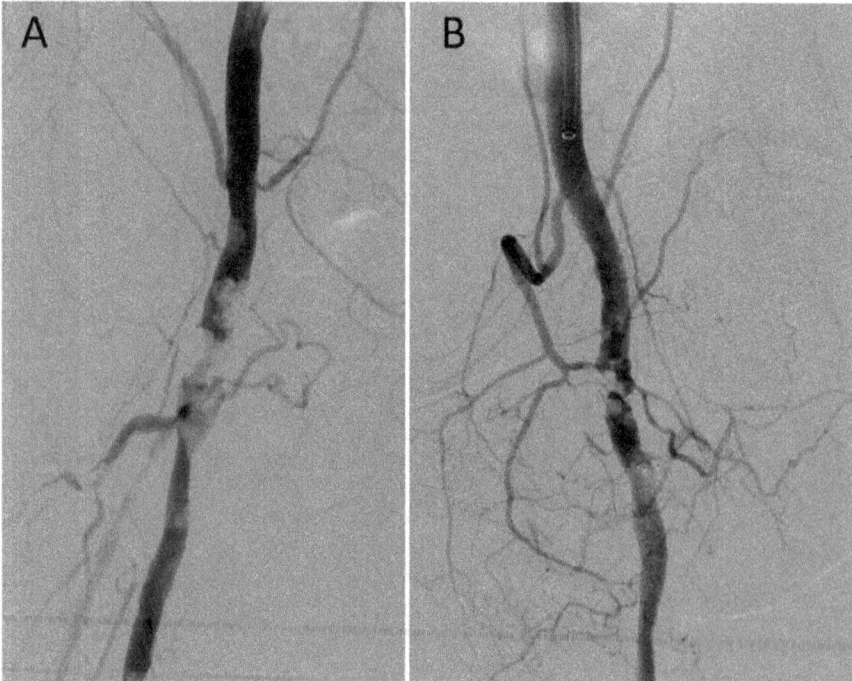

Figure 14. CFA disease with typical coral-like calcification disease on (A) right and (B) left.

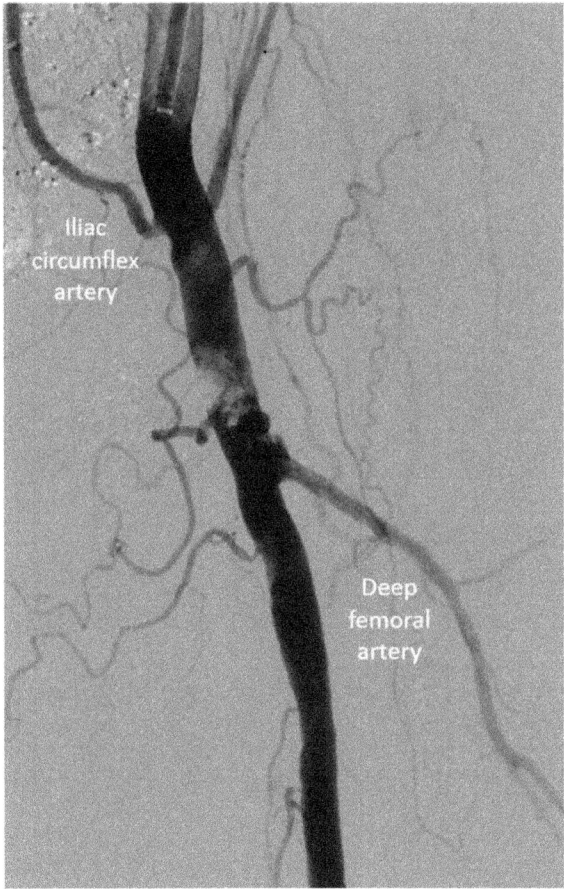

Figure 15. Identification of circumflex iliac artery and deep femoral artery bifurcation by left anterior oblique view.

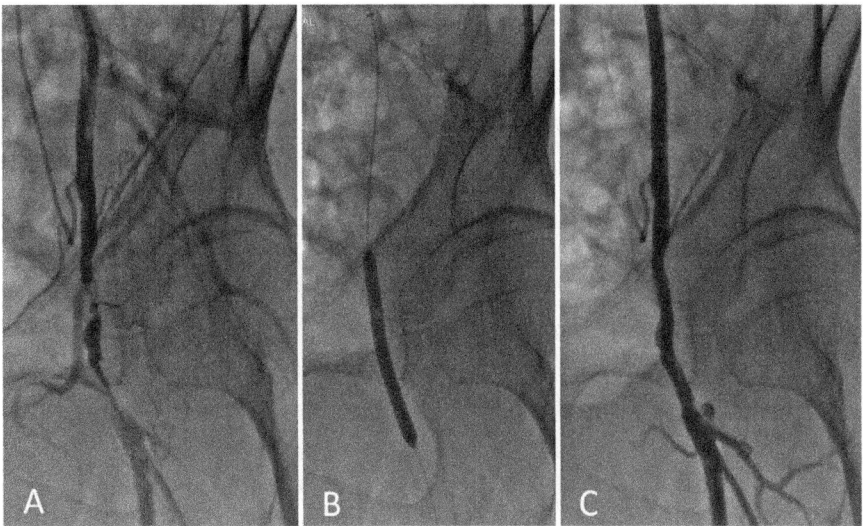

Figure 16. Balloon angioplasty for CFA lesions. (A) Preprocedure shows tight stenosis of left CFA; (B) balloon angioplasty by 5 × 40 mm balloon; (C) postprocedure shows successful angioplasty with minor dissection.

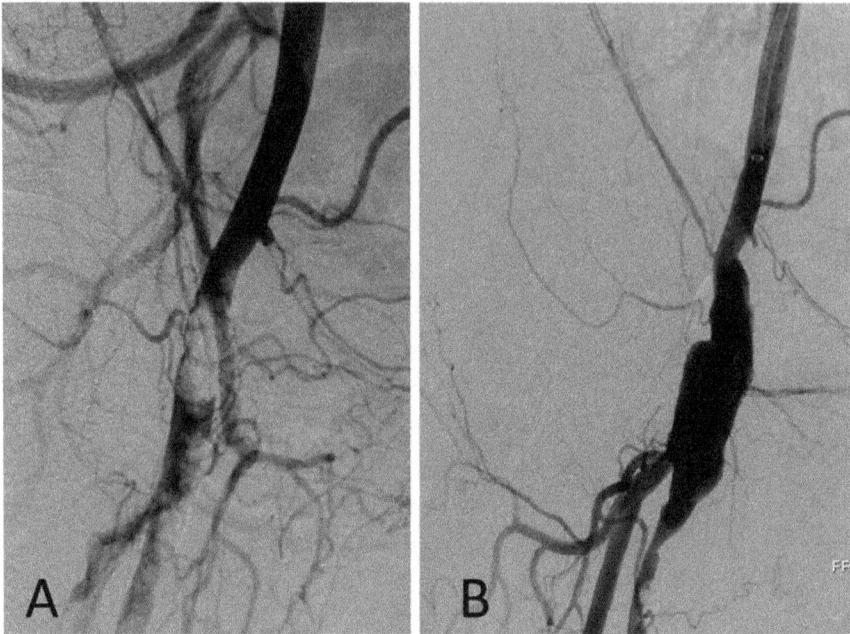

Figure 17. Endarterectomy with patch angioplasty. (A) Presurgical repair. (B) Postsurgical repair.

4. Evaluation of SFA disease

The etiology of SFA disease varies depending on such factors as fibromuscular dysplasia, repetitive occupational trauma, external compression, and inflammatory disease. However, most SFA lesions are a manifestation of arteriosclerosis and its clinical symptoms are induced by stenosis and occluded lesions. Evaluation of SFA disease includes lesion length, morphology, location, calcification, and pattern of restenosis in cases of reintervention.

4.1. Lesion length measurements

Lesion length and morphology can be classified according to the TASC II guidelines [7]. It provides the standard indications of either interventional treatment or bypass surgery. **Figure 18A** shows a single focal lesion of less than 10 cm in length and did not involve SFA origins. This lesion is classified into type A. **Figure 18B** is a single chronic total occlusion (CTO) lesion of less than 15 cm and considered to be type B. **Figure 18C** shows multiple stenosis of more than 15 cm lesion length and a typical example of type C. **Figure 18D** shows the long CTO and the lesion length is more than 20 cm. This is a typical type D lesion and stenting for this complex type of lesion involves a high risk of restenosis.

For lesion length measurements, a tape measure is attached to the front of the thigh (**Figure 19**).

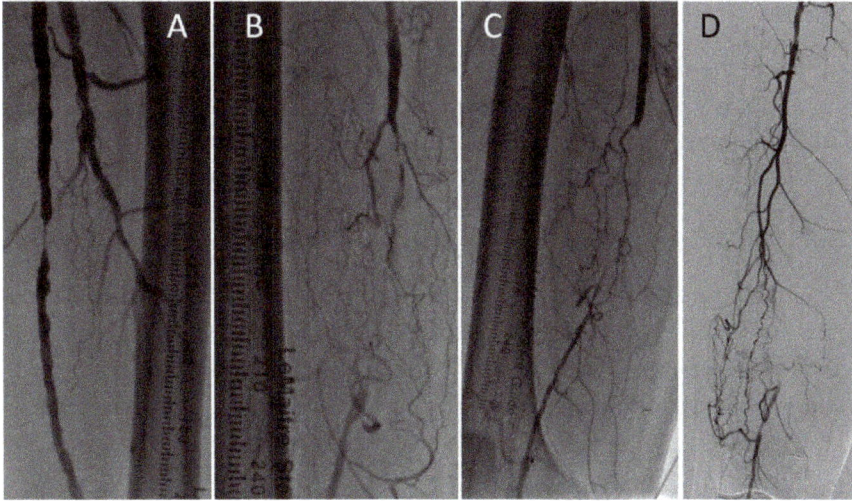

Figure 18. Focal lesion was measured at 1 cm (A). Short CTO was measured at 10 cm (B). Short CTO and stenosis measured at over 15 cm (C). SFA long CTO was measured at 20 cm (D).

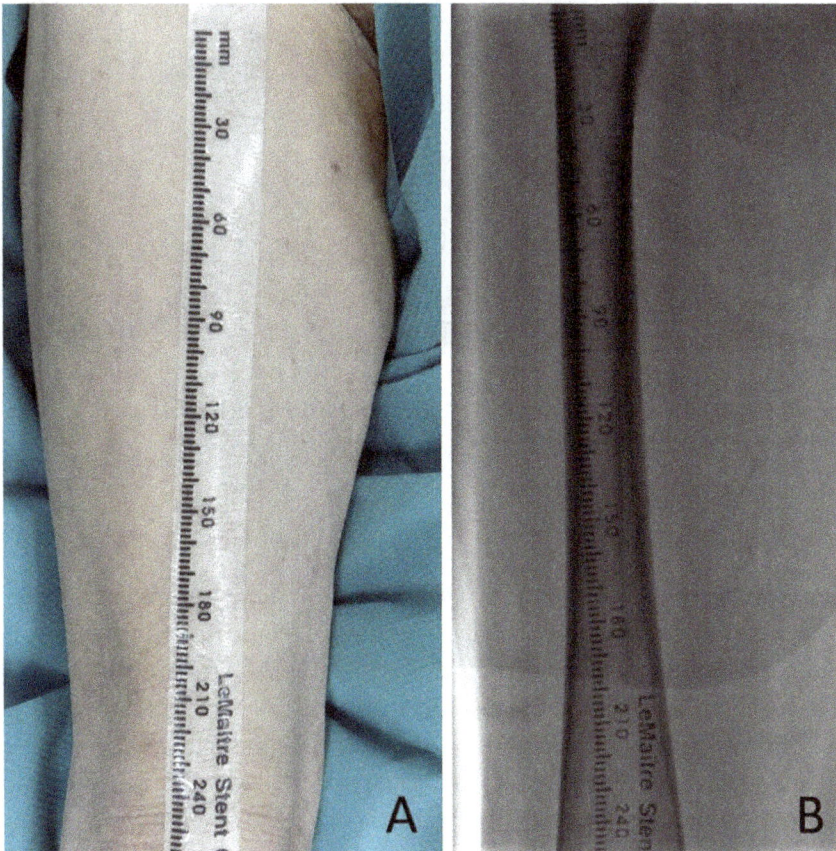

Figure 19. For lesion length measurement, a tape measure is attached to the front of the thigh.

4.2. Lesion location

- Proximal segment: the feasibility of intervention requires assessment not only by TASC ll classifications alone [7]. In a SFA CTO lesion, the initial entry point needs to be clarified. Does the SFA occlusion begin with a proximal stump (**Figure 20A** and **B**) or not (**Figure 20C** and **D**)? This is a key factor for successful wiring in a CTO lesion.

- Distal segment: a distal portion of the SFA lesion needs to be visualized (**Figure 21**).

If antegrade wiring should fail, we may change to a retrograde approach. If we plan to puncture at the distal SFA, the exact location must be clearly identified. To puncture at the distal SFA, the lesion must be collateralized above the popliteal artery (**Figure 22**). If popliteal artery disease is involved, it is contraindicated to puncture at the distal SFA or popliteal artery for the retrograde approach.

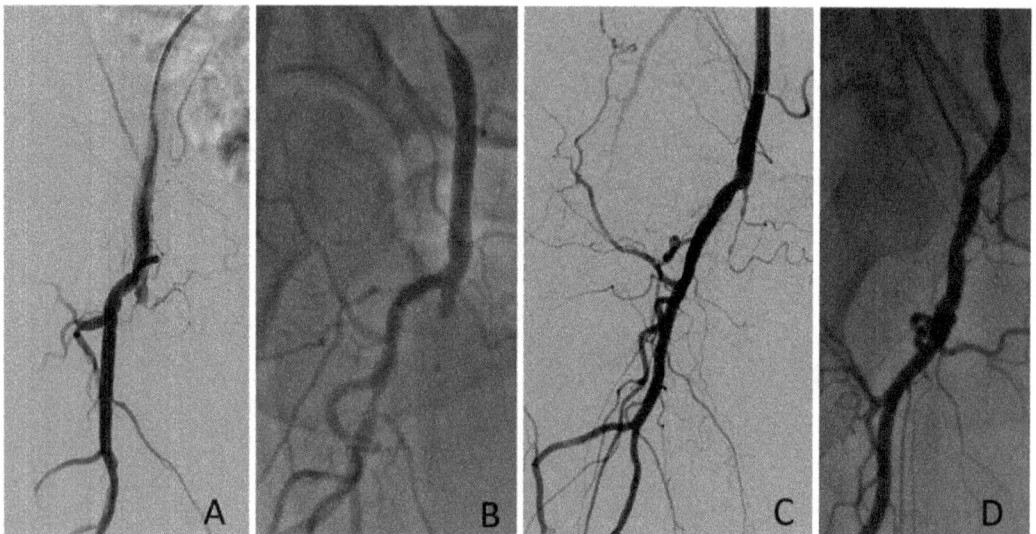

Figure 20. In right anterior oblique view, the stump of SFA ostium occlusion is well visualized by (A) DSA image; (B) DA the stump of SFA ostium occlusion is not well visualized; (C) DSA image; (D) DA.

4.3. Evaluation of calcification

Most endovascular devices are unable to cope with calcified lesions and there is no ideal solution for the treatment of severely calcified lesions. Calcification on the SFA is associated with increased cardiovascular morbidity and mortality [8]. There are two types of calcification, i.e., intimal calcification and media calcification. The first type is associated with stenosis and/or obstruction of the vessel, while the second type is associated with arterial stiffness, increased pulse pressure, and increased cardiac overload. However, current modalities for assessing calcified lesions are limited. From a practical viewpoint, we use only plain X-P and intravascular ultrasound (IVUS) to distinguish between intimal and media calcification in nonoverlapping areas of the vessels. There are two proposed definitions of a calcified lesion. One is the proposed peripheral arterial calcium scoring system (PACSS) diagnosis by

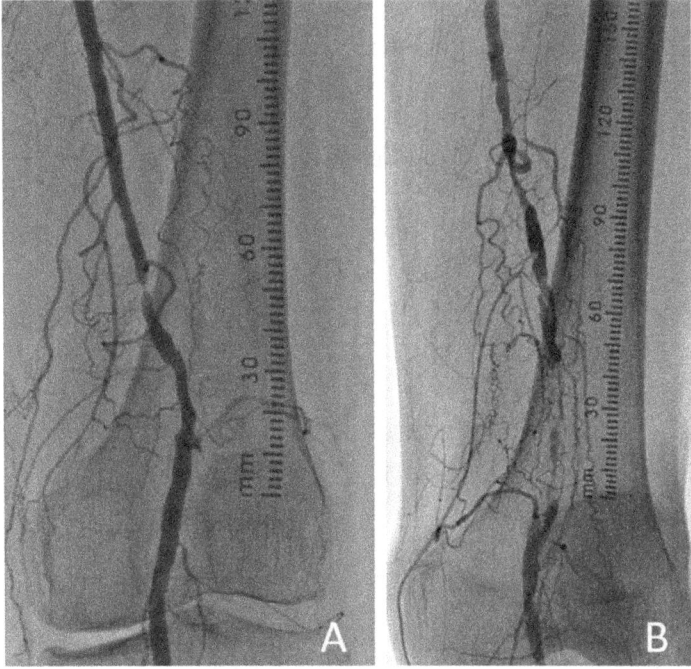

Figure 21. Distal portion of SFA lesion (A) uninvolved popliteal artery and (B) involved proximal popliteal artery.

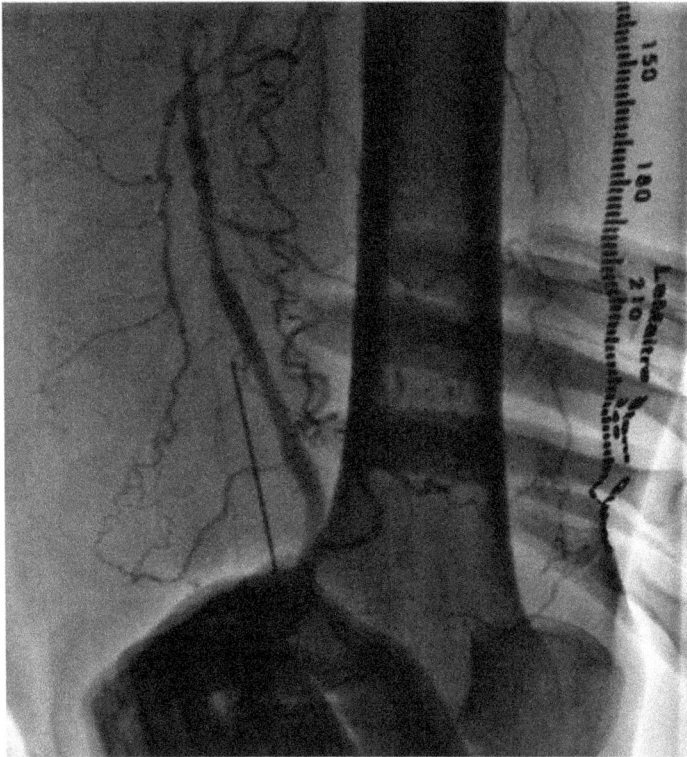

Figure 22. Puncture of distal SFA visualized from collateral flow from PFA.

fluoroscopy [9]. The cut-off value of a severely calcified lesion is defined as more than 5 cm in length. Moreover, a determination of either unilateral or bilateral calcification along with a separation of intimal or medial calcification is required. The second is the calcium burden assessment and less than 3 cm or more than 3 cm has been proposed to determine lesion calcification. Along with the length, assessment of the axial view of the vessel by CT is also recommended. The circumferential distribution of calcification by plain CT is analyzed [10]. Both criteria are based on calcified lesion length and measurement of the calcified angle in the axial section. **Figure 23** shows severe calcification in a lesion evaluated by fluoroscopy. As for the calcified arc, IVUS is more practical in actual clinical situations. However, the meaning and usefulness of this modality are as yet not well known.

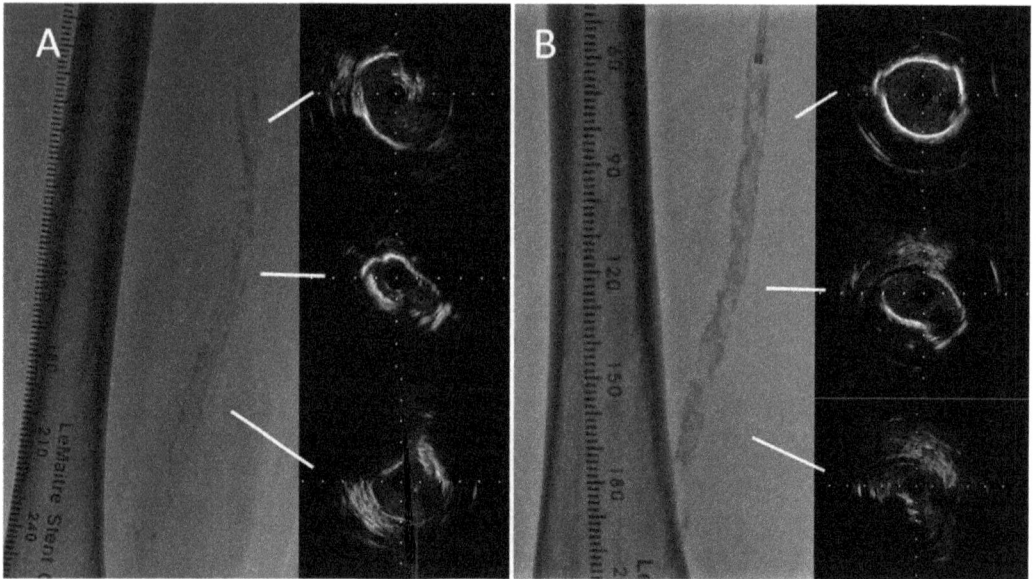

Figure 23. (A) Severe calcification of SFA in mid-portion (>15 cm) evaluated by fluoroscopy and IVUS. (B) Super severe calcification of SFA mid-portion (>10 cm) evaluated by fluoroscopy and IVUS.

4.4. Stent fracture

Over the past decade, stent technologies, which may offer improved clinical outcomes over balloon alone procedure, have been developed. This fact was proved by recent randomized trials demonstrating its superiority over simple percutaneous angioplasty. However, nitinol self-expanding stents are subject to both axial and bending deformation when implanted into the SFA, and stent fracture in SFA is a growing concern. In most cases, stent fracture is not related to restenosis (**Figure 24**).

The stent fracture is classified according to types 1–5 [11]. In a severe form of fracture, aneurysm formation was observed (**Figure 25**). The recent development of nitinol stents, which are more flexible in structure, is expected to lead to a lesser degree of stent fracture, but data for its long-term use are lacking and careful observation and assessment are still required.

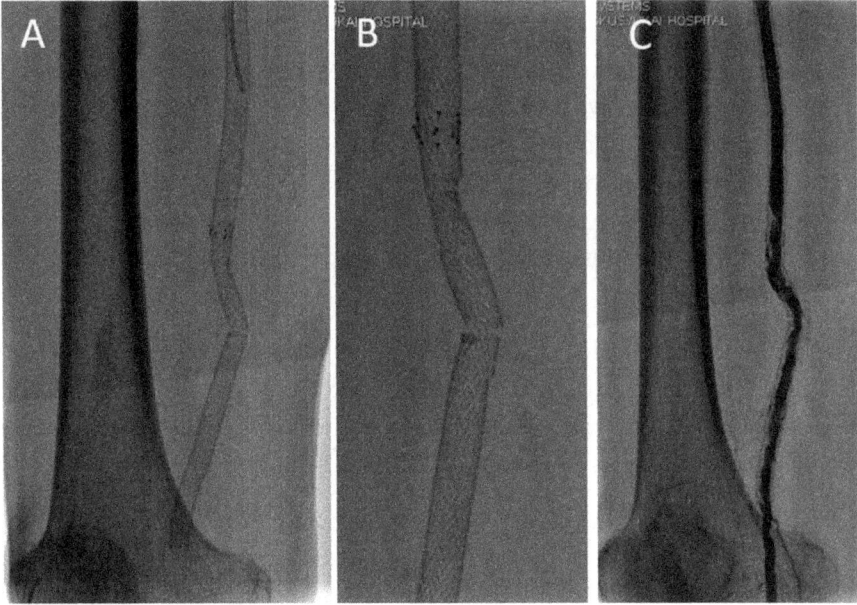

Figure 24. Stent showed complete traverse liner separation without displacement. (A and B) Type 3 stent dissection; (C) no restenosis observed at fracture site.

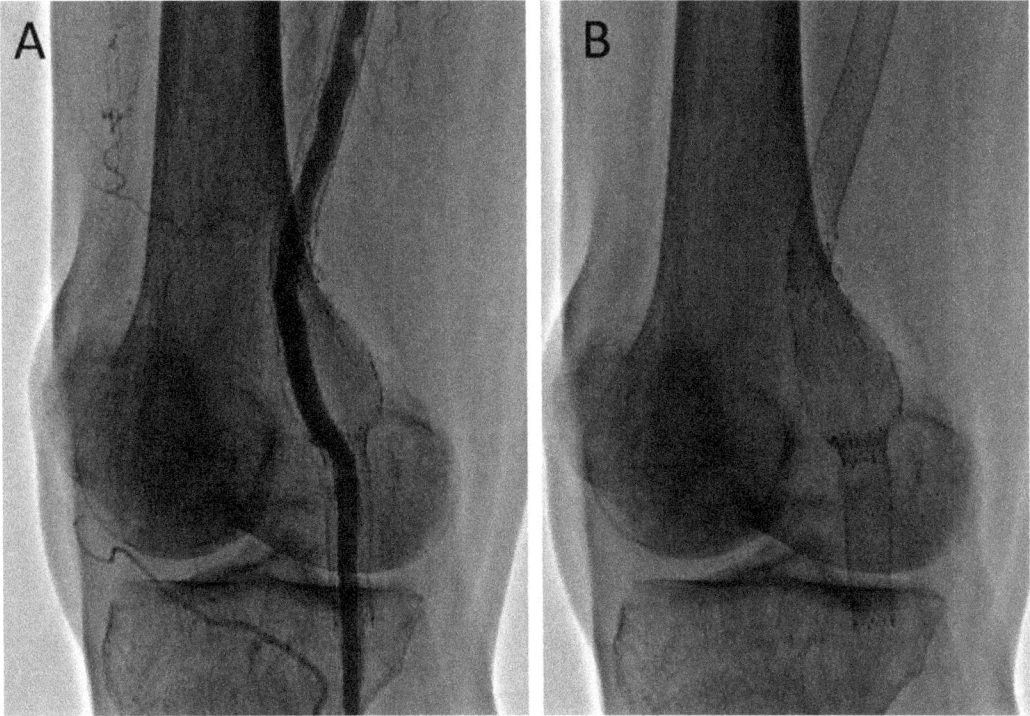

Figure 25. Complete stent fracture at distal right SFA to proximal popliteal artery. (A) The stent showed no restenosis; however, (B) complete break at SFA distal portion with aneurysm formation.

4.5. Stent restenosis

As far as primary patency is concerned, the superiority of stents over balloon angio-plasty has been evidenced by various studies. However, although nitinol stents can be implanted for primary use, stent restenosis is still a serious issue in primary stenting. The SFA long CTO lesion originates from the SFA ostium, and successful recanalization was obtained by stenting. However, angiography at 6 months revealed not only SFA stent restenosis with but also new stenosis in the profound femoral artery initiated by the SFA stent (**Figure 26**).

There are three types of restenotic patterns: Class I includes focal lesions (<50 mm in length, **Figure 27A**); Class II includes diffuse lesions (>50 mm in length, **Figure 27B**); and Class III includes totally occluded in-stent restenosis (ISR) (**Figure 27C**). Restenotic patterns after FP stenting are significant predictors of recurrent ISR and occlusion [12].

Moreover, neointimal hyperplasia is the decisive factor for the restenosis of the SFA stent. However, careful observation shows another cause associated with restenosis. In **Figure 28**, no in-stent restenosis is observed but edge restenosis, showing that the stent edge initiated hyperplasia.

Figure 29 shows the case of short occlusion in the SFA (A). A successful recanalization was performed by stenting (B), but restenosis was found at the site of the original occluded seg-ment, and an eccentric calcified lesion is seen (C). In this restenosis, the calcified lesion is the main cause of restenosis. As shown in these cases, SFA stent restenosis is multifactorial and multifaceted, accounting for the high rate of restenosis in SFA stents and no single solution at present.

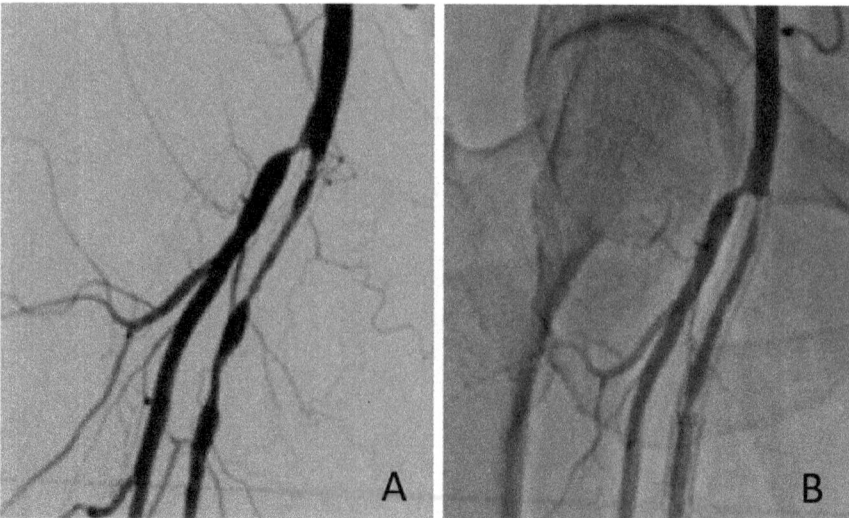

Figure 26. (A) Nitinol stent restenosis. After 6 months stent implantation angiography showed SFA stent restenosis with new stenosis in profunda femoral artery. (B) This restenosis is clearly seen in nonsubtracted angiogram.

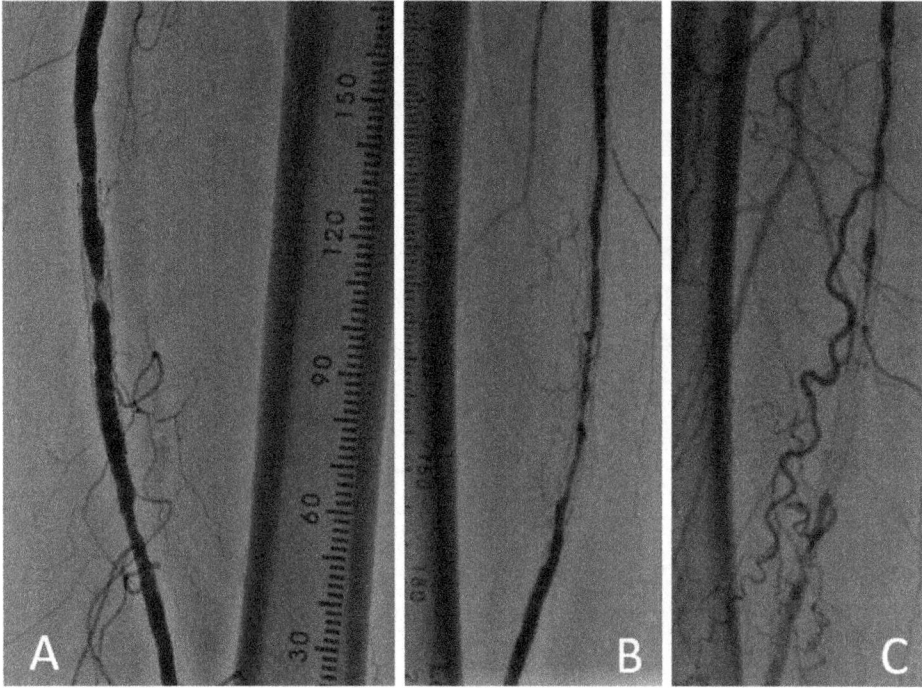

Figure 27. ISR lesions were classified by visual estimate on angiography: Tosaka class I, the focal ISR group (<50 mm in length), included lesions positioned at the stent body, stent edge, or a combination of these sites (A). Tosaka class II, the diffuse ISR group (>50 mm in length), includes not only stent body lesions but also stent edge lesions (B). Tosaka class III is the totally occluded ISR group (C).

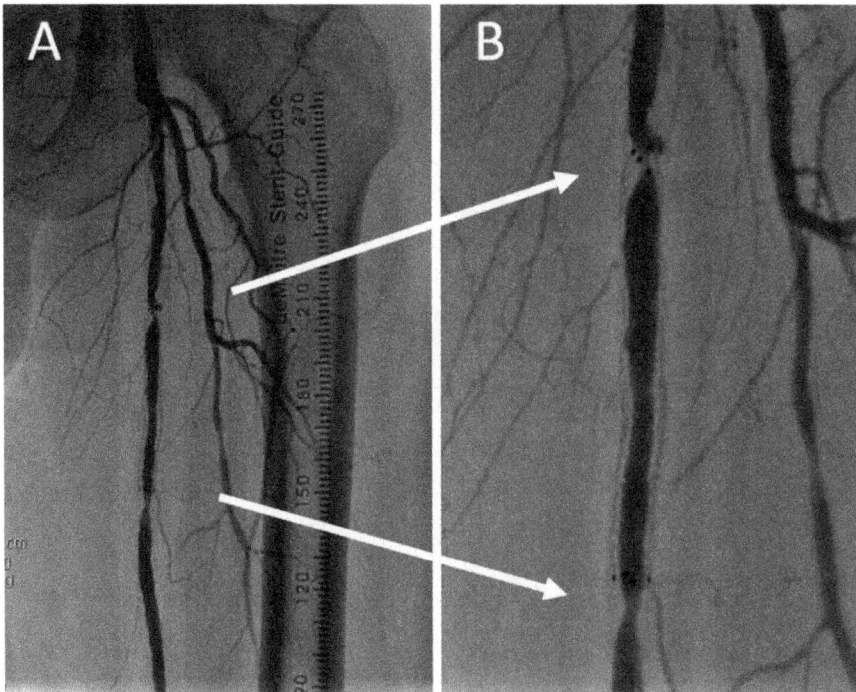

Figure 28. The case of stent edge initiated hyperplasia without in-stent restenosis.

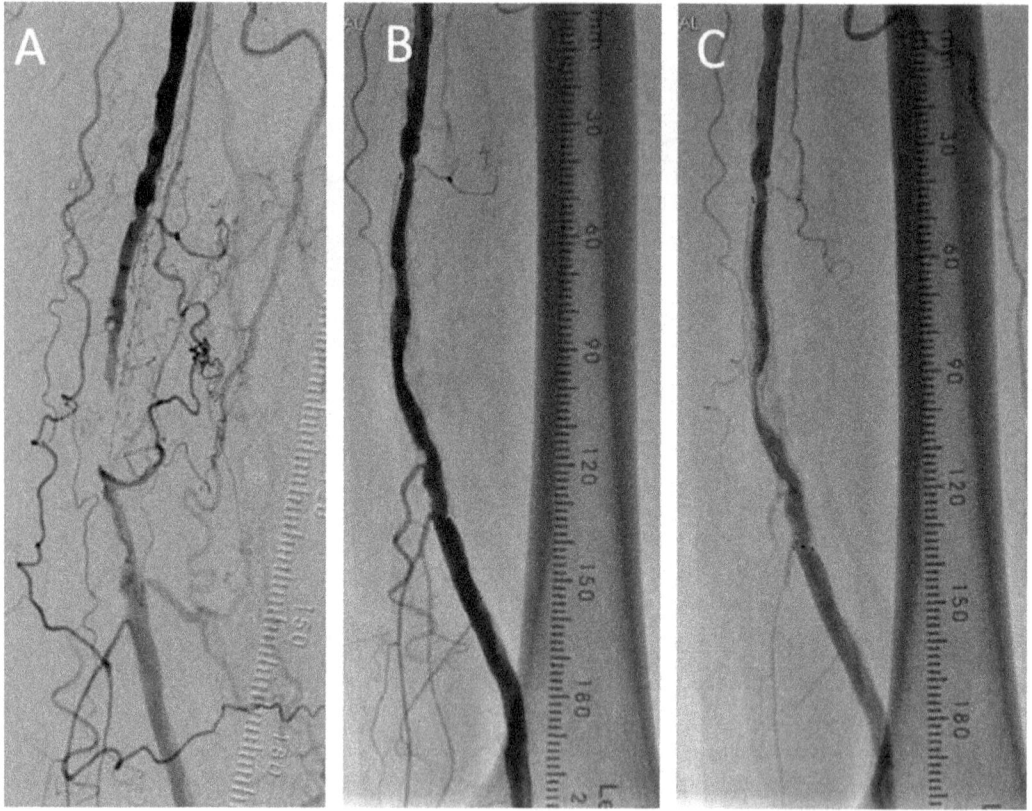

Figure 29. The case of short calcified occlusion in the SFA (A). A successful recanalization was performed by stenting (B). Restenosis was found at the site of the original occluded segment, and an eccentric calcified lesion (C).

5. Endovascular treatment for SFA disease

Endovascular therapy is indicated in the treatment of disabling claudication despite optimal medical therapy or critical limb ischemia. The benefit of revascularization is thought to correspond to the severity of ischemia or the presence of other risk factors for limb loss such as wound and infection severity. Otherwise, retaining the patency rate is yet an unsolved issue. However, there are several options in SFA recanalization (**Figure 30**).

5.1. Balloon angioplasty and nitinol stent implantation

In femoropopliteal artery disease, conventional balloon angioplasty is considered to be the standard approach for solitary lesions. However, balloon angioplasty alone does not have sustained benefits. In the 1990s, many stent trials were started. Stainless steel stents did not show acceptable long-term durability [13], but nitinol stents have shown good results in simple SFA lesions compared to conventional balloon angioplasty [14]. Based on these trials, the world trend has shifted from balloon alone to the era of nitinol stents. Thus, until recently, nitinol stent implantation was the main treatment option for SFA revascularization. However, as mentioned earlier, it became known that nitinol stents showed fracturing mid to long term and a low patency rate in complex lesions. In 2011, the Zilver PTX nitinol stent (COOK Medical,

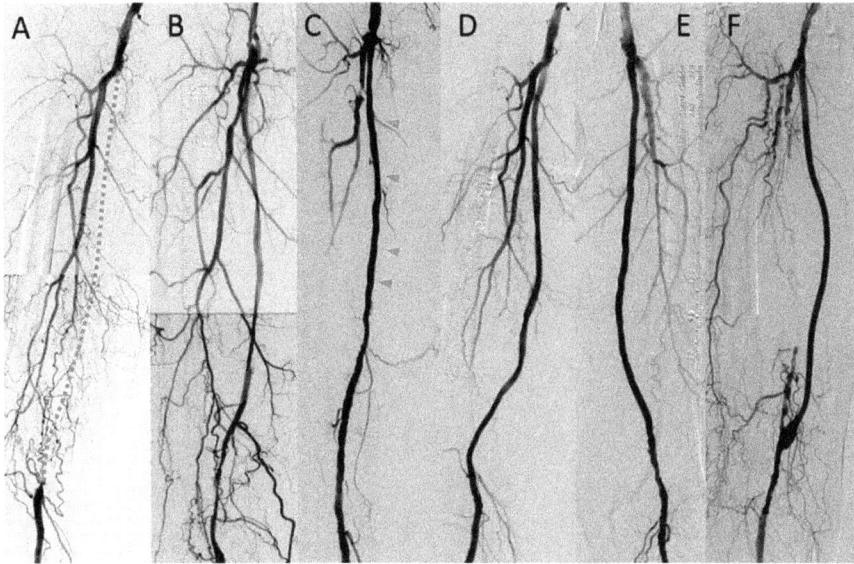

Figure 30. Different techniques to intervene in (A) long SFA disease including (B) balloon angioplasty, (C) spot stenting with short nitinol stent, (D) full cover nitinol stent implantation, (E) stent grafting, and (F) bypass surgery.

Bloomington, Indiana) became the first polymer-free paclitaxel-coated nitinol stent (drug-eluting stent; DES) approved for the treatment of SFA disease. A pivotal randomized controlled trial (RCT) conducted in 2011 reported that the use of a drug-eluting stent (DES) resulted in a higher patency rate of 83.1% at 12 months over percutaneous transluminal balloon angioplasty (PTA) [15]. In short lesions, the initial approach is still balloon angioplasty (**Figure 31**).

The angiogram of postballoon angioplasty shows acceptable results. However, in reality, most of the lesions required stent implantation. **Figure 32** shows a typical 5 cm stenotic lesion and balloon angioplasty was performed.

Balloon dilatation resulted in dissection and bail-out stenting was performed. Nitinol stent implantation could seal the dissection with no residual stenosis. Although such pivotal trials proved the superiority of stents over the balloon, the results could not be extrapolated to real-world cases. First, these studies excluded patients with backgrounds of complex risk factors such as kidney dysfunction. Second, long lesions classified as TASC (II) C/D lesions were also excluded. The real-world population study did not prove the expected patency using DES [16]. From our experience, we are aware that long-segment stent implantation has many disadvantages included stent fracture and thrombosis. Only the covered stent, VIABAHN (Gore, Flagstaff, AZ, USA) showed acceptable results in long lesions (**Figure 33**) [17]. However, the application of covered stents in the SFA is still not well known so a cautious approach should be taken in VIABAHN implantation.

5.2. Drug-coated balloon and atherectomy devices

Since a drug-coated balloon (DCB) was first introduced, there have been many arguments about primary stenting. DCB trials proved to be safe and effective in SFA lesions with better outcomes

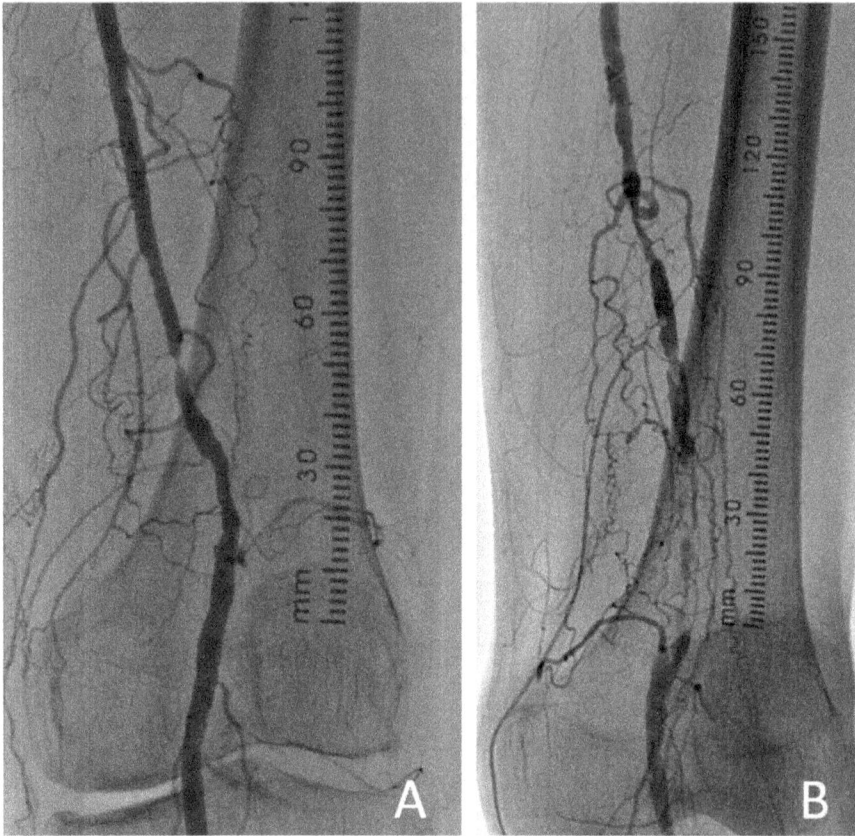

Figure 31. In a short lesion, initial approach is (A) balloon angioplasty; (B) short focal lesion in distal SFA; and (C) balloon angioplasty performed with 5 × 40 mm balloon. Postballoon angioplasty showed residual stenosis of less than 50% at ballooning site.

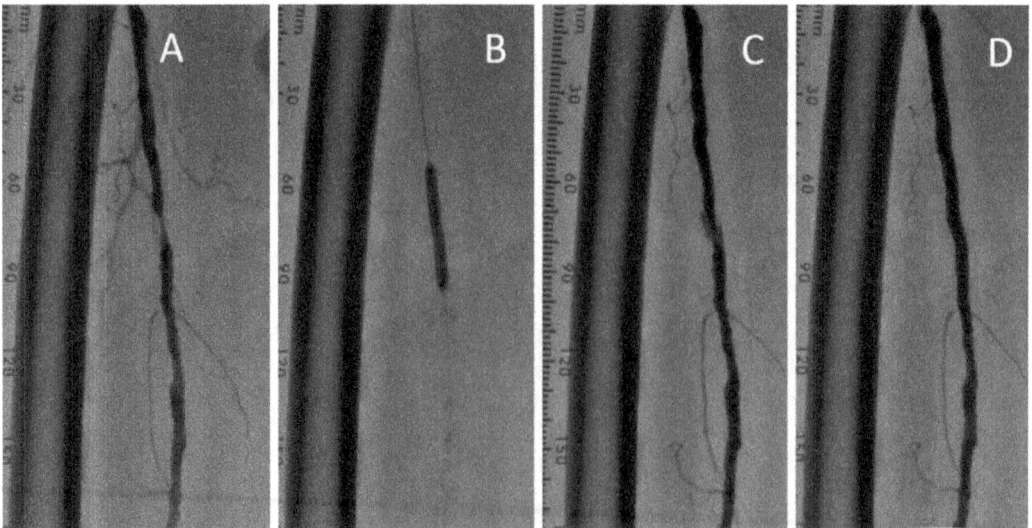

Figure 32. Bail out stenting post balloon angioplasty procedure of (A) 3 cm stenotic lesion; (B) balloon angioplasty performed; (C) dissection; (D) nitinol stenting for bail out purpose successful in sealing dissection.

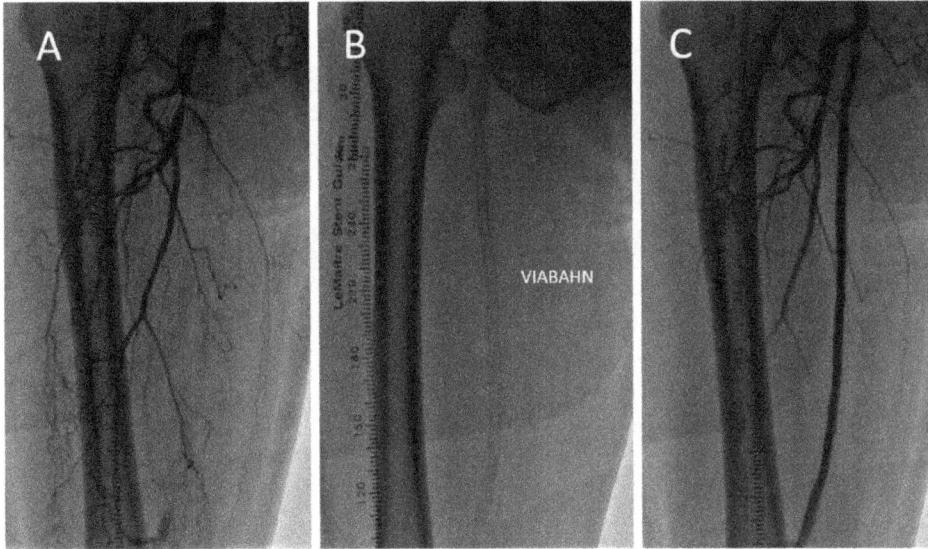

Figure 33. (A) Covered stent implantation for long right SFA CTO lesion; (B) CTO length is over 20 cm lesion; (C) VIABAHN (Gore, Flagstaff, AZ, USA) 6 × 250 mm stenting after balloon angioplasty.

over conventional balloon angioplasty in simple lesions (IN.PACT DCB, Medtronic Inc., Santa Rosa, CA, USA and Lutonix DCB, Bard Peripheral Vascular; Tempe, AZ, USA) (**Figure 34**) [18–20].

Furthermore, various atherectomy devices are being developed. At present, there are two types of atherectomy devices: one is a rotational cutting device (JETSTREAM, Boston Scientific, Cambridge, MA, USA [21, 22] (**Figure 35**) and Diamondback, Cardiovascular Systems,

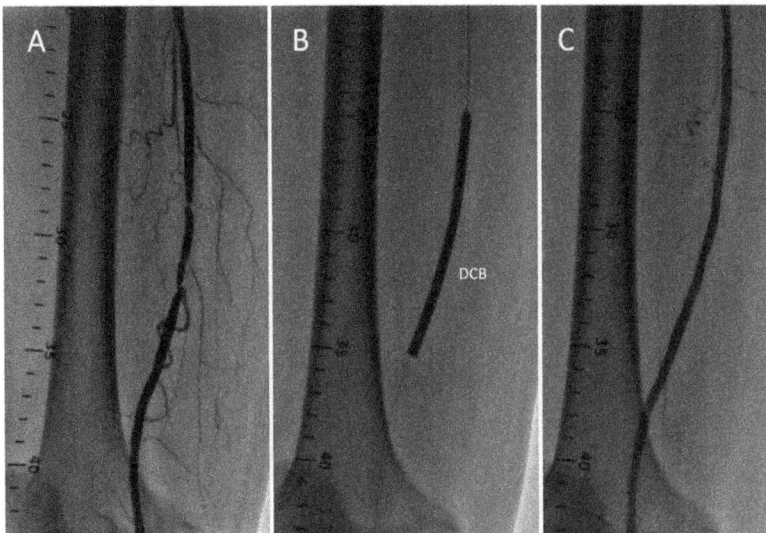

Figure 34. DCB angioplasty procedure. (A) Short focal lesion in mid-SFA; (B) after conventional balloon angioplasty and drug coated balloon angioplasty with LUTONIXX DCB (Bard Peripheral Vascular; Tempe, AZ) 5 × 100 mm balloon; (C) postballoon angioplasty showed residual stenosis of less than 50% at ballooning site.

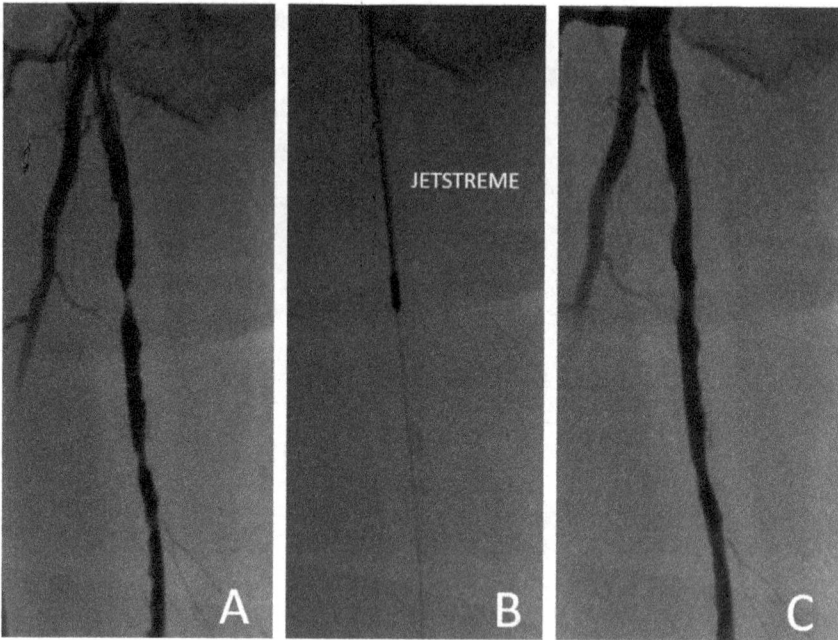

Figure 35. Atherectomy device. (A) Short focal lesion in mid-SFA; (B) atherectomy with JETstreme (Boston Scientific, Cambridge, MA, USA) atherectomy device; (C) postprocedure.

Inc., St. Paul, MN, USA 360 [23]), and the other is a directional cutting device (TurboHawk (**Figure 36**), Silverhawk, Medtronic Inc., Santa Rosa, CA, USA) [24, 25]. However, although solid data on the efficacy of atherectomy devices are still lacking, the worldwide trend toward the "nothing left behind" approach favors these treatment options.

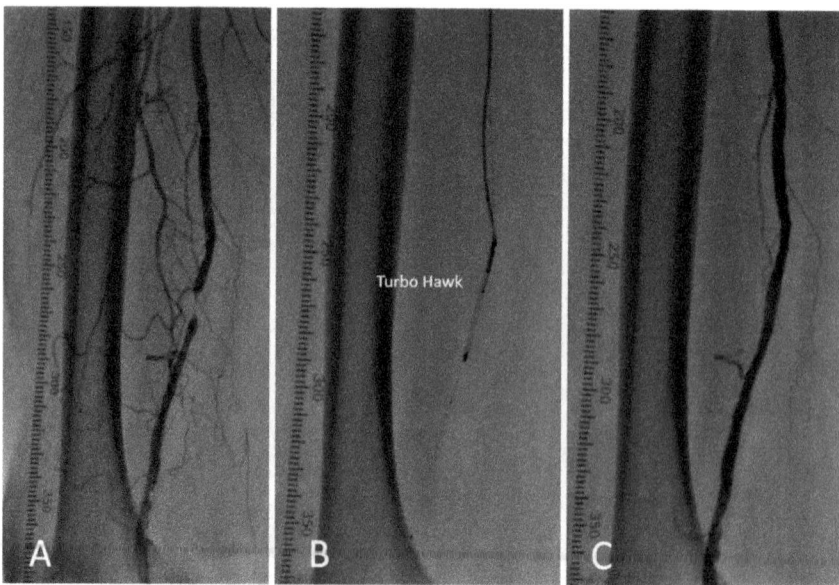

Figure 36. Atherectomy device. (A) Short focal lesion in mid-SFA; (B) atherectomy with TurboHawk (Medtronic Inc, Santa Rosa, CA) atherectomy device; (C) postprocedure.

6. Approach to complex femoropopliteal artery disease

Recanalization of complex SFA lesions is still challenging. In particular, the approach to a chronic total occlusion (CTO) lesion is not yet standardized and technically more demanding.

6.1. Approach site

In general, a contralateral CFA approach is the standard procedure mainly because the puncture site is not on the ischemic limb side, and the proximal SFA and DFA can be safely approached. However, to intervene in a complex lesion, deft manipulation of the wiring is vital, and for that reason, some interventionists prefer the antegrade approach as the initial step. Furthermore, a recent advance in SFA intervention is the use of the bidirectional approach. The distal puncture sites presently being employed are the distal SFA, popliteal artery, and dorsal pedis artery. The bidirectional approach has a higher chance of recanalization compared to a unidirectional approach. However, the safety of employing these new puncture sites is not well elucidated so that a cautious approach is necessary.

6.2. Wire

The antegrade approach via ipsilateral or contralateral CFA access is the standard approach. First, we try to cross the lesion with 0.035 inch guidewires. Subintimal tracking with a 0.035 inch J-loop wire and support catheter is the traditional method of CTO recanalization (**Figure 37**).

When crossing the CTO by the antegrade approach fails, a bidirectional approach with a distal puncture should be attempted. Suitable points for the distal approach include the popliteal, distal SFA, and tibial puncture sites (**Figure 38**).

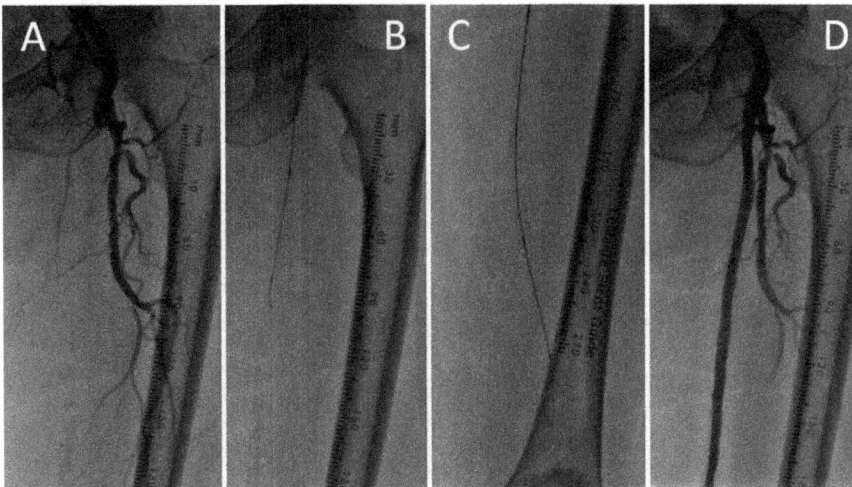

Figure 37. Antegrade approach with 0.018 inch guidewire. (A) SFA long total occlusion from proximal SFA to distal portion; (B) 0.018 inch J-type guidewire with support catheter into CTO lumen; (C) guidewire passage to distal true lumen; (D) final angiography after nitinol stent implantation.

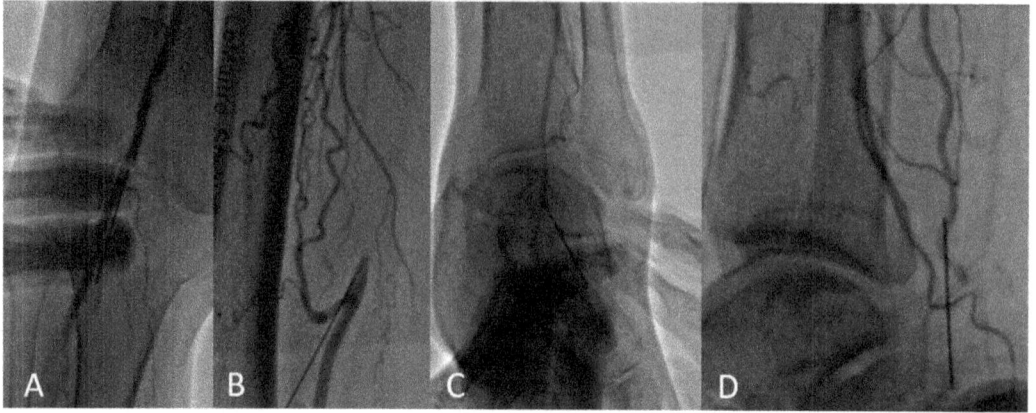

Figure 38. Retrograde access with distal puncture to recanalize SFA total occlusion lesion. (A) Popliteal artery puncture; (B) distal SFA puncture; (C) distal anterior tibial artery puncture; and (D) distal posterior tibial artery.

6.3. CTO crossing devices

CTO crossing devices are being approved, but the safety and efficacy of these devices have not yet been proven. Two types of CTO crossing devices are used broadly: first is a reentry device and the Outback (Cordis Endovascular, Bridgewater, NJ, USA) [26] (**Figure 39**), Pioneer (Medtronic Inc., Santa Rosa, CA, USA) [27], and OffRoad (Boston Scientific, Cambridge, MA, USA) [28] devices are categorized in this group while the other includes devices for true lumen crossing such as the Crosser (Bard Peripheral Vascular; Tempe, AZ, USA) [29] (**Figure 40**),

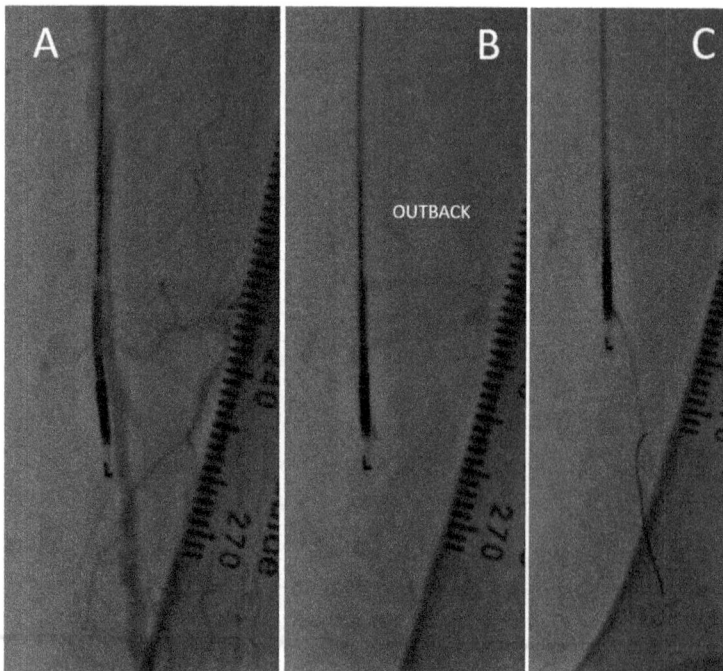

Figure 39. Outback reentry device (Cordis Endovascular, Bridgewater, NJ, USA). (A) Outback reentry device was placed in subintimal space of SFA mid portion. (B) Deploying the cannula from subintimal space to true lumen. (C) Wire crossing.

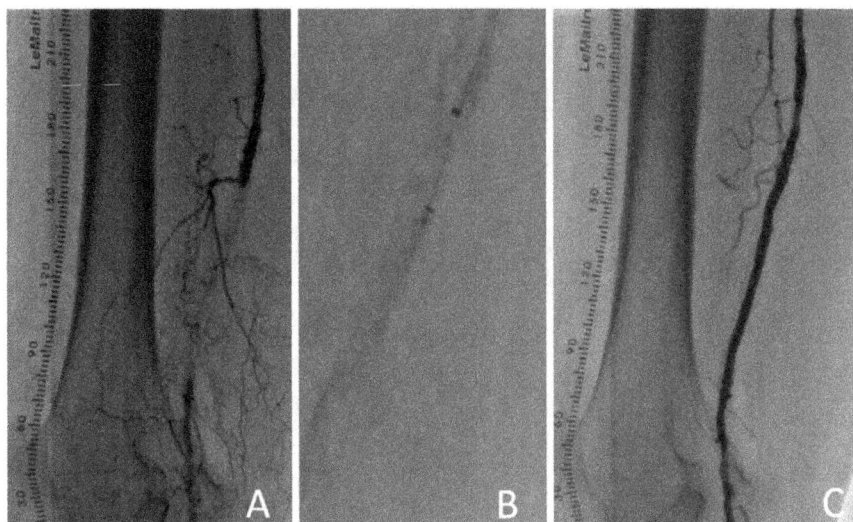

Figure 40. CTO crossing device. (A) Heavy calcified occlusive disease at distal SFA portion; (B) Crosser CTO crossing device (Bard Peripheral Vascular; Tempe, AZ) advanced without guidewire; (C) after crossing device, nitinol stent implantation.

TruePath (Boston Scientific, Cambridge, MA, USA) [30], Frontrunner (Cordis Endovascular, Bridgewater, NJ, USA), and Wildcat (Avinger, Redwood City, CA, USA).

7. Complications in femoropopliteal artery intervention

The rate of complications varies depending on how they are defined. In addition, the operator's experience contributes to the complication rate. Serious complications in femoropopliteal artery intervention are less frequent in experienced hands. Most important is to foresee unexpected events in order to prevent an adverse outcome. The factors most related to complications are complex lesions, long procedure times, the use of many catheters, and excessive long wire manipulation. The other factors are patient related such as obesity, evidence of critical limb, hemodialysis dependence, etc. Understanding such potential risks is essential for those engaging in interventional procedures.

7.1. Vessel perforation

Perforations occur in femoropopliteal artery interventions from various causes. The common causes of femoropopliteal artery perforations have been divided into four types. First is puncture-related perforation. **Figure 41A** shows a puncture-related vessel perforation by the antegrade approach at the CFA. In a retrograde approach, the popliteal artery was perforated by a puncture (**Figure 41B**).

Figure 42 shows the CFA perforation caused by the crossover sheath.

The second are guidewire perforations. Guidewire perforation is usually of little consequence since they are typically small and rarely result in significant or continuous bleeding. They

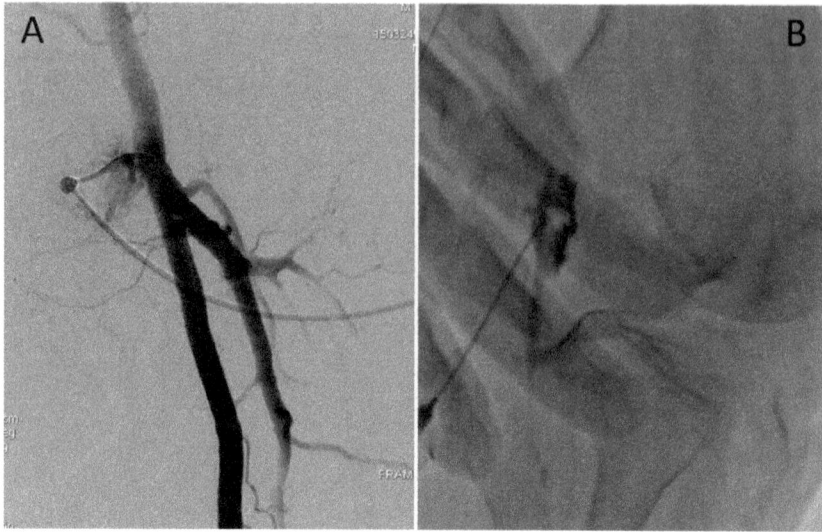

Figure 41. Puncture site vessel perforation. (A) Antegrade approach via CFA puncture; (B) retrograde approach via popliteal artery.

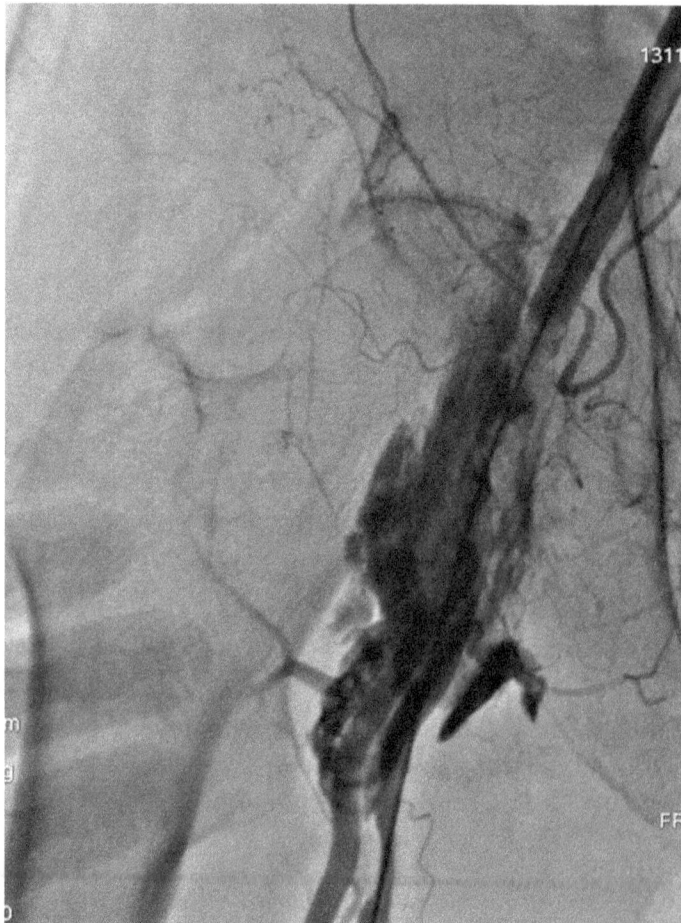

Figure 42. Procedure-related vessel perforation: vessel perforation occurred by cross-over sheath from contra lateral CFA puncture access.

usually occur when the wire is advanced into an occlusion site (**Figure 43A**) or migrate into small side branches (**Figure 43B**). In SFA intervention, after successful wire passage, the tip of the guidewire is not visible due to the long SFA vessel and the distal tip of the wire may advance deeply to perforate the below the knee arteries (**Figure 43C**). The third type is atherectomy or CTO crossing device-induced perforation. These perforations occur due to the direct cutting or mechanical penetration of the adventitial layer. CTO crossing devices have a perforation rate of 1–6% [29, 30].

Figure 44 shows the vessel perforation caused by the Crosser device. Atherectomy devices have a perforation rate of between 0.5 and 2.2% [20–24]. Although atherectomy and CTO-crossing device-related perforation rates are relatively low, interventionists should have a definite strategy to cope with these complications. The last is balloon angioplasty-related perforation. The mechanism of balloon dilatation is to disrupt the intima and media of the vessel wall to obtain an increased luminal area. When the area up to the adventitia is penetrated, vessel perforation occurs. Heavy calcification, high-pressure ballooning, and the use of oversized balloons are the potential risks of balloon perforation.

Figure 45 shows the vessel perforation after balloon angioplasty with or without stent implantation.

7.2. Acute thrombosis and distal emboli

Acute arterial thrombosis is another common problem seen in femoropopliteal interventions. This complication may occur after EVT as a result of the erosion or rupture of the atherosclerotic plaque, and distal emboli. There are not many reports on acute or subacute stent occlusion by drug-eluting stent or balloon, but this paclitaxel-coated device has the potential risk of thrombotic occlusion. When intervening for in-stent-occlusion, there is a high risk of distal emboli during the procedure (**Figure 46**).

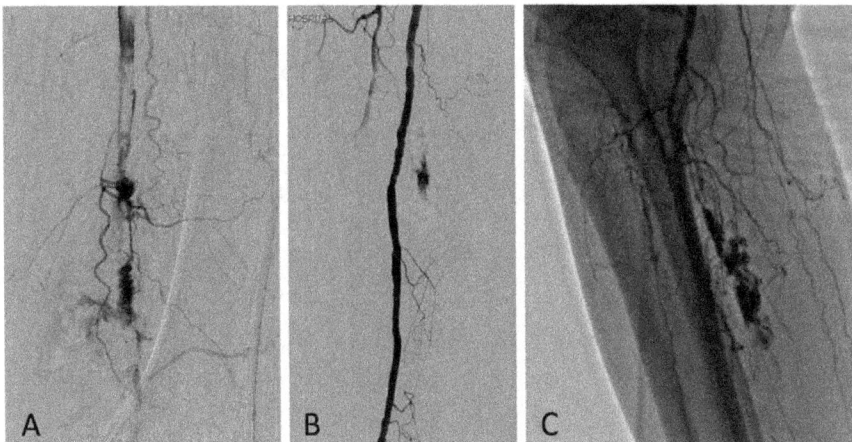

Figure 43. Vessel perforation: (A) caused by hard guidewire advanced into total occlusion portion; (B) aberration to small SFA side branches; (C) too deeply advanced guidewire to below the knee arteries.

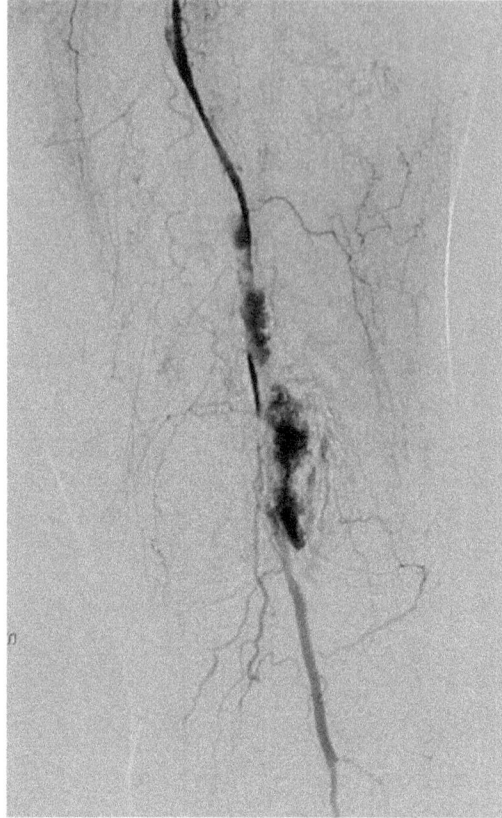

Figure 44. CTO crossing device related vessel perforation: vessel perforation by Crosser device at SFA mid-portion occlusive disease.

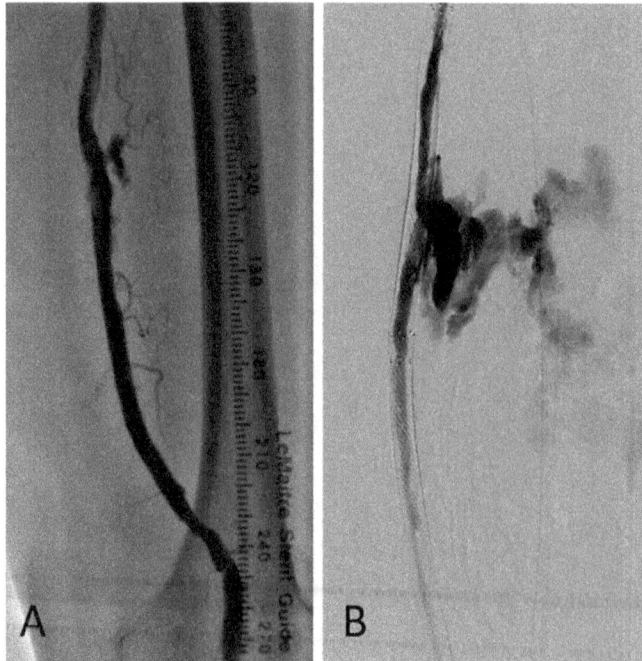

Figure 45. Balloon dilatation related vessel perforation (A) and (B).

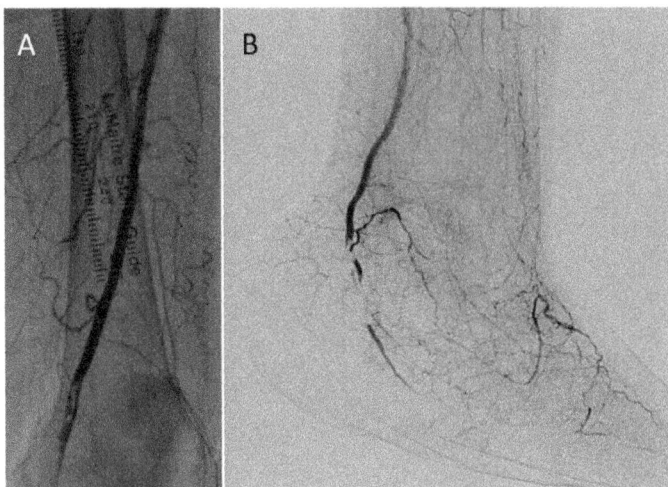

Figure 46. Distal emboli after femoropopliteal intervention. (A) Total occlusion of popliteal artery caused by distal emboli after SFA stent implantation; (B) distal emboli into PTA distal portion.

7.3. Arterial-venous fistula

Arterial-venous communications, which are often seen after subintimal angioplasty, are the least concerning. Irregular AV communications usually represent a series of microperforations between the artery and adjacent vein (**Figure 47**).

Most of these cases may be shielded by balloon or stent implantation (**Figure 48**). In case when balloon shielding is unsuccessful, the covered stent may be the next option.

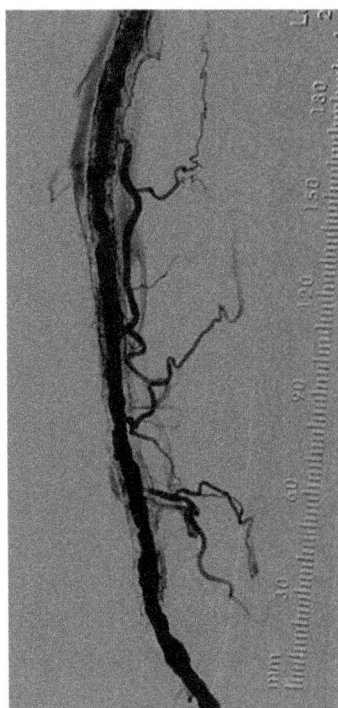

Figure 47. AV fistula: occurred after balloon angioplasty.

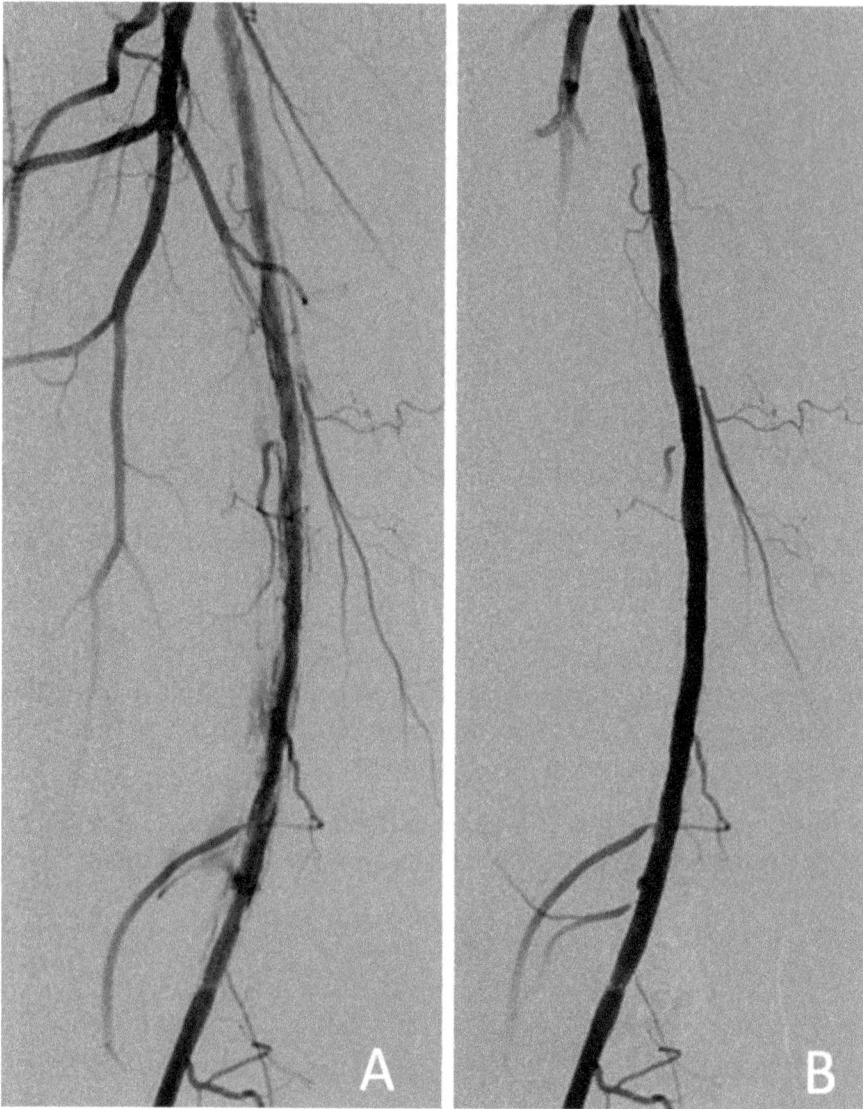

Figure 48. Stent implantation can repair the AV fistula in most cases. (A) Balloon angioplasty performed and resulted in AV fistula; (B) nitinol stenting for bail out purpose succeeded in sealing AV fistula.

8. Popliteal artery disease

The popliteal artery is a deeply placed continuation of the femoral artery after it passes through the adductor hiatus or opening in the distal portion of the adductor magnus muscle. It courses through the popliteal fossa and ends at the lower border of the popliteus muscle, where it branches into the anterior and tibio-peroneal trunk. In the popliteal artery, there are various types of arterial disease such as atherosclerosis stenosis or occlusion, popliteal aneurysms, popliteal artery entrapment syndrome, cystic adventitial disease, and Buerger's disease. The ideal angiographic image is provided by a contralateral view (**Figure 49**).

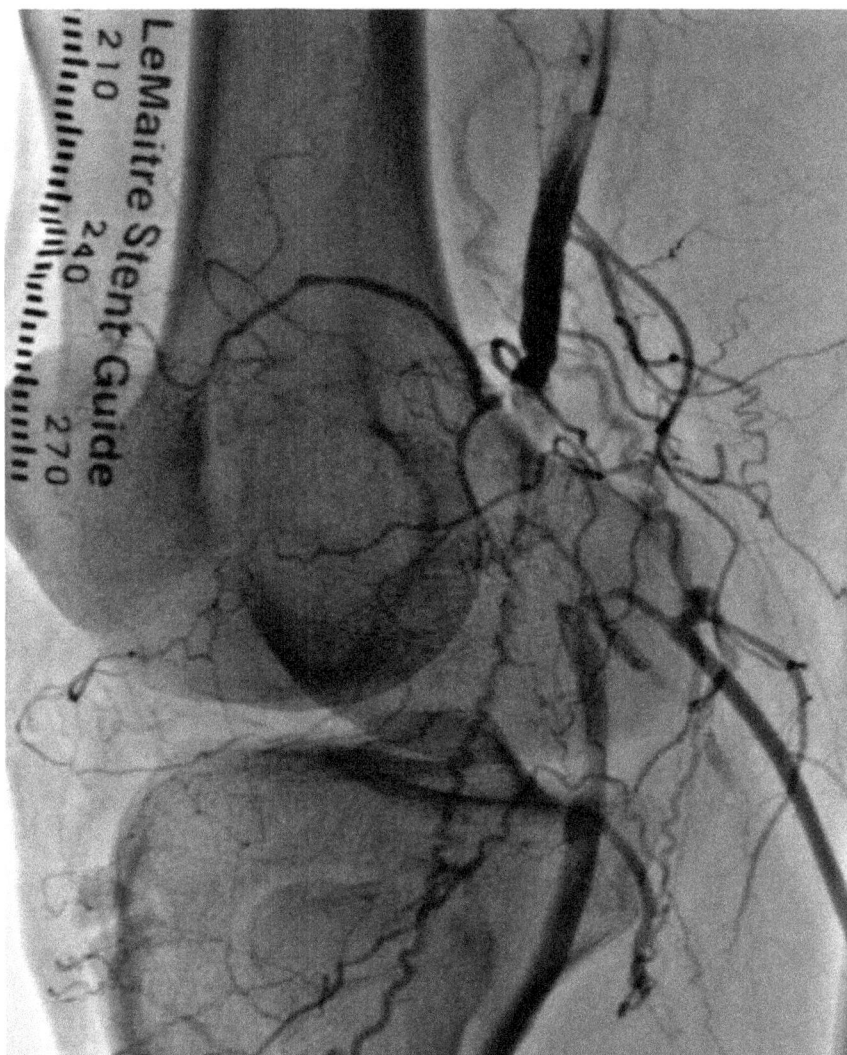

Figure 49. Popliteal artery disease; clear image by contra-lateral angled view.

Surgical therapy for popliteal artery occlusion involves a bypass of the occlusion, which can be achieved with grafts, including the great saphenous vein or PTFE grafts (**Figure 50**).

Endovascular therapy is a less invasive intervention in the treatment of popliteal artery occlusive disease. It is indicated for short and noncalcified lesions. The popliteal artery is a non-stenting zone and stent implantation should be avoided (**Figure 51**).

Some studies have suggested that the use of drug-coated balloons is safe and effective for proximal popliteal disease, especially for preventing restenosis [16–18]. Recently, the SUPERA (Abott Vascular, Santa Clara, California, USA) stent, which is a high kink and fracture-resistant stent, has been introduced and evaluated for primary treatment of the proximal popliteal artery for its flexibility [31].

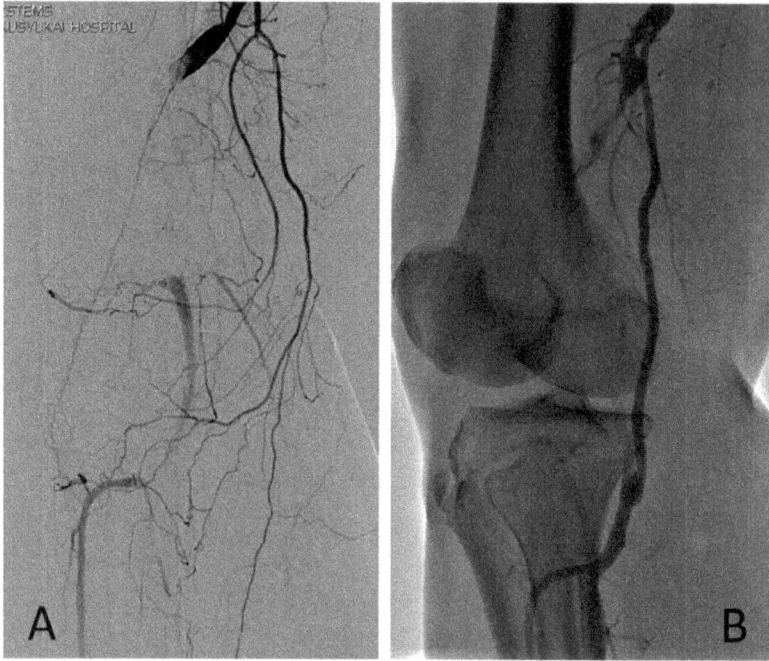

Figure 50. Popliteal artery aneurysm case (A) preprocedure; (B) after surgical therapy with SVG bypass.

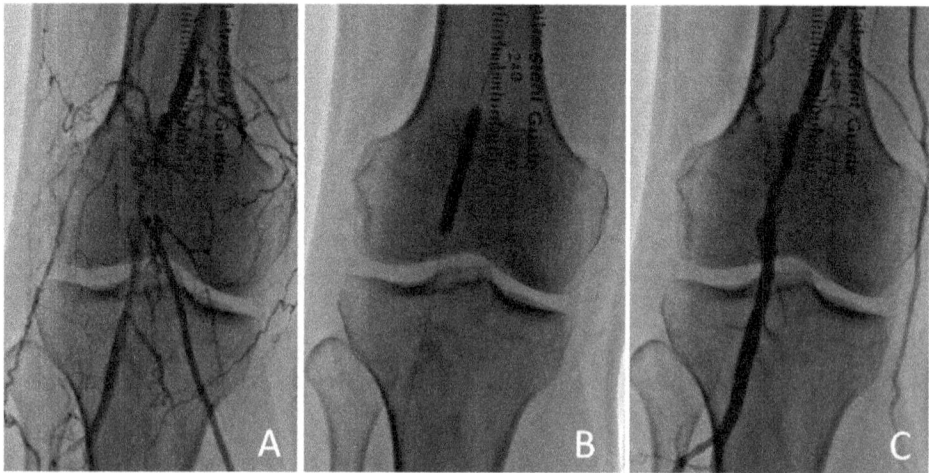

Figure 51. In short popliteal lesion. (A) Short focal lesion in mid-popliteal artery; (B) balloon angioplasty performed with 5 × 40 mm balloon; (C) postballoon angioplasty showed residual stenosis of less than 50% at ballooning site.

Author details

Masahiko Fujihara

Address all correspondence to: masahiko-fujihara@themis.ocn.ne.jp

Kishiwada Tokushukai Hospital, Osaka, Japan

References

[1] Fontaine R, Kim M, Kieny R; Kim, K. Surgical treatment of peripheral circulation disorders. Helvetica Chirurgica Acta 1954; 21 (5/6):499–533.

[2] Rutherford RB, Becker GJ. Standards for evaluating and reporting the results of surgical and percutaneous therapy for the peripheral arterial disease. J Vasc Interv Radiol. 1991; 2:169–74.

[3] Goodney PP, Beck AW, Nagle J, Welch HG, Zwolak RM. National trends in lower extremity bypass surgery, endovascular interventions, and major amputations. J Vasc Surg. 2009; 50(1):54–60.

[4] Scheinert D, Scheinert S, Sax J, Piorkowski C, Bräunlich S, Ulrich M, Biamino G, Schmidt A. Prevalence and clinical impact of stent fractures after femoropopliteal stenting. J Am Coll Cardiol. 2005; 45(2):312–5.

[5] Ho-Young Ahn, et al. Assessment of the Optimal Site of Femoral Artery Puncture and Angiographic Anatomical Study of the Common Femoral Artery. J Korean Neurosurg Soc 2014; 56(2):91–7.

[6] Scheinert D, Werner M, Scheinert S, Paetzold A, Banning-Eichenseer U, Piorkowski M, Ulrich M, Bausback Y, Bräunlich S, Schmidt A. Treatment of complex atherosclerotic popliteal artery disease with a new self-expanding interwoven nitinol stent: 12-month results of the Leipzig SUPERA popliteal artery stent registry. JACC Cardiovasc Interv. 2013; 6(1):65–71.

[7] Norgren L, Hiatt WR, Dormandy JA, Nehler MR, Harris KA, Fowkes FG, Bell K, Caporusso J, Durand-Zaleski I, Komori K, Lammer J, Liapis C, Novo S, Razavi M, Robbs J, Schaper N, Shigematsu H, Sapoval M, White C, White J, Clement D, Creager M, Jaff M, Mohler E 3rd, Rutherford RB, Sheehan P, Sillesen H, Rosenfield K, TASC II Working Group. Inter-society consensus for the management of peripheral arterial disease (TASC II). Eur J Vasc Endovasc Surg 2007; 33(suppl 1):S1–75.

[8] London GM, Guerin AP, Marchais SJ, Metivier F, Pannier B, Adda H. Arterial media calcification in end-stage renal disease: impact on all-cause and cardiovascular mortality. Nephrol Dial Transplant 2003; 18:1731–40.

[9] Rocha-Singh KJ, Zeller T, Jaff MR. Peripheral arterial calcification: prevalence, mechanism, detection, and clinical implications. Catheter Cardiovasc Interv. 2014;83(6):E212–20.

[10] Fanelli F, Cannavale A, Gazzetti M, Lucatelli P, Wlderk A, Cirelli C, d'Adamo A, Salvatori FM. Calcium burden assessment and impact on drug-eluting balloons in peripheral arterial disease. Cardiovasc Intervent Radiol. 2014; 37(4):898–907.

[11] Jaff M, Dake M, Pompa J, Ansel G, Yoder T. Standardized evaluation and reporting of stent fractures in clinical trials of noncoronary devices. Catheter Cardiovasc Interv. 2007; 70(3):460–2.

[12] Tosaka A, Soga Y, Iida O, Ishihara T, Hirano K, Suzuki K, Yokoi H, Nanto S, Nobuyoshi M. Classification and clinical impact of restenosis after femoropopliteal stenting. J Am Coll Cardiol. 2012; 59(1):16–23.

[13] Zdanowski Z, Albrechtsson U, Lundin A, Jonung T, Ribbe E, Thörne J, Norgren L. Percutaneous transluminal angioplasty with or without stenting for femoropopliteal occlusions? A randomized controlled study. Int Angiol. 1999;18(4):251–5.

[14] Laird JR, Katzen BT, Scheinert D, Lammer J, Carpenter J, Buchbinder M, Dave R, Ansel G, Lansky A, Cristea E, Collins TJ, Goldstein J, Jaff MR, RESILIENT Investigators. Nitinol stent implantation versus balloon angioplasty for lesions in the superficial femoral artery and proximal popliteal artery: twelve-month results from the RESILIENT randomized trial. Circ Cardiovasc Interv. 2010; 3(3):267–76.

[15] Dake MD, Ansel GM, Jaff MR, Ohki T, Saxon RR, Smouse HB, Zeller T, Roubin GS, Burket MW, Khatib Y, Snyder SA, Ragheb AO, White JK, Machan LS, Zilver PTX Investigators. Paclitaxel-eluting stents show superiority to balloon angioplasty and bare metal stents in femoropopliteal disease: twelve month Zilver PTX randomized study results. Circ Cardiovasc Interv 2011; 4:495–504.

[16] Iida O, Takahara M, Soga Y, Nakano M, Yamauchi Y, Zen K, Kawasaki D, Nanto S, Yokoi H, Uematsu M, ZEPHYR Investigators. 1-Year Results of the ZEPHYR Registry (Zilver PTX for the Femoral Artery and Proximal Popliteal Artery): predictors of restenosis. JACC Cardiovasc Interv. 2015; 8(8):1105–12.

[17] Lammer J, Zeller T, Hausegger KA, Schaefer PJ, Gschwendtner M, Mueller-Huelsbeck S, Rand T, Funovics M, Wolf F, Rastan A, Gschwandtner M, Puchner S, Ristl R, Schoder M. Heparin-bonded covered stents versus bare-metal stents for complex femoropopliteal artery lesions: the randomized VIASTAR trial (Viabahn endoprosthesis with PROPATEN bioactive surface [VIA] versus bare nitinol stent in the treatment of long lesions in super-ficial femoral artery occlusive disease). J Am Coll Cardiol. 2013; 62(15):1320–7.

[18] Tepe G, Laird J, Schneider P, Brodmann M, Krishnan P, Micari A, Metzger C, Scheinert D, Zeller T, Cohen DJ, Snead DB, Alexander B, Landini M, Jaff MR, IN.PACT SFA Trial Investigators. Drug-coated balloon versus standard percutaneous transluminal angio-plasty for the treatment of superficial femoral and popliteal peripheral artery disease: 12-month results from the IN.PACT SFA randomized trial. Circulation. 2015; 131(5):495–502.

[19] Rosenfield K, Jaff MR, White CJ, Rocha-Singh K, Mena-Hurtado C, Metzger DC, Brodmann M, Pilger E, Zeller T, Krishnan P, Gammon R, Müller-Hülsbeck S, Nehler MR, Benenati JF, Scheinert D, LEVANT 2 Investigators. Trial of a paclitaxel-coated bal-loon for femoropopliteal artery disease. N Engl J Med. 2015; 373(2):145–53.

[20] Zeller T, Beschorner U, Pilger E, Bosiers M, Deloose K, Peeters P, Scheinert D, Schulte KL, Rastan A, Brodmann M. Paclitaxel-coated balloon in infrapopliteal arteries: 12-month results from the BIOLUX P-II randomized trial (BIOTRONIK'S-First in Man study of the Passeo-18 LUX drug releasing PTA Balloon Catheter vs. the uncoated Passeo-18 PTA balloon catheter in subjects requiring revascularization of infrapopliteal arteries). JACC Cardiovasc Interv. 2015; 8(12):1614–22.

[21] Zeller T, Krankenberg H, Steinkamp H, Rastan A, Sixt S, Schmidt A, Sievert H, Minar E, Bosiers M, Peeters P, Balzer JO, Gray W, Tübler T, Wissgott C, Schwarzwälder U, Scheinert D. One-year outcome of percutaneous rotational atherectomy with aspiration in infrainguinal peripheral arterial occlusive disease: the multicenter pathway PVD trial. J Endovasc Ther. 2009;16(6):653–62.

[22] Maehara A, Mintz GS, Shimshak TM, Ricotta JJ 2nd, Ramaiah V, Foster MT 3rd, Davis TP, Gray WA. Intravascular ultrasound evaluation of JETSTREAM atherectomy removal of superficial calcium in peripheral arteries. EuroIntervention. 2015; 11(1):96–103.

[23] Shammas NW, Lam R, Mustapha J, Ellichman J, Aggarwala G, Rivera E, Niazi K, Balar N. Comparison of orbital atherectomy plus balloon angioplasty vs. balloon angioplasty alone in patients with critical limb ischemia: results of the CALCIUM 360 randomized pilot trial. J Endovasc Ther. 2012; 19(4):480–8.

[24] Ramaiah V, Gammon R, Kiesz S, Cardenas J, Runyon JP, Fail P, Walker C, Allie DE, Chamberlin J, Solis M, Garcia L, Kandzari D; TALON Registry. Midterm outcomes from the TALON Registry: treating peripherals with SilverHawk: outcomes collection. J Endovasc Ther. 2006; 13:592–602.

[25] Roberts D, Niazi K, Miller W, Krishnan P, Gammon R, Schreiber T, Shammas NW, Clair D, DEFINITIVE Ca^{++} Investigators. Effective endovascular treatment of calcified femoropopliteal disease with directional atherectomy and distal embolic protection: final results of the DEFINITIVE Ca^{++} trial. Catheter Cardiovasc Interv. 2014; 84(2):236–44.

[26] Kitrou P, Parthipun A, Diamantopoulos A, Paraskevopoulos I, Karunanithy N, Katsanos K. Targeted true lumen re-entry with the outback catheter: accuracy, success, and complications in 100 peripheral chronic total occlusions and systematic review of the literature. J Endovasc Ther. 2015; 22(4):538–45.

[27] Scheinert D, Bräunlich S, Scheinert S, Ulrich M, Biamino G, Schmidt A. Initial clinical experience with an IVUS-guided transmembrane puncture device to facilitate recanalization of total femoral artery occlusions. EuroIntervention. 2005; 1(1):115–9.

[28] Schmidt A, Keirse K, Blessing E, Langhoff R, Diaz-Cartelle J, European Study Group. Offroad re-entry catheter system for subintimal recanalization of chronic total occlusions in femoropopliteal arteries: primary safety and effectiveness results of the re-route trial. J Cardiovasc Surg (Torino). 2014; 55(4):551–8.

[29] Laird J, Joye J, Sachdev N, Huang P, Caputo R, Mohiuddin I, Runyon J, Das T. Recanalization of infrainguinal chronic total occlusions with the crosser system: results of the PATRIOT trial. J Invasive Cardiol. 2014; 26(10):497–504.

[30] Bosiers M, Diaz-Cartelle J, Scheinert D, Peeters P, Dawkins KD. Revascularization of lower extremity chronic total occlusions with a novel intraluminal recanalization device: results of the ReOpen study. J Endovasc Ther. 2014; 21(1):61–70.

[31] Scheinert D, Grummt L, Piorkowski M, Sax J, Scheinert S, Ulrich M, Werner M, Bausback Y, Braunlich S, Schmidt A. A novel self-expanding interwoven nitinol stent for complex femoropopliteal lesions: 24-month results of the SUPERA SFA registry. J Endovasc Ther. 2011; 18(6):745–52.

9

Extracranial Carotid Atherosclerosis in the Patients with Transient Ischemic Attack

Mei-Ling Sharon Tai, Jun Kit Khoo and
Mohamed Abdusalam Elwaifa

Abstract

Management of transient ischemic attack (TIA) is important because potentially fatal ischemic strokes can be prevented. Detection of extracranial carotid atherosclerosis in these patients is beneficial because medical therapy can be given, and in certain cases, surgery can be performed. In a Chinese study conducted on the patients with TIA, only 19% of them had extracranial carotid atherosclerosis. Another study was conducted to compare the location and the severity of atherosclerotic lesions between Americans and the Japanese who presented with carotid system TIA. This study showed that 85% of the American patients had extracranial carotid stenosis (stenosis ≥50%). However, only 16.7% of the Japanese patients had similar lesions.

Keywords: transient ischemic attack, extracranial, carotid, atherosclerosis, stroke

1. Introduction

In the patients with transient ischemic attack (TIA), ischemic strokes often occur early after the first presenting clinical features especially in the first 7 days [1–4]. Management of TIA is important because potentially fatal ischemic strokes can be prevented [5]. It is important to identify the highest risk patients urgently so that the necessary management can be instituted for appropriate early treatments [6, 7].

Neuroimaging is beneficial to stratify the risk of recurrent stroke [8]. The modalities useful for imaging of the extracranial carotid vessels are ultrasound carotid Doppler with/without enhancement, computed tomography angiography (CTA), magnetic resonance angiography (MRA), and positron emission tomography (PET)/CT [8–14].

With improvements in vascular imaging techniques, it is now possible to risk stratify the patients on the degree of carotid artery stenosis and also on the vulnerability of the plaque to rupture [13]. The risk stratifications are based on the presence of imaging features such as intraplaque hemorrhage (IPH), plaque ulceration, plaque neovascularity, fibrous cap thickness, and presence of a lipid-rich necrotic core (LRNC) [13].

The risk of early recurrent stroke in the patients with TIA is 9.5–20% at 90 days [2, 15, 16].

The risk of early recurrent stroke is highest in patients with large artery atherosclerosis, which consists of extracranial carotid atherosclerosis and intracranial stenosis [9]. Therefore, it is important for urgent ultrasound carotid Doppler and transcranial Doppler (TCD) to be performed in these high-risk patients [9].

The carotid arteries are elastic and are predilection sites for atherosclerosis [17, 18]. Carotid intima media thickening is an indicator for subclinical atherosclerosis, and this frequently occurs earlier than atherosclerosis in coronary arteries and intracranial arteries [17, 18].

The patients who developed a hemispheric TIA due to internal carotid artery (ICA) disease had the greatest risk of ischemic stroke in the first few days after the TIA [9]. Carotid stenosis is associated with recurrent strokes [9, 19]. In the TIA patients, carotid stenosis predicted 90-day stroke [19]. Carotid stenosis is significantly associated with stroke in the short term, and also in the long term for up to 3 years [1].

In a Chinese study conducted on the patients with TIA, only 19% of them had extracranial carotid atherosclerosis [20]. Another study was conducted to compare the location and the severity of atherosclerotic lesions between Americans and the Japanese who presented with carotid system TIA [21]. This study showed that 85% of the American patients had extracranial carotid stenosis (stenosis ≥50%) [21]. However, only 16.7% of the Japanese patients had similar lesions [21]. In another study, the African-Americans had slightly more extracranial carotid atherosclerosis compared to the Caucasians [22].

In a multicenter study on the patients with TIA or minor stroke, 15.5% of the patients (28 out of 85) had at least one stenosis of ≥50% or occlusion [23]. In a recent study, 6.3% of the TIA patients had extracranial carotid artery disease [5]. In that study, 10 (35.7%) patients had moderate stenosis (50–69% stenosis), 8 (28.6%) patients had severe stenosis (70–99% stenosis), and 10 (35.7%) had total occlusion [4]. Five (17.9%) patients had recurrent TIAs before admission [5]. No patient had ischemic stroke within 90 days of TIA onset [5].

In another prospective study on the patients with TIA and minor stroke, extracranial carotid artery occlusion or stenosis ≥50% was found in 9.4% of the patients [8]. In a Japanese study, 21.8% of patients had carotid stenosis [1]. In a study conducted in Ireland, 23.8% of the TIA patients had unilateral carotid stenosis (40.4%, with 50–69% stenosis, 59.6% with ≥70% stenosis or occlusion) [19].

In the study by Coutts et al., 19% of the patients with TIA and minor stroke who developed recurrent stroke had extracranial carotid stenosis ≥50% or occlusion [8]. In comparison, only 9% of the patients with TIA and minor stroke who developed recurrent stroke had similar lesions [8].

A TIA event within 7 days before TIA (dual TIA) is a useful predictive factor for short- and long-term stroke [1]. In addition, ischemic stroke risk is elevated with increasing severity of carotid stenosis [19]. The risk of stroke is 5.4% with <50% carotid stenosis and 17.2% with severe carotid stenosis and occlusion at 90 days after TIA [19].

2. Diagnostic modalities

The advantages and disadvantages of the various imaging modalities are illustrated in **Table 1**. Ultrasound carotid Doppler is easily available, cheap, and noninvasive [19]. The sensitivity in carotid stenosis >70% is 91–95% [11, 24]. The specificity in severe stenosis of more than 70% is 86–97% [11, 24]. Being operator dependent is one of the limitations of ultrasound carotid Doppler [11]. The peak systolic velocity (PSV) analysis on the insonated tortuous vessel is difficult, and the stenosis in internal carotid artery (ICA) at the distal end also is difficult to be examined [11].

The diagnostic criteria for stenosis according to The Society of Radiologists in Ultrasound Consensus Criteria for Carotid Stenosis are used to classify the degrees of stenosis [25]. Carotid stenosis of at least 50% is defined as peak systolic velocity (PSV) ≥ 125 and end-diastolic velocity (EDV) ≥ 40. Carotid stenosis of at least ≥70% is defined as peak systolic velocity (PSV) ≥ 230 and end-diastolic velocity (EDV) ≥ 100 [25].

Contrast-enhanced ultrasound is a novel, noninvasive, and cost-effective technique to assess plaque morphology and characteristics [13, 14]. Contrast-enhanced ultrasound assists with the identification of several surrogate markers of vulnerable carotid plaques [14]. The use of ultrasound microbubbles allows a reliable detection of microulcerations [14]. As microbubbles are intravascular tracers, the detection of individual microbubbles inside the plaque signifies intraplaque neovessels [14]. The limitation is the poor sensitivity and specificity for detection of lipid-rich necrotic core and plaque hemorrhage compared with MRI [13].

An early evaluation of the extracranial vessels with computed tomography (CT) and CT angiography (CTA) predicts recurrent stroke and functional outcome in the patients with TIA [8]. In many hospitals especially in the developing countries, CTA is more readily available than magnetic resonance imaging (MRI) due to the cost factor [8]. The doctors will utilize the modality which is more easily and rapidly available in the hospitals [8].

Multislice helical CT scan machines with CTA are widely available in many hospitals [8]. CTA involves the administration of intravenous contrast media to evaluate the extracranial and intracranial vessels with high spatial resolution [8, 26].

Multirow spiral CTA helps with the evaluation of plaques and stenosis [11, 27, 28]. CTA helps to identify large artery atherosclerosis [10, 29]. CT also enables high-resolution imaging and accurately detects ulceration and calcification [13]. The limitation of CTA is the inadequate detection of the morphology of the plaque and its content [11, 27, 28]. In addition, CT is unable to distinguish between lipid-rich necrotic core and intraplaque hemorrhage accurately [13].

There is a technological advancement in the imaging of extracranial carotid atherosclerotic lesions with high-resolution MRI and MRA [11]. Presently, MRI is the gold standard in the imaging of carotid plaque [13]. MRI has high resolution and high sensitivity for assessment of intraplaque hemorrhage, ulcerated plaque, and lipid-rich necrotic core [30]. The limitation of MRI is time factor [13].

Careful examination of these lesions with high-resolution bright-blood and black-blood MRI analysis of the extracranial carotid vessels accurately evaluates the contents in the plaques [11]. This is performed using the 3.0-Tesla MRI machine [11, 31, 32]. The advantage is the high spatial resolution [11, 31, 32].

The time-of-flight sequence bright-blood technique demonstrates calcified plaques [11, 33]. Black-blood technique is the MRI technique in which the imaging of vessel wall adjacent to the intravascular space is clearer [11, 33]. The bright-blood and black-blood techniques are highly correlated with the diagnosis of contrast-enhanced MRA in the degree of stenosis [11]. The sensitivity and specificity of using MRI technique to detect stenosis of ≥50% are 88.9 and 100%, respectively [11]. The accuracy of MRI diagnosis of similar degree of stenosis is 97.9% [11].

The fibrous cap is isointense in T1-weighted image (T1WI) and hyperintense in proton density weighted image (PDWI) and T2-weighted image (T2WI) [11]. The lipid core is isointense or hyperintense (mild) in T1WI [11]. It is isointense, hyperintense, or hypointense in PDWI and hypointense in T2WI [11].

Ulcerative plaques are characterized by irregular intravascular space surface in the black-blood sequences [11]. In addition, the black hypointensity band is not observed in three-dimensional time-of-flight MRA [11]. The hypointensity band is not continuous, and the intrusion of hyperintensities into the plaques can be picked up [11].

In a recent study on extracranial carotid atherosclerosis with MRI, visual and quantitative analyses demonstrated that the border between the plaque and vessel lumen was better delineated on three-dimensional (3-D) T1-weighted turbo-spin echo black-blood (TSEBB) MRI than on 3-D T1-turbo field-echo black-blood (TFEBB) MRI [12]. Three-dimensional T1-TSEBB MRI was superior to 3-D T1-TFEBB MRI for delineating carotid plaques [12]. But the high signal plaques were underestimated on 3-D T1-TSEBB MRI [12]. In another recently conducted study, 7.0-Tesla MRI enables adequate evaluation to determine luminal and vessel wall areas [34]. Signal hyperintensity in 7.0-Tesla MRI images was inversely proportional to calcification [34].

Positron emission tomography (PET)/CT is an effective modality to evaluate active inflammation in the plaque [13]. However, PET/CT does not allow for assessment of anatomy, ulceration, intraplaque hemorrhage, and lipid-rich necrotic core [13]. In addition, a combination of [18] F-fluorodeoxyglucose (FDG) positron emission tomography (PET) and MRI are complementary to predict high-risk carotid plaque, such as lipid-rich or hemorrhagic plaque [35]. FDG-PET accurately evaluates the lipid-rich and inflamed plaque [35]. MRI is valuable to identify unstable plaque with a large intraplaque hemorrhage [35].

Digital subtraction angiography (DSA) was the gold standard for the assessment of intracranial and extracranial vasculature before the era for MRI [11, 36]. This investigation method has numerous limitations [11, 36]. Firstly, DSA is invasive [11, 36]. Secondly, the sensitivity is only 46% and the specificity is 74% [11, 36].

Higher levels of cystatin C are independently associated with symptomatic extracranial internal carotid artery (ICA) stenosis, in patients with noncardioembolic stroke [37]. Cystatin C is a biomarker and it is a protein with low molecular weight of 13 kDa [38]. Cystatin C is a cysteine proteinase inhibitor [38].

Cystatin C is an independent risk factor for cardiovascular events and all-cause death in the elderly patients with a normal estimated glomerular filtration rate (eGFR) [39, 40]. It has been suggested that cystatin C levels are associated with inflammation and atherosclerosis [41].

The association between cystatin C and the risk of cardiovascular events is observed in the patients with asymptomatic carotid atherosclerosis, thus ultrasound carotid Doppler can be ordered to detect the carotid abnormalities early [38] (**Table 1**).

	Advantages	Disadvantages
Conventional ultrasound carotid Doppler [11, 24]	• Easily available • Cheap • Noninvasive	• Operator dependent
Contrast-enhanced ultrasound [13, 14]	• Noninvasive • Cost-effective • Detection of microulcerations	• Poor sensitivity and specificity for detection of lipid-rich necrotic core and plaque hemorrhage
CT/CTA brain and carotid [8, 13, 26–28]	• More easily and rapidly available in the hospitals due to lower cost • High spatial resolution	• Administration of contrast media, therefore can cause allergy • Inadequate detection of the morphology of the plaque and the content • Cannot distinguish between lipid-rich necrotic core and intraplaque hemorrhage accurately
MRI/MRA brain and carotid [11, 13, 30]	• Gold standard in the imaging of carotid plaque • High resolution and high sensitivity to assess intraplaque hemorrhage, ulcerated plaque, and lipid-rich necrotic core	• Time factor • Cost factor
PET/CT [13, 18, 35]	• Evaluates active inflammation in the plaque	• Not good in the assessment of anatomy, ulceration, intraplaque hemorrhage, and lipid-rich necrotic core
Digital subtraction angiography [11, 36]	• Very accurate	• Invasive • Poor sensitivity • Poor specificity

Table 1. Advantages and disadvantages of the various imaging modalities.

3. Therapeutic options

Detection of extracranial carotid atherosclerosis in these patients is beneficial because proper management can be given [32, 42]. The patients with TIA due to extracranial carotid stenosis should be given intensive medical therapy [42]. Intensive medical therapy consists of pharmacological management and lifestyle interventions [42].

The pharmacological management involves antiplatelet therapy and statin use [5, 42]. The antiplatelet therapy which routinely administered is aspirin or clopidogrel [43]. Adequate blood pressure control is necessary with a target blood pressure of less than 140/90 [42]. A reduction in blood pressure to the ideal level slows down the progression of carotid artery stenosis and also reduces the carotid intima media thickness (CIMT) [43]. Identification and treatment of vascular risk factors are important [43].

Lifestyle changes involve Mediterranean-style diet, exercise, and smoking cessation [42, 43]. In addition, lifestyle choices such as unhealthy diet and excessive alcohol intake are modifiable risk factors [43]. The combination of dietary modification, physical exercise, and use of aspirin, statin, and an antihypertensive agent can give a cumulative relative stroke risk reduction of 80% [43]. The antiplatelet therapy and statin use reduce the risk of recurrent stroke in patients with symptomatic extracranial carotid stenosis [5].

4. Carotid endarterectomy and carotid artery stenting

In the patients with carotid stenosis of 70–99%, the revascularization procedures such as carotid endarterectomy (CEA) and carotid artery stenting (CAS) may be considered [5, 42]. The patient with a low-grade stenosis but an ulcerated plaque or intraplaque hemorrhage may benefit more from a revascularization procedure than a patient with a stable 70% asymptomatic stenosis with a thick fibrous cap [13].

5. Carotid endarterectomy and carotid artery stenting in symptomatic extracranial carotid stenosis

Carotid endarterectomy and carotid artery stenting reduce the risk of recurrent stroke in patients with symptomatic extracranial carotid stenosis [5]. The revascularization procedures reduce the 90-day risk of subsequent ischemic stroke in the patients with severe extracranial carotid artery stenosis [5]. While awaiting the revascularization procedures, a combination of aspirin and clopidogrel in recently symptomatic patients with carotid stenosis can be given [43].

MR plaque imaging is useful in identifying revascularization candidates who are better candidates for carotid endarterectomy than carotid artery stenting [13]. This is because high intraplaque signal on time-of-flight imaging is associated with vulnerable plaque and in-creased rates of adverse events in patients undergoing stenting but not carotid endarterectomy [13].

In the recent guidelines, carotid endarterectomy is likely the preferred option for the man-agement of asymptomatic carotid stenosis [44, 45]. Carotid artery stenting has higher risk of periprocedural stroke and mortality [44–46]. Carotid endarterectomy is safer in comparison to carotid artery stenting [44, 45]. The risk of periprocedural stroke and mortality after carotid endarterectomy has declined tremendously throughout the years [47].

However, carotid endarterectomy is associated with an increased risk of periprocedural myo-cardial infarction [44, 45, 48]. To date, the long-term outcomes of these two modalities remain uncertain [44]. In patients with high risk of periprocedural complications, best medical treatment is recommended by the American Heart Association and the Society for Vascular Surgery [32, 44, 49].

6. Conclusion

In conclusion, evaluation of extracranial carotid atherosclerosis in the patients with TIA is very important. There are several modalities which can be employed to investigate for extra-cranial carotid stenosis. Pharmacological and nonpharmacological management can be given to the patients with extracranial carotid atherosclerosis.

Author details

Mei-Ling Sharon Tai*, Jun Kit Khoo and Mohamed Abdusalam Elwaifa

*Address all correspondence to: sharont1990@gmail.com

Division of Neurology, Department of Medicine, Faculty of Medicine, University of Malaya, Malaysia

References

[1] Kiyohara T, Kamouchi M, Kunai Y, Ninomiya T, Hata J, Yoshimura S, et al. ABCD3 and ABCD3-I scores are superior to ABCD2 score in the prediction of short- and long-term risks of stroke after transient ischemic attack. Stroke. 2014;**45**:418-425

[2] Johnston SC, Gress DR, Browner WS, Sidney S. Short-term prognosis after emer-gency department diagnosis of TIA. Journal of the American Medical Association. 2000;**284**:2901-2906

[3] Lisabeth LD, Ireland JK, Risser JM, Brown DL, Smith MA, Garcia NM, et al. Stroke risk after transient ischemic attack in a population-based setting. Stroke. 2004;**35**:1842-1846

[4]   Rothwell PM, Warlow CP. Timing of TIAs preceding stroke: Time window for prevention is very short. Neurology. 2005;**64**:817-820

[5]   Uehara T, Ohara T, Toyoda K, Nagatsuka K, Minematsu K. Clinical, laboratory, and imaging characteristics of transient ischemic attack caused by large artery lesions: A comparison between carotid and intracranial arteries. Cerebrovascular Diseases Extra. Oct 16, 2015;**5**(3):115-123

[6]   Rothwell PM, Giles MF, Chandratheva A, Marquardt L, Geraghty O, Redgrave JN, et al. Effect of urgent treatment of transient ischaemic attack and minor stroke on early recurrent stroke (EXPRESS study): A prospective population-based sequential comparison. Lancet. 2007;**370**:1432-1442

[7]   Lavallee PC, Meseguer E, Abboud H, Cabrejo L, Olivot JM, Simon O, et al. A transient ischaemic attack clinic with round-the-clock access (SOS-TIA): Feasibility and effects. Lancet Neurology. 2007;**6**:953-960

[8]   Coutts SB, Modi J, Patel SK, Demchuk AM, Goyal M, Hill MD, Calgary Stroke Program. CT/CT angiography and MRI findings predict recurrent stroke after transient ischemic attack and minor stroke: Results of the prospective CATCH study. Stroke. 2012;**43**:1013-1017

[9]   Purroy F, Montaner J, Molina CA, Delgado P, Ribo M, Alvarez-Sabín J. Patterns and predictors of early risk of recurrence after transient ischemic attack with respect to etiologic subtypes. Stroke. 2007;**38**:3225-3229

[10] Lovett JK, Coull AJ, Rothwell PM. Early risk of recurrence by subtype of ischemic stroke in population-based incidence studies. Neurology. 2004;**62**:569-573

[11] Li M, Le WJ, Tao XF, Li MH, Li YH, Qu N. Advantage in bright-blood and black-blood magnetic resonance imaging with high-resolution for analysis of carotid atherosclerotic plaques. Chinese Medical Journal. Sep 20, 2015;**128**(18):2478-2484

[12] Inoue K, Maeda M, Umino M, Takase S, Yamahata T, Sakuma H. Cervical carotid plaque evaluation using 3D T1-weighted black-blood magnetic resonance imaging: Comparison of turbo field-echo and turbo spin-echo sequences. European Journal of Radiology. May 2016;**85**(5):1035-1039

[13] Brinjikji W, Huston 3rd J, Rabinstein AA, Kim GM, Lerman A, Lanzino G. Contemporary carotid imaging: From degree of stenosis to plaque vulnerability. Journal of Neurosurgery. Jan 2016;**124**(1):27-42

[14] Alonso A, Artemis D, Hennerici MG. Molecular imaging of carotid plaque vulnerability. Cerebrovascular Diseases. 2015;**39**(1):5-12

[15] Hill MD, Yiannakoulias N, Jeerakathil T, Tu JV, Svenson LW, Schopflocher DP. The high risk of stroke immediately after transient ischemic attack: A population-based study. Neurology. 2004;**62**:2015-2020

[16] Coull AJ, Lovett JK, Rothwell PM. Population based study of early risk of stroke after transient ischaemic attack or minor stroke: Implications for public education and organisation of services. British Medical Journal. 2004;**328**:326

[17] Nomura M, Kasami R, Ohashi M, Yamada Y, Abe H. Significantly higher incidence of carotid atherosclerosis found in Japanese type 2 diabetic patients with early nephropathy. Diabetes Research and Clinical Practice. 2004;66(Suppl 1):S161-S163

[18] Frauchiger B, Schmid HP, Roedel C, Moosmann P, Staub D. Comparison of carotid arterial resistive indices with intima-media thickness as sonographic markers of atherosclerosis. Stroke. 2001;32:836-841

[19] Sheehan OC, Kyne L, Kelly LA, Hannon N, Marnane M, Merwick A, et al. Population-based study of ABCD2 score, carotid stenosis, and atrial fibrillation for early stroke prediction after transient ischemic attack: The North Dublin TIA study. Stroke. 2010;41:844-850

[20] Huang YN, Gao S, Li SW, Huang Y, Li JF, Wong KS, Kay R. Vascular lesions in Chinese patients with transient ischemic attacks. Neurology. Feb 1997;48(2):524-525

[21] Nishimaru K, McHenry Jr LC, Toole JF. Cerebral angiographic and clinical differences in carotid system transient ischemic attacks between American Caucasian and Japanese patients. Stroke. Jan–Feb 1984;15(1):56-59

[22] Ryu JE, Murros K, Espeland MA, Rubens J, McKinney WM, Toole JF, Crouse JR. Extracranial carotid atherosclerosis in black and white patients with transient ischemic attacks. Stroke. Sep 1989;20(9):1133-1137

[23] Amarenco P, Lavallée PC, Labreuche J, Albers GW, Bornstein NM, Canhão P, et al. One-year risk of stroke after transient ischemic attack or minor stroke. The New England Journal of Medicine. Apr 21, 2016;374(16):1533-1542

[24] Landwehr P, Schulte O, Voshage G. Ultrasound examination of carotid and vertebral arteries. European Radiology. 2001;11:1521-1534

[25] Grant EG, Benson CB, Moneta GL, Alexandrov AV, Baker JD, Bluth EI, et al. Carotid artery stenosis: Gray-scale and Doppler US diagnosis. Radiology. Nov 2003;229:340-346

[26] Lima FO, Lev MH, Levy RA, Silva GS, Ebril M, de Camargo EC, et al. Functional contrast-enhanced CT for evaluation of acute ischemic stroke does not increase the risk of contrast-induced nephropathy. AJNR. American Journal of Neuroradiology. 2010;31:817-821

[27] Nandalur KR, Baskurt E, Hagspiel KD, Phillips CD, Kramer CM. Calcified carotid atherosclerotic plaque is associated less with ischemic symptoms than is noncalcified plaque on MDCT. American Journal of Roentgenology. 2005;184:295-298

[28] Wintermark M, Jawadi SS, Rapp JH, Tihan T, Tong E, Glidden DV, et al. High-resolution CT imaging of carotid artery atherosclerotic plaques. American Journal of Neuroradiology. 2008;29:875-882

[29] Chimowitz MI, Lynn MJ, Howlett-Smith H, Stern BJ, Hertzberg VS, Frankel MR, et al. Comparison of warfarin and aspirin for symptomatic intracranial arterial stenosis. The New England Journal of Medicine. 2005;352:1305-1316

[30] Kernan WN, Ovbiagele B, Black HR, Bravata DM, Chimowitz MI, Ezekowitz MD, et al. Guidelines for the prevention of stroke in patients with stroke and transient ischemic

attack: A guideline for healthcare professionals from the American Heart Association/ American Stroke Association. Stroke. 2014;**45**:2160-2236

[31] Hinton DP, Cury RC, Chan RC, Wald LL, Sherwood JB, Furie KL, et al. Bright and black blood imaging of the carotid bifurcation at 3.0T. European Journal of Radiology. 2006;**57**:403-411

[32] Anumula S, Song HK, Wright AC, Wehrli FW. High-resolution black-blood MRI of the carotid vessel wall using phased-array coils at 1.5 and 3 Tesla. Academic Radiology. 2005;**12**:1521-1526

[33] Hatsukami TS, Ross R, Polissar NL, Yuan C. Visualization of fibrous cap thickness and rupture in human atherosclerotic carotid plaque in vivo with high-resolution magnetic resonance imaging. Circulation. 2000;**102**:959-964

[34] de Rotte AA, Koning W, Truijman MT, den Hartog AG, Bovens SM, Vink A, et al. Seven-tesla magnetic resonance imaging of atherosclerotic plaque in the significantly stenosed carotid artery: A feasibility study. Investigative Radiology. Nov 2014;**49**(11):749-757

[35] Saito H, Kuroda S, Hirata K, Magota K, Shiga T, Tamaki N, et al. Validity of dual MRI and F-FDG PET imaging in predicting vulnerable and inflamed carotid plaque. Cerebrovascular Diseases. 2013;**35**(4):370-377

[36] Streifler JY, Eliasziw M, Fox AJ, Benavente OR, Hachinski VC, Ferguson GG, et al. Angiographic detection of carotid plaque ulceration. Comparison with surgical observations in a multicenter study. North American Symptomatic Carotid Endarterectomy Trial. Stroke. 1994;**25**:1130-1132

[37] Umemura T, Kawamura T, Mashita S, Kameyama T, Sobue G. Higher levels of cystatin C are associated with extracranial carotid artery steno-occlusive disease in patients with noncardioembolic ischemic stroke. Cerebrovascular Diseases Extra. Jan 20, 2016;**6**(1):1-11

[38] Hoke M, Amighi J, Mlekusch W, Schlager O, Exner M, Sabeti S, et al. Cystatin C and the risk for cardiovascular events in patients with asymptomatic carotid atherosclerosis. Stroke. 2010;**41**:674-679

[39] Shlipak MG, Sarnak MJ, Katz R, Fried LF, Seliger SL, Newman AB, et al. Cystatin C and the risk of death and cardiovascular events among elderly persons. The New England Journal of Medicine. 2005;**352**:2049-2060

[40] Ix JH, Shlipak MG, Chertow GM, Whooley MA. Association of cystatin C with mortality, cardiovascular events, and incident heart failure among persons with coronary heart disease: Data from the Heart and Soul Study. Circulation. 2007;**115**:173-179

[41] Salgado JV, Souza FL, Salgado BJ. How to understand the association between cystatin C levels and cardiovascular disease: Imbalance, counterbalance, or consequence? Journal of Cardiology. 2013;**62**:331-335

[42] Wabnitz AM, Turan TN. Symptomatic carotid artery stenosis: Surgery, stenting, or medical therapy? Current Treatment Options in Cardiovascular Medicine. Aug 2017;**19**(8):62

[43] Cheng SF, Brown MM. Contemporary medical therapies of atherosclerotic carotid artery disease. Seminars in Vascular Surgery. Mar 2017;**30**(1):8-16

[44] Moresoli P, Habib B, Reynier P, Secrest MH, Eisenberg MJ, Filion KB. Carotid stenting versus endarterectomy for asymptomatic carotid artery stenosis: A systematic review and meta-analysis. Stroke. Aug 2017;**48**(8):2150-2157

[45] Kakkos SK, Kakisis I, Tsolakis IA, Geroulakos G. Endarterectomy achieves lower stroke and death rates compared with stenting in patients with asymptomatic carotid stenosis. Journal of Vascular Surgery. Aug 2017;**66**(2):607-617

[46] Liu ZJ, Fu WG, Guo ZY, Shen LG, Shi ZY, Li JH. Updated systematic review and meta-analysis of randomized clinical trials comparing carotid artery stenting and carotid endarterectomy in the treatment of carotid stenosis. Annals of Vascular Surgery. 2012;**26**:576-590

[47] Lokuge K, de Waard DD, Halliday A, Gray A, Bulbulia R, Mihaylova B. Meta-analysis of the procedural risks of carotid endarterectomy and carotid artery stenting over time. The British Journal of Surgery. Jan 2018;**105**(1):26-36

[48] Sardar P, Chatterjee S, Aronow HD, Kundu A, Ramchand P, Mukherjee D, et al. Carotid artery stenting versus endarterectomy for stroke prevention: A meta-analysis of clinical trials. Journal of the American College of Cardiology. 2017;**69**:2266-2275

[49] Ricotta JJ, Aburahma A, Ascher E, Eskandari M, Faries P, Lal BK, Society for Vascular Surgery. Updated Society for Vascular Surgery guidelines for management of extracranial carotid disease: Executive summary. Journal of Vascular Surgery. 2011;**54**:832-836

10

Angiography and Endovascular Therapy for Aortoiliac Artery Disease

Keisuke Fukuda

Abstract

The treatment of aortoiliac occlusive disease has shifted to endovascular therapy. Even in complex lesion, precise angiography enables successful treatment in endovascular work. However, complications-related endovascular intervention of these lesions is catastrophic. Accurate angiographic assessment is mandatory to complete the procedure. This article reviews angiographic approach for aortoiliac artery disease in diagnosis, endovascular intervention, and complications.

Keywords: aortoiliac occlusive disease, TASC II classification, access

1. Introduction

Aortoiliac occlusive disease results from the common cardiovascular condition atherosclerosis, accounting for approximately one-third of all symptomatic peripheral artery disease (PAD) [1]. Most cases of aortoiliac artery disease presents with lower limb claudication and can potentially progress to critical limb ischemia. In revascularization for aortoiliac disease, endovascular therapy is increasingly being employed instead of surgical bypass. Even in complex aortoiliac artery diseases such as bifurcation disease, long segment occlusion, and aortic occlusion, endovascular therapy is being employed with the application of stents [2, 3]. The most commonly quoted classification of iliac lesions has been set forth by the Trans-Atlantic Inter-Society Consensus (TASC II) group with recommended treatment options [4]. These classifications of their morphology have finally been defined by assessment in accurate detail with angiography. Therefore, precise angiographic assessment is vital to success in aortoiliac artery interventions. This article reviews an angiographic approach to aortoiliac artery disease presenting various detailed images and analyses pre- and postrevascularization.

2. Angiographic technique for the aortoiliac artery

2.1. Vascular anatomy of the aortoiliac artery

A solid understanding of the vascular anatomy of the aortoiliac artery in angiography is indispensable to diagnostic or interventional work. The vasculature within range from the infra-renal artery to the common femoral artery is shown in **Figure 1**.

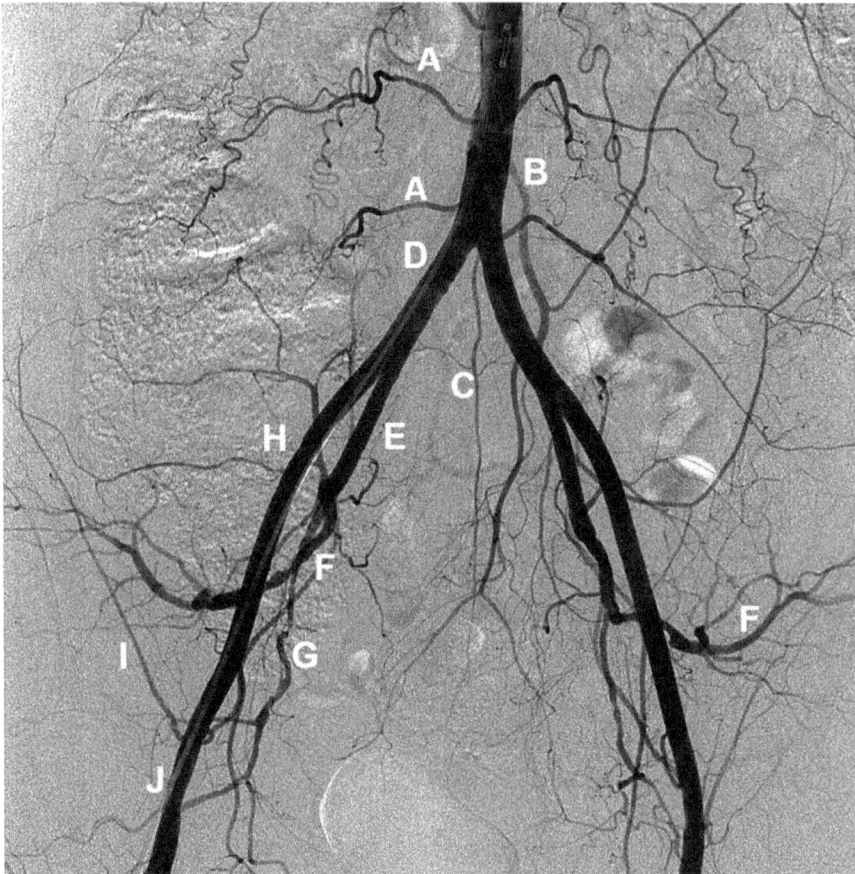

Figure 1. Anatomy in aortoiliac artery angiography. Aortoiliac angiography image includes abdominal aorta, lumber branch (A), inferior mesenteric artery (B), median sacral artery (C), common iliac artery (D), internal iliac artery (E), superior (F) and inferior (G) gluteal arteries, external iliac artery (H), deep circumflex iliac artery, (I) and common femoral artery (J).

Commonly, the aortoiliac angiographic image includes the abdominal aorta, lumber branch, inferior mesenteric artery, median sacral artery, common iliac artery (CIA), internal iliac artery (IIA), superior and inferior gluteal arteries, external iliac artery (EIA), deep circumflex iliac artery, and common femoral artery (CFA). Safe and successful procedures are accomplished by meticulous manipulation of a wire and/or catheter to a target vessel. Particularly, in the case of complex aortoiliac disease with total occlusion or calcification, a wire or catheter is more likely to stray unintentionally into unexpected vessels. Therefore, a thorough understanding of the vasculature including a normal vasculature, anomalies, and complex collateral networks is required before any intervening procedure.

2.2. Image size and optimal view

To visualize aortoiliac disease, an image field of more than 30 cm is required. Information on the vessel size and lesion length is needed as well. The wide 30 cm image could not confirm the precise morphology of the lesion, while a 20 cm image was better suited (**Figure 2**).

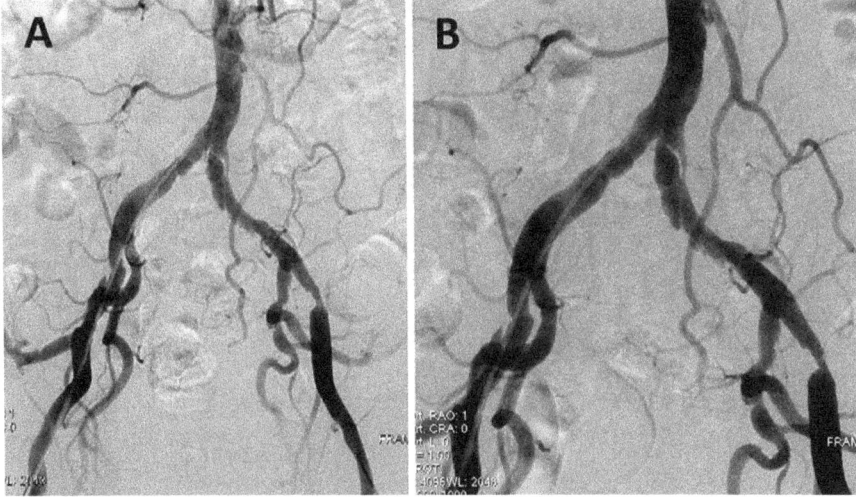

Figure 2. Aortoiliac artery angiography by 30 and 20 cm image size. (A) By 30 cm DSA image, whole aortoiliac disease is visualized. (B) By 20 cm DSA image, the precise morphology of left common iliac artery ulcerated lesion and tight stenosis of left external iliac artery are well visualized.

Unlike femoropopliteal or below the knee arteries, the aortoiliac arteries are located in the intraperitoneal space and form three-dimensionally from the terminal aorta to the common femoral artery (**Figure 3**).

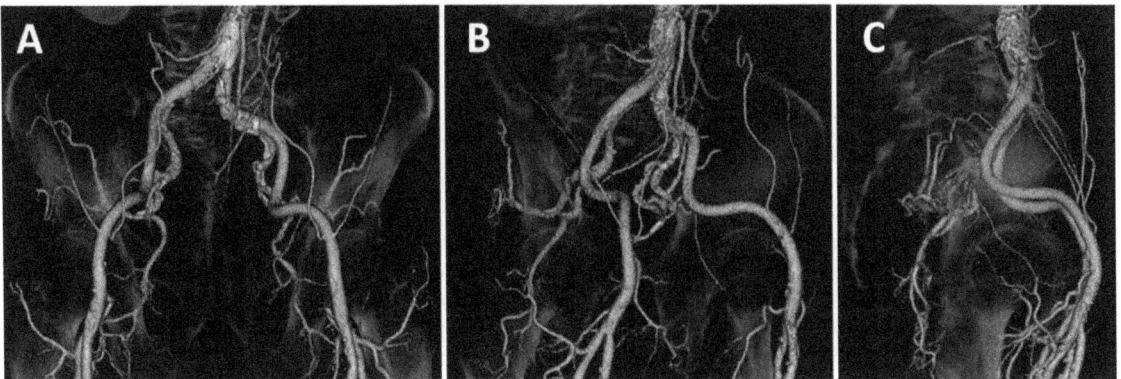

Figure 3. Aortoiliac artery by 3D CT angiography. (A) AP view, (B) RAO 45° view, (C) lateral view. RAO view and lateral view show that aortoiliac arterial system located in intraperitoneal space with three-dimensional CT angiography.

Multidirectional projection in angiography is also useful to achieve successful endovascular revascularization. The optimal view for interventional work is commonly obtained by magnification and various oblique projections. Not only anterior-posterior views but also a contralateral view is important (**Figure 4**).

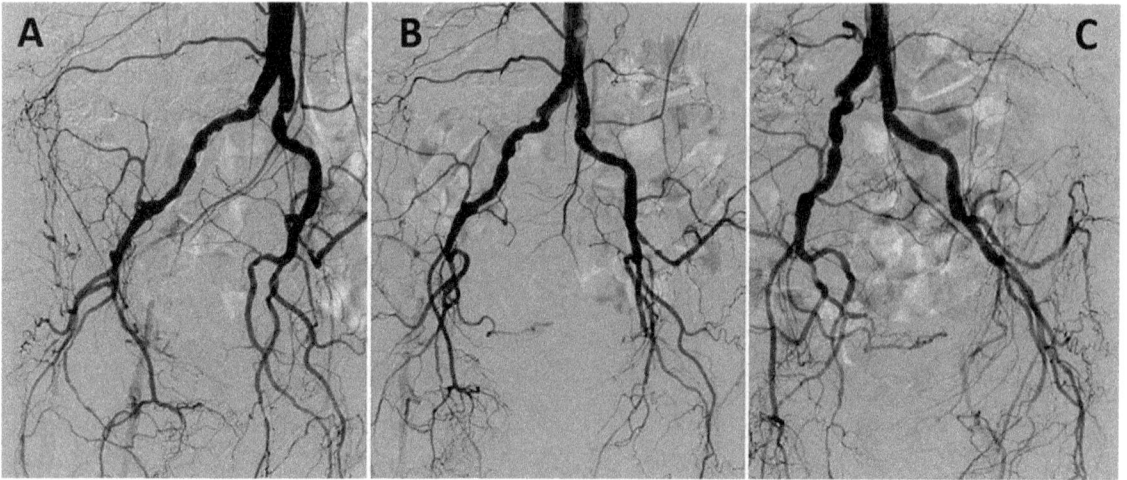

Figure 4. Basic three aortographic views. (A) DSA in LAO view. (B) DSA in AP view. (C) DSA in RAO view.

If a lesion could not be identified or is not well visualized, angiography should be performed using a contralateral oblique (20°–30°) projection. Particularly in EIA lesions, this angled view is imperative in obtaining accurate information on a lesion (**Figure 5**).

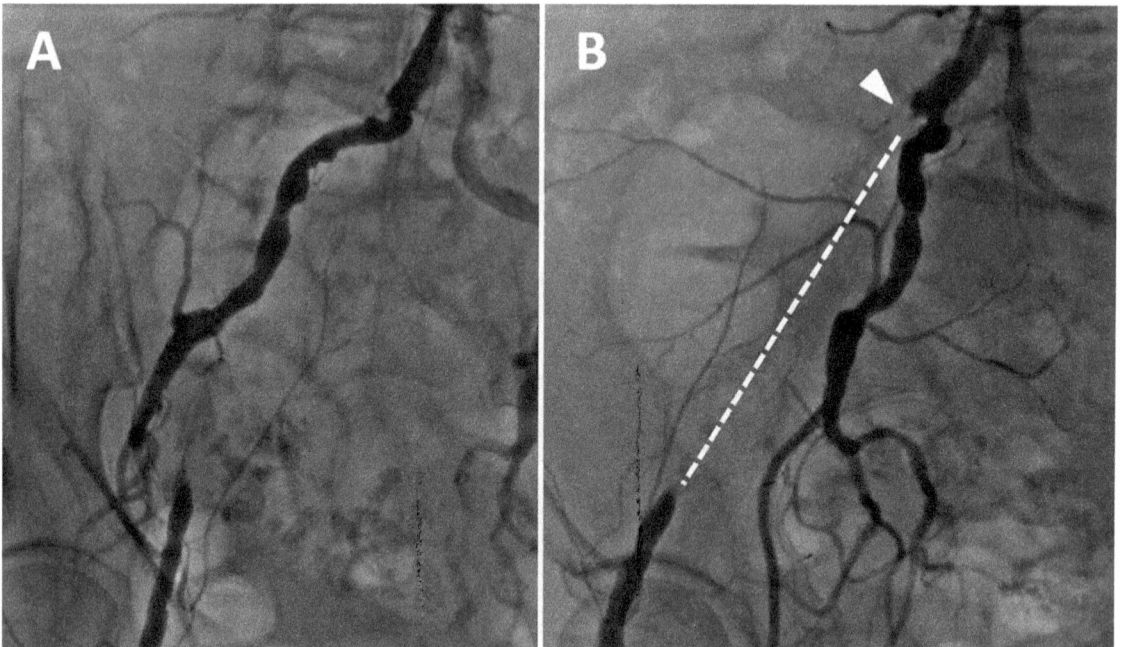

Figure 5. Right EIA occlusion in LAO and RAO views. (A): in LAO view, stump is hidden and occluded lesion overlaps with internal iliac artery. (B): In RAO view, stump (arrow head) can be clearly visualized and occluded lesion is well-isolated (white dot line).

Digital subtracted angiography (DSA) images are considered to be the standard modality for iliac artery disease, but visualization of the pelvic vessels is often interfered by bowel movement and gas in a 30 cm image. Breath holding during contrast injection is requested in conscious patients. With recent advanced digital angiography (DA), similar images to DSA can be obtained. Moreover, to take excellent images for diagnostic angiography, the 5-Fr pigtail catheter is preferred over a 4-Fr system. Decisions for intervention are thus made after diagnostic angiography. We exchange to a 6-Fr system if intervention is indicated.

2.3. Access

2.3.1. Antegrade upper limb access

Upper limb access including the brachial or radial artery has several advantages compared to conventional femoral access in terms of anatomical reasons, fewer bleeding complications, and/or patient preference [5]. In common iliac artery disease, the contralateral femoral artery approach may encounter difficulty when crossing the contralateral common iliac artery lesion. Left brachial or radial artery access can be employed for aortography [6]. This approach is useful in cases with suspected or known total occlusion in aortoiliac artery lesions [7]. Generally speaking, the left brachial or radial artery approach is anatomically suited to reach the terminal aorta through the aortic arch due to the shorter length and more linear route from the access site to the terminal aorta, so that catheter manipulation of the catheter and wire is much easier as compared to the right upper limb approach (**Figure 6**).

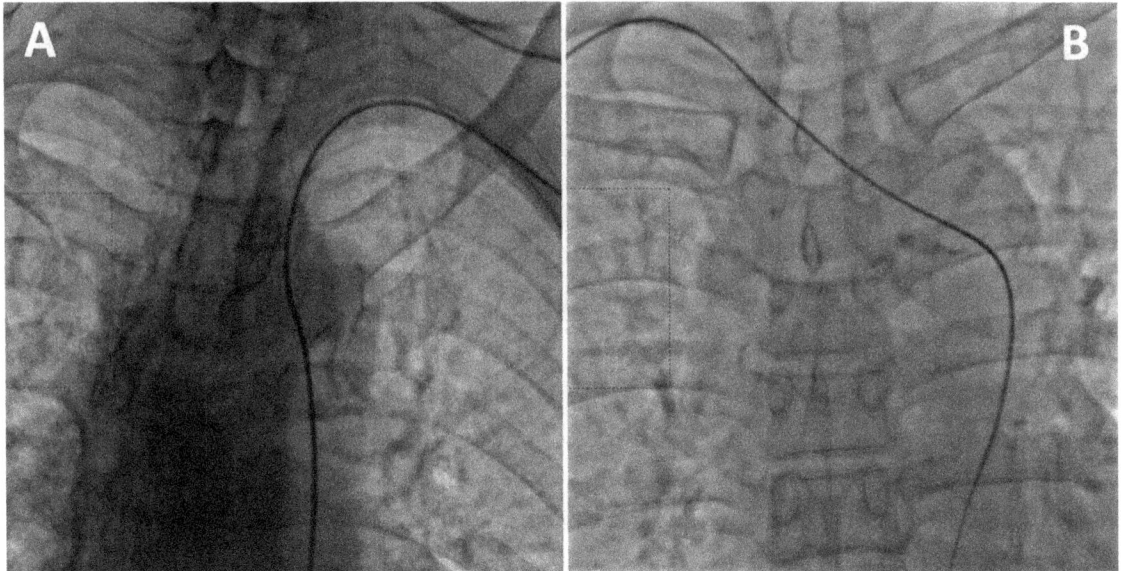

Figure 6. Difference between left and right upper limb approach. (A) From left arm approach, the shape of the wire is in linear form with shorter length. (B) From right arm approach, the wire and catheter have to pass through the aortic arch.

In complex aortic bifurcation or proximal CIA occlusions, the antegrade approach is necessary and effective in conjunction with the femoral approach for successful intervention. Additionally, this approach is vital in cases when the crossover technique cannot be employed due to previous kissing stenting at the aortic bifurcation or when CFA access is hindered due to severe stenosis or anastomosis for a bypass graft. A lesion may be easily crossed with a wire through a 6-Fr-long sheath from the left brachial artery, and ballooning or stenting can then be performed by this approach. In recent endovascular devices for PAD, there are systems with long shafts of between 130 and 150 cm in length and these devices enable an upper limb approach. However, these are limited to balloons and stents. Large diameter size devices such as those for atherectomy are not advised for a brachial or radial artery approach.

2.3.2. Retrograde ipsilateral CFA access

The retrograde ipsilateral CFA approach is most frequently used as a standard technique. For a precise CFA puncture, we routinely use echo with fluoroscopy guidance. After confirming no CFA disease, an ipsilateral approach is selected for iliac artery intervention. If there is no CFA disease, we advance a 4-Fr or 5-Fr pigtail catheter to the terminal aorta. By power injection of the contrast dye at the terminal aorta, we inject 13 cc/s for a total of 26 cc by a 4-Fr pigtail and 16–18 cc/s for a total of 25 cc by a 5-Fr pigtail catheter. Manual contrast injection is not recommended at the aortoiliac artery. In TASC ll A or B lesions, retrograde sheath injection can be performed. In bilateral iliac lesions, if a contralateral CIA ostial lesion is not involved, treatment can proceed by a retrograde and crossover antegrade technique at one femoral artery access site (**Figure 7**).

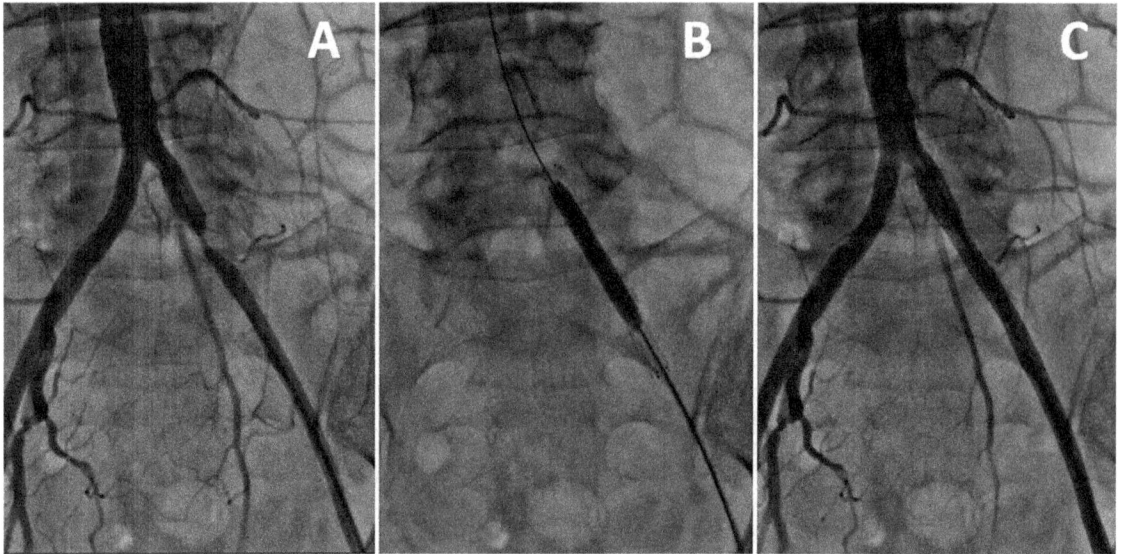

Figure 7. Angiography and treatment from ipsilateral CFA sheath. (A) Angiography from retrograde sheath injection shows severe stenosis of left EIA. (B) Ballooning and stenting performed from retrograde sheath. (C) Completion of angiography from retrograde sheath shows good results.

In intervention for total occlusion of the common iliac artery with or without distal EIA disease, a bidirectional wiring technique is the key to successful recanalization. Therefore, ipsilateral retrograde intervention in conjunction with an antegrade approach from the contralateral femoral side or from the brachial or radial artery is essential for successful wiring.

2.3.3. Retrograde contralateral CFA access

Retrograde contralateral CFA access is an indispensable technique for interventions of peripheral artery disease at each level of the lower extremity, including the iliac, femoropopliteal, and below the knee arteries. For interventions from the iliac artery to below the knee, the crossover technique is requisite. Mastering the crossover technique is required of every interventionist since, in patients with CFA, proximal SFA, and/or distal EIA disease, this approach is mainly selected. Operators who are experienced and skillful in this technique can freely select any access site, leading to safer procedures and more successful outcomes. Total occluded iliac artery interventions commonly require a bidirectional approach from both CFA access sites. To cross the guidewire to the contralateral iliac artery, we generally use a JR diagnostic (4 or 5 Fr) catheter placed to the bifurcation of the terminal aorta. If there is an acute angle at the bifurcation of the iliac artery, the 4-Fr IMA catheter can be used. We do not use a pigtail catheter for crossover purposes since the movement of the wire is unpredictable and may damage the vessel wall. Exchange to a stiff guidewire was performed to advance the crossover sheath (5 or 6 Fr). In the case of heavily tortuous or calcified CIA, it is very difficult to advance the sheath to the contralateral side. In such a case, the balloon anchor technique is helpful to crossover the sheath (**Figure 8**) [8].

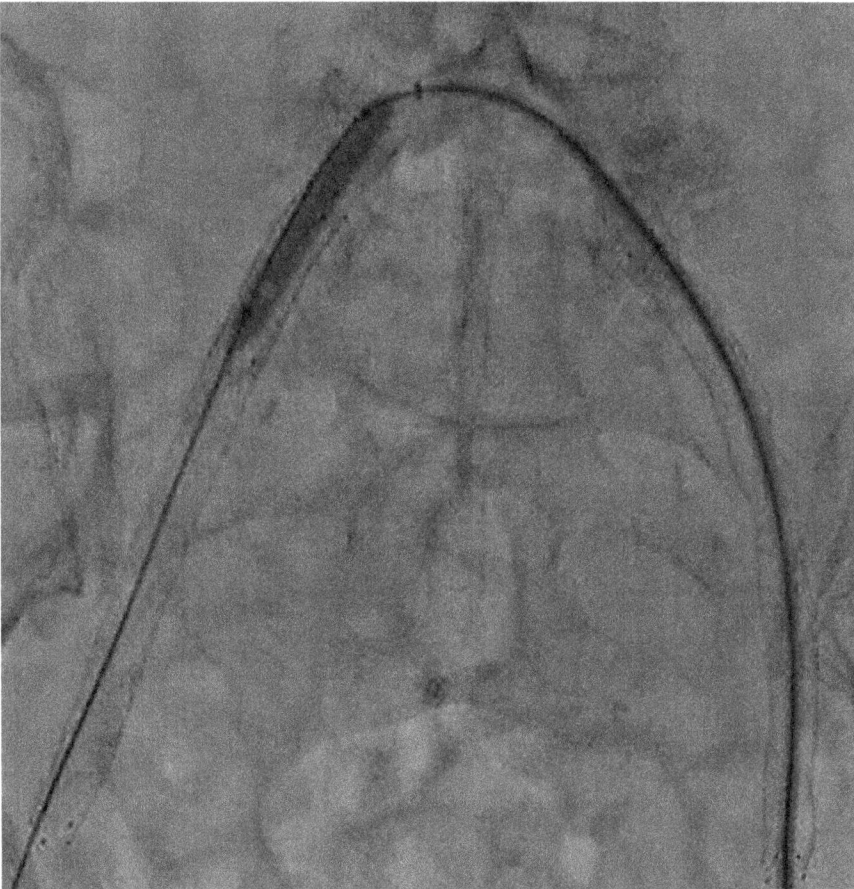

Figure 8. Using balloon anchor technique, the crossover sheath was advanced to contralateral iliac artery.

However, there are some cases when crossover at the bifurcation is not possible (**Figure 9**), for example, with a sharp-angled isthmus, poststent graft, or postkissing stent. Therefore, detailed reinterventional planning is essential.

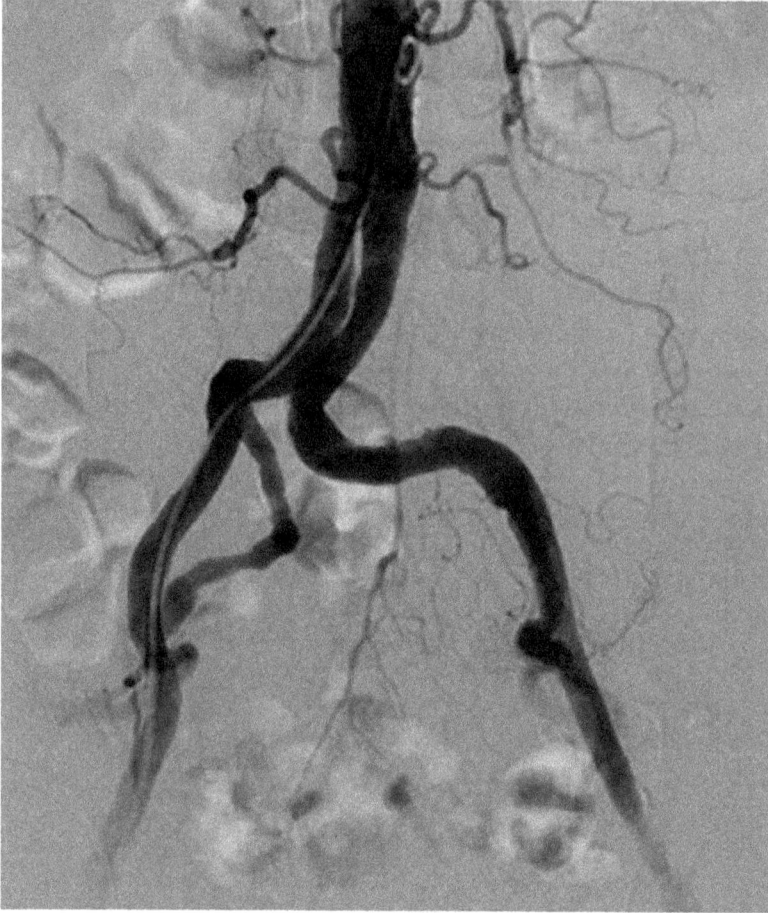

Figure 9. Crossover technique is not indicated in the case of sharp-angled isthmus, poststent graft, or postkissing stent.

3. Aortic stenosis and aortic occlusion

Many studies have demonstrated that endovascular therapy for extensive aortoiliac occlusive disease shows better long-term patency and clinical outcomes [9–11]. The main strategy of endovascular therapy for this field has increasingly shifted to primary stenting [12–14]. Balloon expandable stents, self-expanding stents, or covered stents are basic treatment options. In iliac artery stenting, a self-expandable stent is preferred to a balloon expandable system. The self-expandable stent is compatible with a 6-Fr sheath, and sizes up to 10–12 mm are available. Selection of the stent type may be left to the operator based on lesion location and characteristics. In the treatment of aortic occlusion, catastrophic complications may occur. Operators need to keep in mind the risks of rupture, dissection or emboli to the renal, mesenteric artery or distally to the pelvic arteries, or lower limb arteries. There are reports that aortic occlusion can be treated with an endovascular technique using the three way access sites including the upper limb or both CFAs [15–18].

Infra-renal aortic stenosis of less than 3 cm and a focal lesion is classified as TASC ll B which is considered a good indication for endovascular intervention as first line therapy. Isolated infra-renal aortic stenosis is shown in **Figure 10A**. To clearly visualize and identify aortic stenosis, a lateral view is useful (**Figure 10B**) and measurement of the pressure gradient across the lesion is a factor in making the final decision.

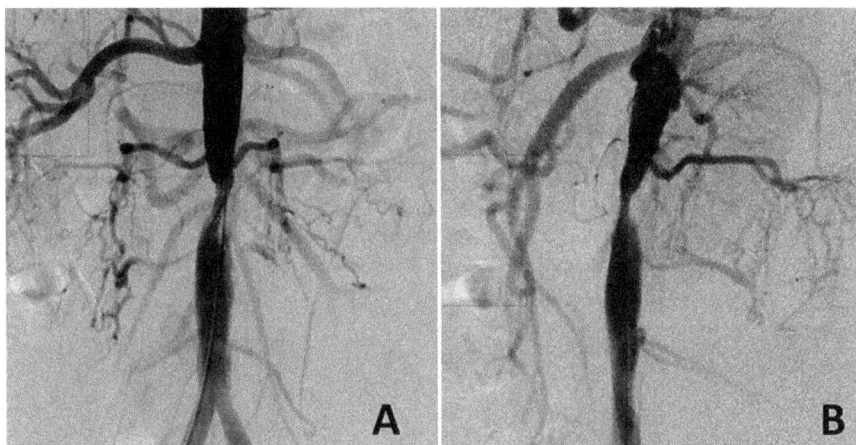

Figure 10. Isolated infra-renal aortic stenosis. (A) DSA image in AP view shows aortic stenosis of less than 3 cm. (B) In lateral view, stenosis is more visible.

Aortic stenosis is mostly treated with a self-expandable stent and postdilatation because of the large vessel size (**Figure 11**).

Aggressive postdilatation is not recommended in order to avoid the above mentioned complications. Even if moderate residual stenosis remains, reducing the pressure gradient across the lesion (<10 mmHg) is acceptable. In the case of aortoiliac occlusion involving bilateral CIAs (**Figure 12A**), upper limb and bilateral CFA access is required. Wiring is performed from the upper limb through a long sheath with simultaneous retrograde angiography from the CFA to guide the direction of the wiring (**Figure 12B**). Kissing stent insertion and kissing ballooning resulted in excellent recanalization on this complex occlusion at the terminal aorta (**Figure 12C** and **D**). Stenting above the aortic bifurcation combined with the kissing stent technique can be considered an effective alternative option to open surgical reconstruction for extensive aortoiliac occlusive disease.

Complex distal aortic occlusive disease often involves either the CIA or EIA (**Figure 13A**). A retrograde 0.035 wire carefully passed through the bifurcation to the abdominal aorta, and initial stent was placed at the aorta (**Figure 13B**). After the first stenting, the next wire was carefully crossed inside the aortic stent from the other side of the CFA access. After the two wires were crossed inside the aortic stent, a kissing stent technique was performed (**Figure 13C**), and the final angiogram was taken (**Figure 13D**). In this poststenting DSA, care must be taken to check for any perforations or residual thrombi.

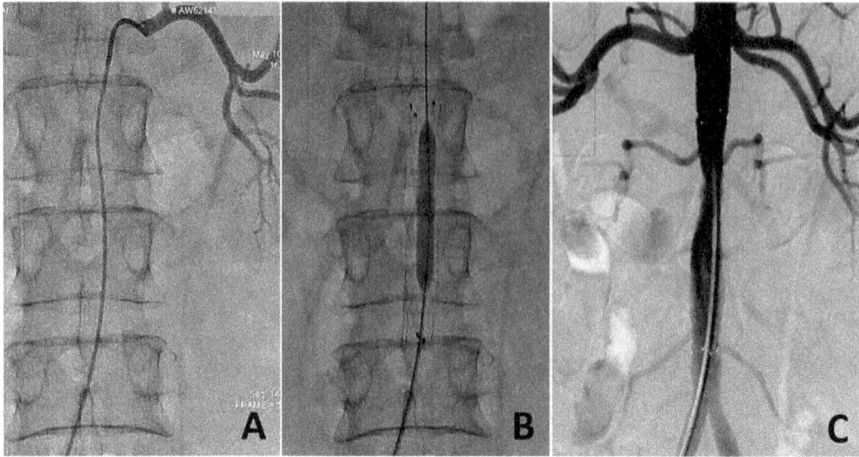

Figure 11. EVT for isolated infra-renal aortic stenosis. (A) Ostium of renal artery is confirmed by selective renal artery angiography. (B) After stenting, postdilatation is performed by lower diameter balloon at relatively lower pressure. (C) Final angiography shows acceptable dilatation of the lesion and no complications.

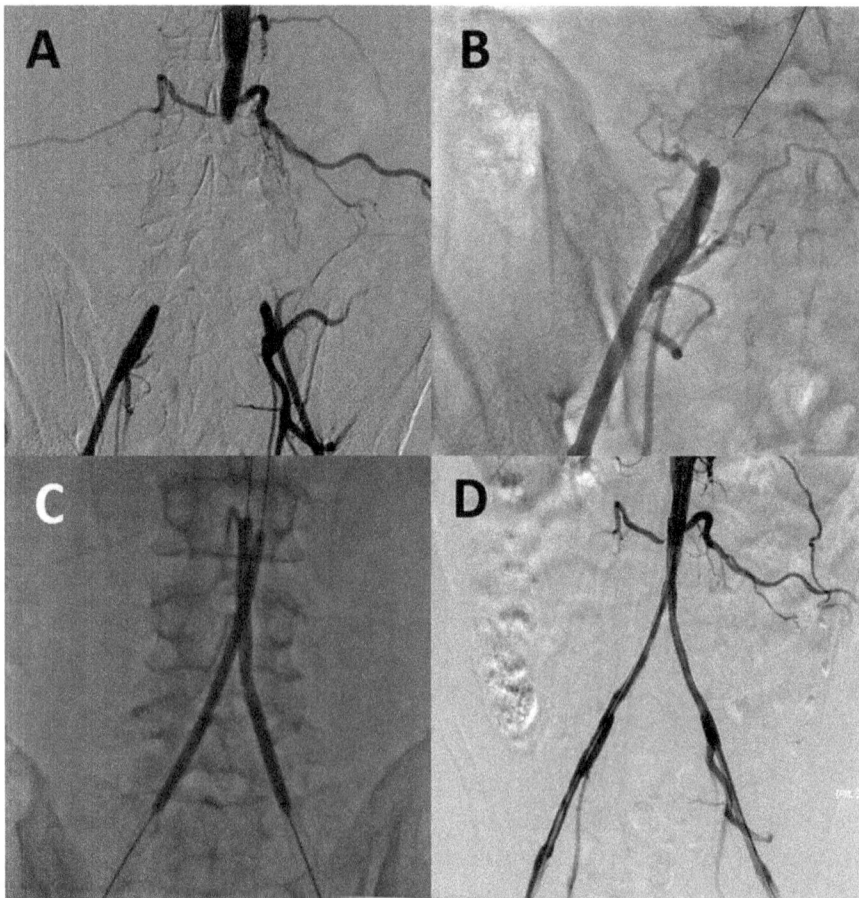

Figure 12. Aortic occlusion involving bilateral CIA. (A) DSA injected from three ways access can clearly visualize total occlusion of aortic bifurcation. (B) Simultaneous retrograde angiography from CFA in order to direct wiring from upper limb. (C) Kissing stent technique and kissing postdilatation are performed from bilateral CFA. (D) Completion of DSA angiography shows excellent recanalization.

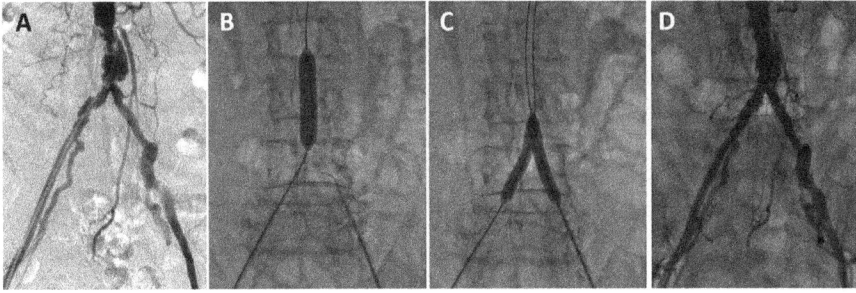

Figure 13. Complex distal aortic occlusive disease involving either CIA or EIA. (A) The 30 cm DSA image shows aortic stenosis extending to both CIAs and the left EIA. (B) Final angiogram is taken in DA, which shows complete recanalization. (C) Initial stent is placed at aorta, and postdilatation at lower pressure was performed. (D) After two wires are carefully crossed inside the initial stent from both CFA sheaths, a kissing stent is implanted.

4. Iliac artery disease: TASC ll A-C

Endovascular treatment has become a major part of revascularization of iliac artery occlusive disease [19–21]. Among the various interventional devices, stent is main stay of treatment strategy. From TASCII A to TASCII C, the stent implantation is now the standard technique and shows reasonable good long-term outcome with low reinterventions rate. In TASCII D, the basic strategy is considered to be surgical approach. However, recent development of endovascular technique enabled endovascular first approach, and in experienced hands, fairly high success rate can be achieved.

The iliac stent choice can be largely categorized into choosing either a balloon expandable or self-expanding stent based on lesion characteristics. It depends on introducer size, access site, vessel tortuosity, and lesion location. However, we are using self-expandable stent in every iliac artery lesion. Newer-generation nitinol self-expanding stents exhibit minimal foreshortening and have a more predictable length with 12 mm in size by 6-Fr sheath.

In image size for iliac artery intervention, 20 cm size with DA image is preferred to 30 cm image because position adjustment and determination of stent size or length. In recanalization of aortoiliac occlusive lesion, measurement of pressure gradient across the lesion should be checked pre- and postprocedure. This hemodynamic assessment can be helpful to make the final decision to terminate the procedure even after angiographic moderate stenosis remained [22]. This section shows that typical TASCII A-C iliac artery lesion underwent endovascular therapy.

4.1. TASC II A lesion

Case 1: In **Figure 14A**, a typical lesion of the left CIA is presented. The DSA image (30 cm) of aortography with a 5-Fr pigtail catheter is taken from a 6-Fr sheath placed at the ipsilateral left CFA. Isolated severe stenosis with ulceration of the left CIA can be observed. For intervention of this lesion, a DA image by a contralateral right anterior oblique (RAO) view with a 20 cm image size is employed as the standard method (**Figure 14B**). Compared to a 30 cm image, more precise information on lesion characteristics can be obtained. After diagnostic angiography, the lesion was crossed by a 0.035-inch wire through a diagnostic pigtail catheter. After visual reference of the bony landmarks on the DA image, a self-expanding stent was implanted followed by postdilatation by balloon (**Figure 14C**). The final angiogram is shown in **Figure 14D**. To avoid vessel rupture and dissection, aggressive postdilatation is not recommended. We usually use a smaller balloon of up to 7 or 8 mm in diameter and inflation with lower pressure. When considering a balloon size of more than 8 mm for postdilatation, careful vessel size assessment is required.

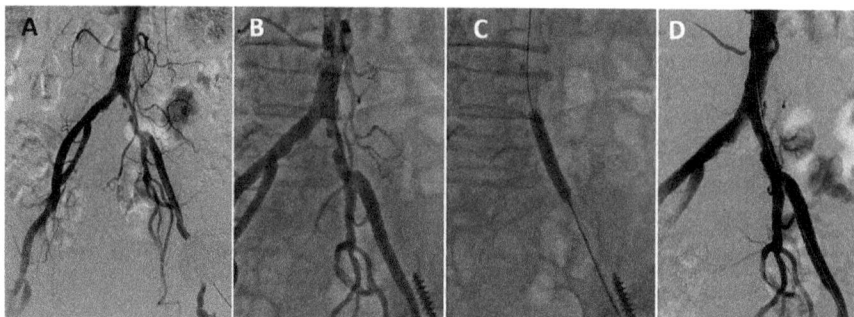

Figure 14. Left CIA stenosis classified as TASCII type A. (A) DSA image in 30 cm size of aortography in AP view shows unilateral left CIA stenosis. (B) DA in larger size (20 cm) and in contralateral oblique (RAO) view more clearly revealed lesion. (C) Stenting and ballooning are performed in reference to visual bony landmark. (D) Final angiogram shows complete recanalization.

Case 2: Aortography of a bilateral short EIA lesion is shown in **Figure 15A**. However, this 30 cm image size and AP projection failed to visualize the precise characteristics of each EIA lesion. The 20 cm size image with contralateral oblique angiography could identify the EIA lesions (**Figure 15B** and **C**). Endovascular intervention was performed by the right CFA approach. First, from the right CFA sheath, a 0.035-inch guidewire was used to cross the right EIA lesion followed by stenting and ballooning. After confirmation of a good expanded stent on the right EIA lesion, a crossover approach was introduced to treat the left EIA lesion. For the left EIA lesion, a RAO view is generally taken. This left lesion was also treated by stenting and ballooning (**Figure 15D** and **E**). These views could clearly visualize the lesion in high tortuosity in the EIA. Generally, a TASC II A lesion is treated from only one access site by employing a crossover approach. The advantage of this technique is that both the right and left lesions can be treated through a single-access site, minimizing access site complications.

4.2. TASC II B lesion

Case.3: EIA stenosis between 3 and 10 cm not extending into the CFA (TASC II B) could be treated by an endovascular technique (**Figure 16A**). In cases of EIA lesions, either an antegrade crossover approach or retrograde sheath approach is taken. Selecting the approach site depends on the distance from the lesion to the CFA and/or configuration of the terminal aorta when unable to use a crossover technique. When both approaches are not feasible, radial or brachial access is another option. The CFA is a so-called no stenting zone. To avoid CFA stenting, angiography should include the femoral head. Intervention should be performed based on the final control angiogram (**Figure 16B** and **C**). When we see the reference angiogram, the table should not be moved until stent expansion. The antegrade approach allows the stent to be placed more accurately close to the CFA as compared to the retrograde approach.

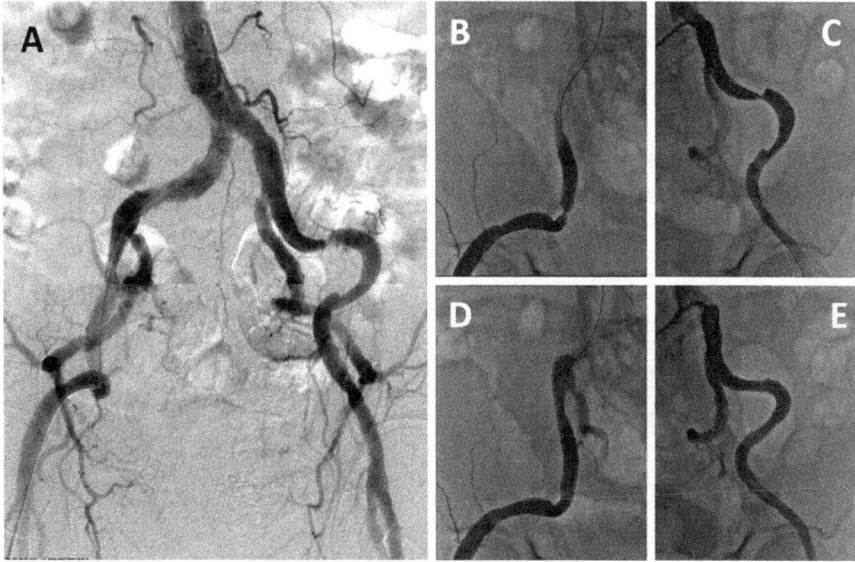

Figure 15. Bilateral short EIA lesion. (A) DSA in AP view could not reveal bilateral EIA stenosis due to severe iliac tortuosity. (B and C) Angiography in deep LAO (B) and RAO (C) can precisely reveal right EIA stenosis and left EIA stenosis, respectively. (D and E) Both lesions can be treated with stent placement using crossover technique from one access site.

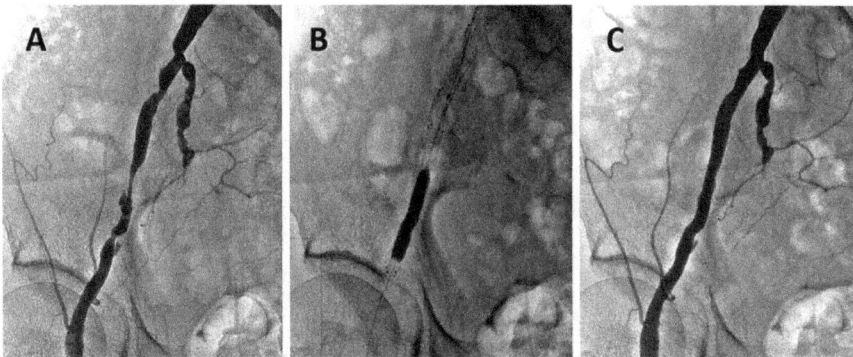

Figure 16. Multiple EIA lesions treated without changing the working view. In the crossover approach from the left CFA, angiography shows multiple stenotic lesions of the right EIA not extending to the right CFA (A). Keeping working view including the femoral head, the stent position is carefully determined so as not to implant in "no stenting zone" (B). Final result also confirmed with this view (C).

Case 4: Unilateral CIA occlusion is classified as TASC II B (**Figure 17A**). This aortography is performed from the left brachial artery and shows occlusion of the left CIA orifice. Seemingly, the total occluded part looks quite long; however, delayed-phase angiography revealed a patent external iliac artery, and only occlusion of the CIA was found (**Figure 17B**). Viewing up to the delayed phase, in particular for total occlusion, is very important to identify the actual occluded segment. The ipsilateral left CFA was punctured by echo guidance, and a 6-Fr sheath was positioned. Angiography by a 20 cm image was performed by simultaneous injection from the terminal aortography with hand injection from the left CFA sheath, more clearly revealing an image of the target lesion (**Figure 17C**). From the left CFA sheath, a 0.035-inch wire with a 5-Fr multipurpose catheter is carefully advanced with the knuckle wire technique (**Figure 17D**). After crossing the CTO lesion, a self-expandable stent was implanted, followed by postdilatation at low pressure with the same size balloon as predilatation. The final angiogram from the terminal aorta shows successful and complete recanalization of the total occlusion of the CIA (**Figure 17E**). Finally, we checked the pressure gradient between the left CFA and aorta. No pressure gradient was found across the stented segments.

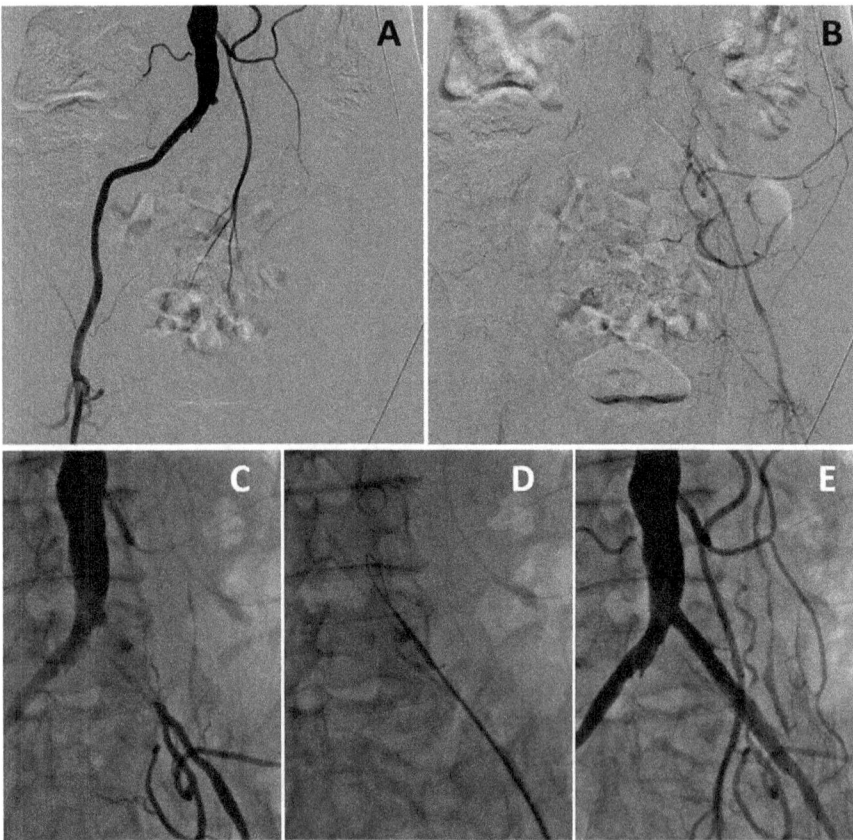

Figure 17. Left CIA occlusion. (A) Unilateral CIA occlusion is clearly found in angiogram from upper limb access. (B) Delayed phase of this angiogram reveals patent EIA supplied from collateral vessels. (C) DA (20 cm) performed by simultaneous injection from terminal aorta, while left CIA sheath reveals more precise lesion characteristics. (D) From left CFA sheath, 0.018-inch wire by knuckle wire technique supported with 5-Fr multipurpose catheter successfully used to pass the lesion. (E) Final angiography from terminal aorta shows successful recanalization.

4.3. TASC II C lesion

Case 5: Long total occlusion of the EIA with CFA involvement is classified as TASC II C which is relatively safe and can be effectively treated with endovascular therapy. For successful recanalization, angiographic work plays a crucial role. The first image to understand is the whole view of both iliac arteries with a 30 cm DSA image (**Figure 18**).

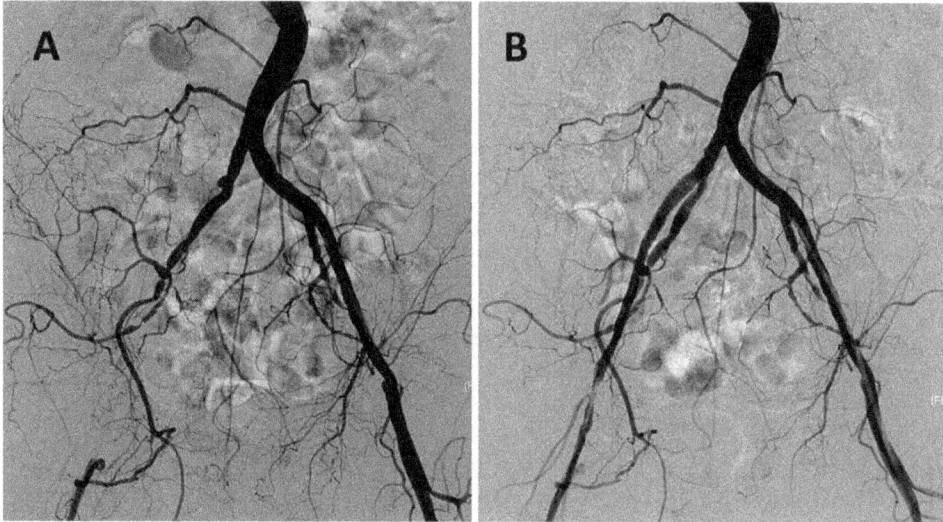

Figure 18. Long total occlusion of right EIA with involvement of CFA. (A) 30 cm DSA shows long EIA occlusion with involvement of CFA. (B) Complete recanalization is shown compared to initial diagnostic angiography.

In the delayed phase, the left CFA is visualized. After confirmation of an occluded EIA, the 20 cm contralateral DA image was positioned for working view. A 20 cm DA image in a contralateral left anterior oblique (LAO) view is actually used for interventions (**Figure 19**).

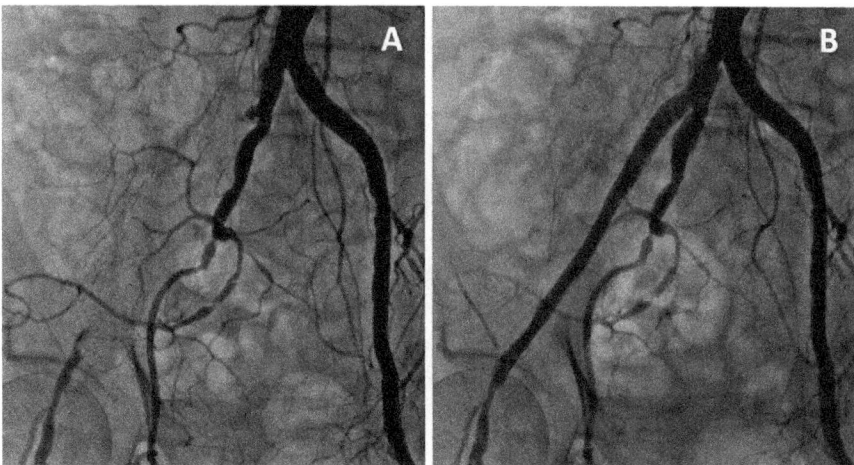

Figure 19. EVT for long total occlusion of right EIA with involvement of CFA. (A) 20 cm DA image in contralateral LAO view is actually used for interventions. (B) Final angiography is taken in working view.

For the bidirectional approach, an ipsilateral CFA puncture is performed under angiographic guidance where the 6-Fr sheath is placed (**Figure 20A**). From the crossover sheath, a 0.035-inch J-tip wire supported with a 5-Fr diagnostic catheter is advanced by antegrade access with the knuckle wire technique through the lesion (**Figure 20B**). Generally speaking, a bidirectional approach has a higher chance of wire crossing than a one way approach. When the antegrade wire fails to cross the lesion, retrograde wiring is the next step. After successfully crossing the occlusion, the wire position should constantly be monitored to see that it is in the distal true lumen. Predilatation should be performed by an undersized balloon, and a self-expandable stent should be placed. Careful attention is necessary to confirm that the distal stent does not extend to the CFA (**Figure 20C**). Adjunctive postdilatation by balloon at lower pressure was performed and the completion of angiography achieved.

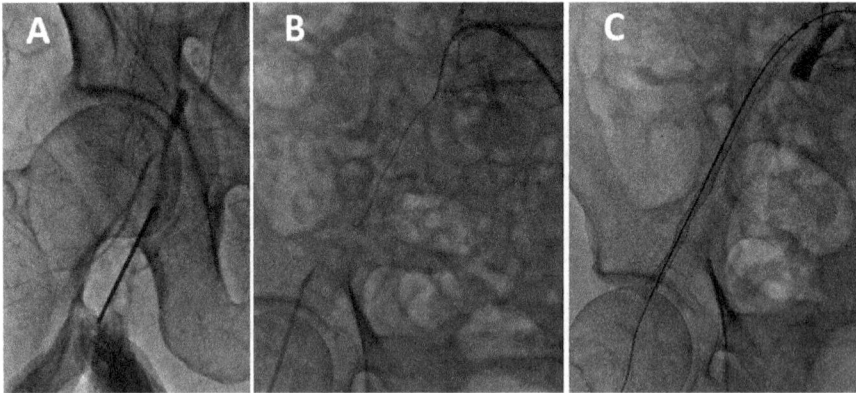

Figure 20. Long total occlusion of right EIA with involvement of CFA. (A) Ipsilateral CFA puncture is performed under angiographic guidance for bidirectional approach. (B) 0.035-inch J-tip wire supported with 5-Fr diagnostic catheter advanced with knuckle wire technique from the crossover sheath. (C) Self-expanded stent is carefully implanted not to cover the CFA.

5. Approach to complex iliac artery disease

Advanced atherosclerotic disease of the iliac artery oftentimes involves an abdominal aortic aneurysm or extensive aortic bifurcation with or without unilateral or bilateral long total occlusions of the iliac artery. Most cases are classified as TASC II D, and in some cases, no TASC classification can be applied. Moreover, patients with these complex iliac artery diseases are commonly not candidates for surgical revascularization due to comorbidities. These patients benefit by an endovascular approach by employing various tools or angiographic techniques. In some medical centers, endovascular therapy for TASC II D is considered to be first line revascularization with safe and effective treatment by experienced interventionists [23–25]. When total occlusion is involved, aortography should be performed up to the delayed phase in which the distal patent flow could be visualized through the collateral flow (**Figure 21**). Additionally, angiography taken from multiple angles is important to navigate the guidewire correctly.

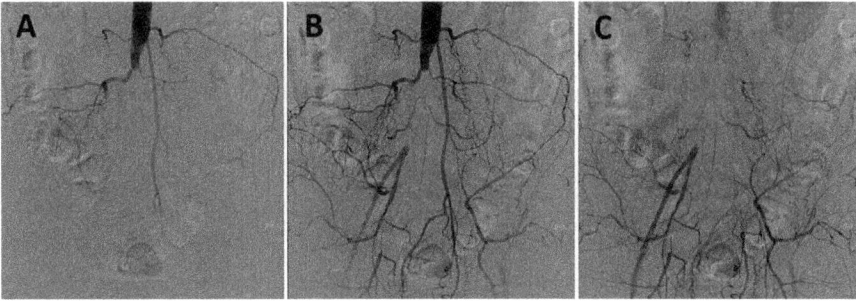

Figure 21. Aortography of aortic occlusion in the early phase (A), middle phase (B), and delayed phase (C), which can visualize distal arterial flow via collateral vessels.

Case 6: This patient has right EIA occlusion and left severe EIA stenosis. Both the right EIA occlusion and left EIA stenosis could be treated with a contralateral crossover technique from left CFA access. Both EIA lesions were successfully treated by only the left anterior oblique (LAO) projection as the working image. First, aortography revealed right EIA total occlusion and left EIA stenosis (**Figure 22A**). In the delayed phase, the right CFA is slightly visible (**Figure 22B**). **Figure 22C** is the angiogram for simultaneous injection from the terminal aorta and right CFA sheath in the LAO projection. In this image, the occluded lesion can be visualized precisely. From the left CFA, a 6-Fr crossover sheath is advanced to the right CIA after a 0.035-inch J-tip Radifocus wire is used to cross the right internal iliac artery. The 0.035-inch J-tip wire with a 4-Fr support catheter could cross the occluded EIA to the right superficial femoral artery (SFA) (**Figure 22D**). Predilatation by a balloon was performed followed by the implantation of a self-expandable stent (**Figure 22E**). Postdilatation was performed by the same balloon and successful recanalization was confirmed by angiography from the crossover sheath. After opening the occluded right EIA, stenting and ballooning were performed for the left EIA stenosis (**Figure 22F**) and the final angiogram showed complete revascularization of both EIA lesions (**Figure 22G**).

Case 7: In **Figure 23A**, aortography shows an infra-renal aortic aneurysm, heavily calcified stenosis of the right CIA, and moderate stenosis of the left CIA. From the right CFA, a 0.035-inch J-tip wire was advanced, however, this wire could not cross the right CIA stenosis and was exchanged to a 0.014-inch wire. This 0.014-inch wire succeeded in crossing the lesion. The 4-Fr diagnostic catheter was gently advanced through the aneurysm, and the 0.014-inch wire was then exchanged to a 0.035-inch spring wire. After predilatation by a balloon at the right CIA, kissing stenting with a self-expandable stent was performed (**Figure 23B** and **C**). The final angiography in 20 cm DSA shows excellent results (**Figure 23D**) and pressures at both CFA sheaths showed equalized systemic arterial pressure.

Case 8: Extensive heavily calcified stenosis from the aortic bifurcation to both iliac arteries is treated by endovascular techniques (**Figure 24**). In a heavily calcified lesion, 3D CTA is not suited for diagnosis of the stenosis (**Figure 24D**).

Compared to angiography, these 3D CTA images are completely different. Patients with heavily calcified lesions are at high risk for open surgical treatment, especially those on hemodialysis, and endovascular reconstruction is often required. In this case, an upper limb approach is not available due to the AV shunt and left CFA access is unfeasible because of a pulseless or indeterminable blood flow by ultrasound. Viewing the angiography from the right CFA sheath, left CFA access could be obtained. Wire crossing by a retrograde approach from the right CFA sheath was successful but failed from the left side due to heavily calcified stenosis of the left CIA (**Figure 25A**). Using a snare device to pull the wire into the left sheath, a microcatheter was advanced to the abdominal aorta (**Figure 25B**). Kissing stenting and mild postdilatation was performed, and an adjunctive overlap stent in both iliac arteries was placed (**Figure 25C and D**). Successful recanalization is confirmed in **Figure 25E**.

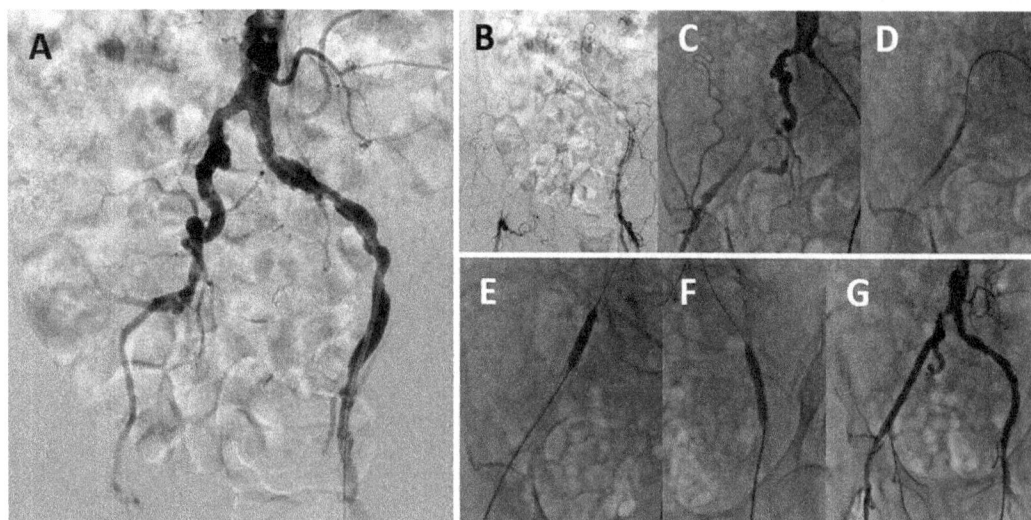

Figure 22. Right EIA occlusion with diffuse stenosis from right CIA to EIA. (A) Initial diagnostic DSA reveals right EIA total occlusion and multiple stenosis from left CIA to EIA. (B) In delayed phase, right CFA is slightly visible. (C) Simultaneous angiography from terminal aorta and right CFA sheath in deeper LAO view used for intervention, clearly revealing lesion morphology. (D) 0.018-inch wire with 4-Fr support catheter could cross the occluded EIA. (E) Stenting for distal EIA is performed from crossover sheath and, for proximal CIA, stenting is performed from retrograde ipsilateral CFA sheath. (F) After treatment for right iliac lesion, left side lesions are treated with stenting and ballooning. (G) Final angiogram shows complete revascularization of both CIA and EIA.

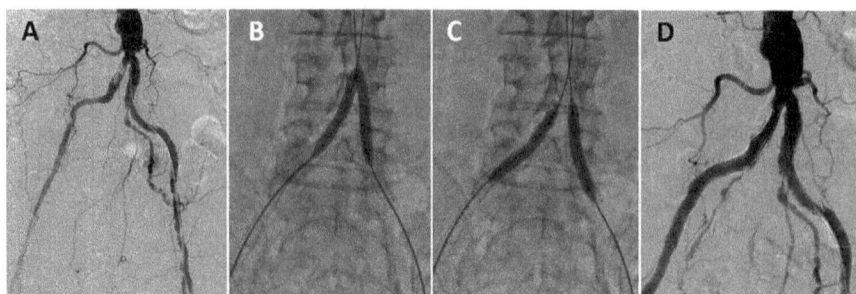

Figure 23. CIA stenosis with severe calcification and abdominal aortic aneurysm. (A) Aortography shows infra-renal aortic aneurysm, heavily calcified stenosis of right CIA, and moderate stenosis of left CIA. (B and C) Kissing stenting at aortic bifurcation (B) and postdilatation of both CIA (C) are carefully performed due to heavily calcified lesion. (D) Final angiography taken in DSA and 20 cm image shows good expansion and no complications such as rupture, dissection, or embolism.

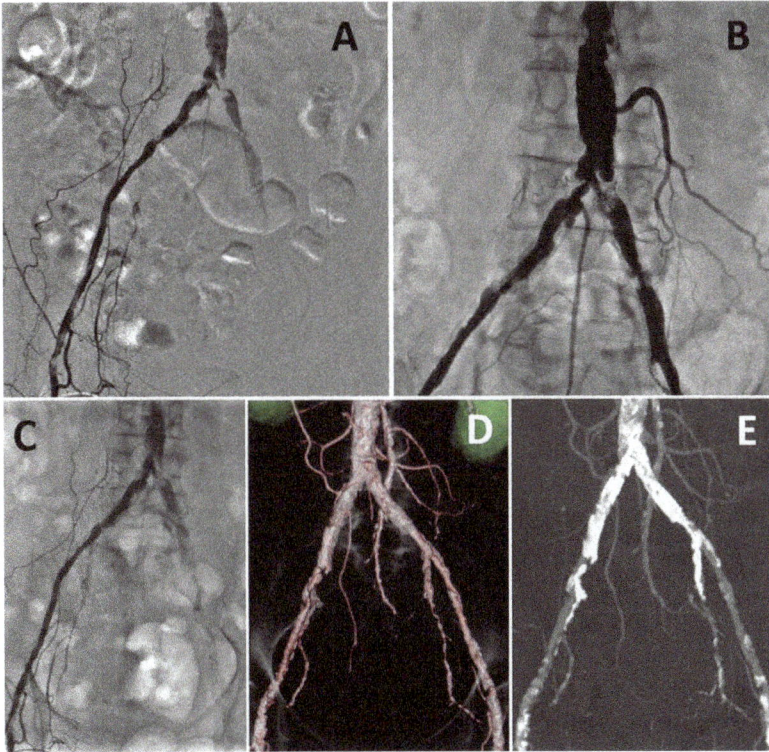

Figure 24. Heavily calcified aortic bifurcation disease involving orifices of bilateral CIA. (A) Extensive heavily calcified stenosis from aortic bifurcation to both CIAs is shown in 30 cm DSA. (B) More precise information of lesion can be obtained from 20 cm DA. (C–E) In case with severe calcification, CT angiogram is not suited as diagnostic or assessment tool since details of intravascular conditions due to calcification not visualized.

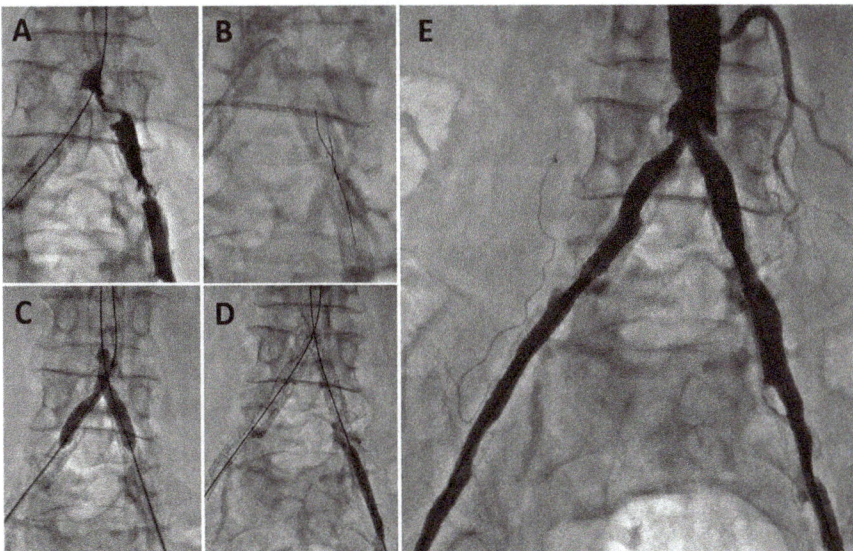

Figure 25. Heavily calcified aortic bifurcation disease involving orifices of bilateral CIA. (A) Wire crossing by retrograde from right CFA sheath is successful but due to heavily calcified stenosis of left CIA, unable to cross the wire. (B) Snare device pulls the wire from right iliac artery into the left CFA sheath. (C) Kissing stenting and mild postdilatation are performed at aortic bifurcation. (D) Adjunctive overlapping stents placed in both iliac arteries. (E) Successful recanalization is clearly visualized in final angiography.

6. Complications related to aortoiliac artery intervention

Complications in iliac artery intervention, especially bleeding due to perforation, are the most serious. Iliac artery perforation immediately causes hemorrhagic shock which may result in cardiac arrest. The iliac artery runs in the posterior abdominal cavity, and therefore, bleeding cannot be controlled with manual compression to establish hemostasis. Too much time is required to convert to open surgical repair so this is not a practical solution. Immediate endovascular repair should be attempted, and a covered stent should be positioned at the perforation site [26].

Wire perforation of the EIA is shown in **Figure 26A**. From another angle, the perforation site could not be detected (**Figure 26B**). Extravasation is clearly visualized in DSA. When suspecting perforation, DSA should be taken in several projections. The covered stent should be prepared at the same time as balloon inflation is being carried out to minimize bleeding (**Figure 26C**). After implantation of the covered stent, extravasation is not seen and complete shielding has succeeded (**Figure 26D**). To repair a perforation, aneurysm, or the other vessel injury, the covered stent is the most useful device and should be prepared along with the appropriate catheter.

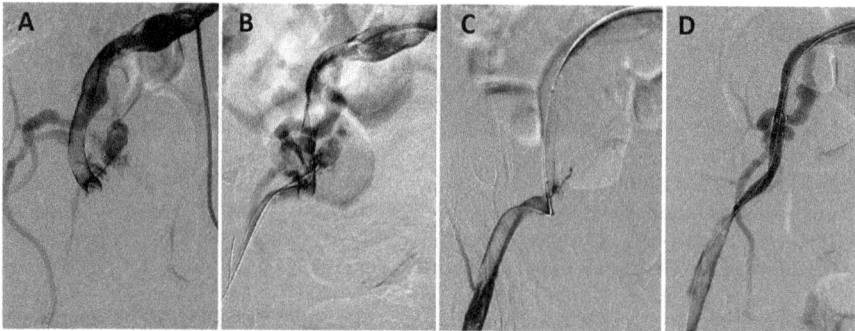

Figure 26. Wire perforation and extravasation. (A) Wire perforation of EIA is clearly detected in DSA. (B) In another angle view, perforation site could not be detected. (C) Balloon inflation can minimize bleeding. (D) After implantation of covered stent, extravasation is not seen in DSA.

Dissection caused by intervention may cause acute occlusion or stop the flow to the distal vessel. In **Figure 27A**, the large dissection is caused by sheath placement due to a tortuous external iliac artery. This dissection was successfully wired to the true lumen and treated by self-expandable stent placement (**Figure 27B**). The dissection could be commonly repaired by a self-expandable stent to support the dissected flap to the vessel wall. After crossing the true lumen, we preferred a 0.014-inch wire since it is more atraumatic compared to a 0.035-inch wire.

In dealing with an aortoiliac artery bifurcation lesion with either ballooning or stenting, the potential complication is plaque shift. Therefore, a kissing stent or balloon technique has been widely employed. **Figure 28A** and **B** is typical images of plaque shift at the aortoiliac bifurcation. A large plaque shifted to the contralateral iliac artery where acute occlusion may cause acute limb ischemia on the contralateral limb. Therefore, precise information on the aortoiliac bifurcation lesion is essential, especially on the inward position of the plaque and/or large plaque burden by various different angled views before interventions.

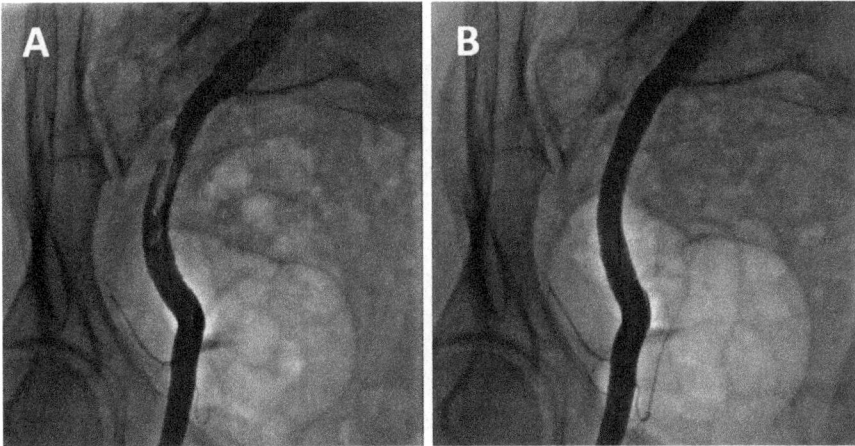

Figure 27. The large dissection caused by sheath. (A) Large dissection by sheath with flap is found in DA. (B) Complete repair is achieved with stent implantation.

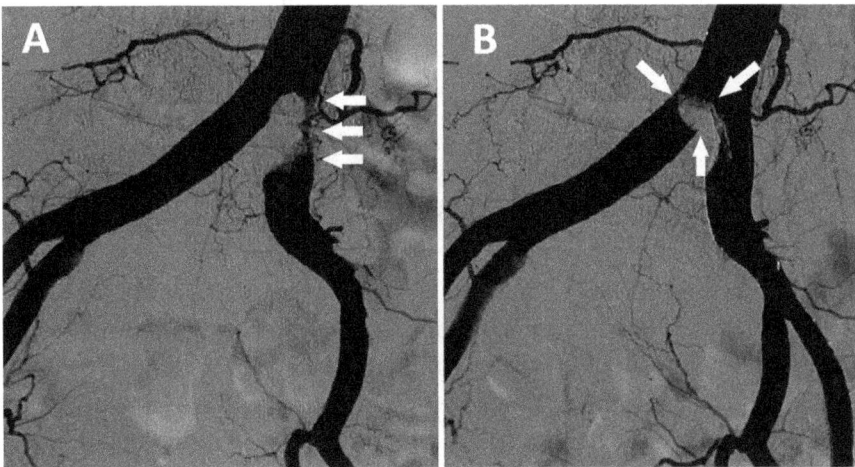

Figure 28. Unfavorable plaque shift. Right CIA stenosis with large burden of plaque (A; white arrow) is shifted to contralateral left CIA (B; white arrow) after ballooning (Special Courtesy by Dr. Yoshito Kadoya).

Recently, transcatheter aortic valve replacement (TAVR) has emerged as a promising procedure, and a transfemoral approach is the standard technique. However, vascular complications, in particular iliac artery injury, are the major clinical problem [27]. A large profile sheath in TAVR often injures the iliac artery. The DSA image clearly visualizes the injured EIA (**Figure 29A**). This complication can immediately cause catastrophic bleeding and shock. In this case, a 0.035-inch wire is carefully advanced from the ipsilateral CFA sheath for TAVR and successfully used to cross the ruptured site of the EIA followed by deployment of a covered stent (**Figure 29B**). Complete and successful repair could be achieved. The final angiogram by DSA showed no extravasation and established a TIMI 3 flow (**Figure 29C**).

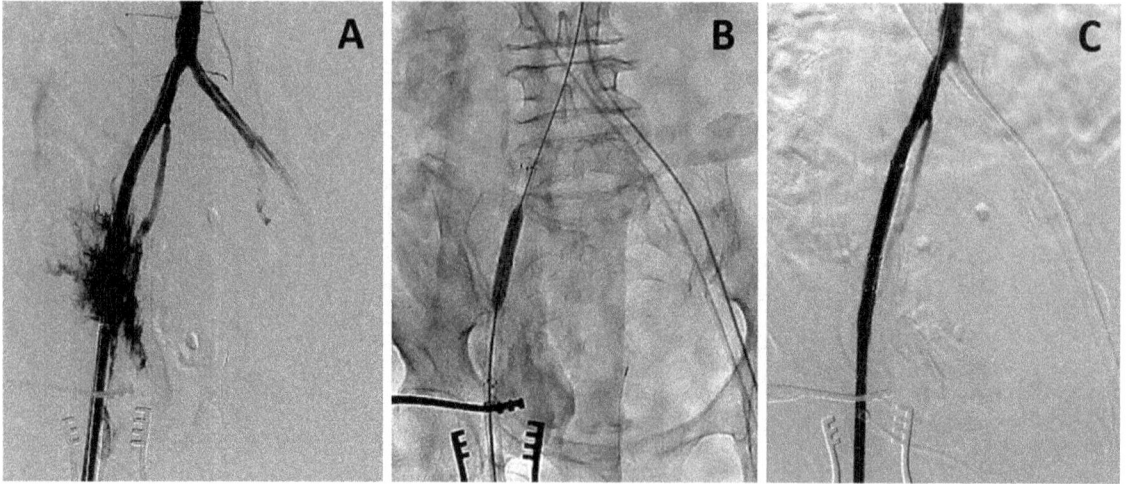

Figure 29. Ruptured EIA in TAVR. (A) DSA image can clearly visualize the ruptured EIA caused by large profile sheath for TAVR. (B) 0.035-inch wire was carefully advanced from ipsilateral sheath for TAVR and successfully crossed the ruptured site of EIA followed by deployment covered stent. (C) Successful endovascular repair is completely achieved. The final angiogram by DSA showed no extravasation and established TIMI 3 flow.

7. Conclusion

No randomized controlled trials (RCTs) have definitively established the magnitude and durability of the benefit of open surgical vs endovascular strategies. However, there has been an increase in the adoption of the endovascular first strategy for even the most complex anatomies up to TASC ll D in clinical practice. In aortoiliac artery disease, a 12-month primary patency for TASC D lesions treated with stents was considered to be fairly high. Therefore, the trend for the "endovascular first" approach will not change in addition to patient preference. And more complex TASC C-D aortoiliac lesions will be treated by stent. To succeed in treating complex lesions, careful angiographic assessment is of vital importance and unless a clear image of the lesion is not obtained, complex aortoiliac artery lesions cannot be revascularized, resulting in high complication rates.

Author details

Keisuke Fukuda

Address all correspondence to: fukudateam54@gmail.com

Kishiwada Tokushukai Hospital, Osaka, Japan

References

[1] Aboyans V, Desormais I, Lacroix P, Salazar J, Criqui MH, Laskar M. The general prognosis of patients with peripheral arterial disease differs according to the disease localization. *J Am Coll Cardiol*. 2010;55:898–903.

[2]   Kashyap VS, Pavkov ML, Bena JF, et al. The management of severe aortoiliac occlusive disease: endovascular therapy rivals open reconstruction. *J Vasc Surg*. 2008;48:1451–1457, 1457.e1–e3.

[3]   Indes JE, Mandawat A, Tuggle CT, Muhs B, Sosa JA. Endovascular procedures for aorto-iliac occlusive disease are associated with superior short-term clinical and economic outcomes compared with open surgery in the inpatient population. *J Vasc Surg*. 2010;52:1173–1179.

[4]   Norgren L, Hiatt WR, Dormandy JA, Nehler MR, Harris KA, Fowkes FG; TASC II Working Group. Inter-Society Consensus for the Management of Peripheral Arterial Disease (TASC II). *J Vasc Surg*. 2007;45 Suppl S:S5–67

[5]   Staniloae CS, Korabathina R, Coppola JT. Transradial access for peripheral vascular interventions. *Catheter Cardiovasc Interv*. 2013;81(7):1194–203

[6]   Stavroulakis K, Usai MV, Torsello G, Schwindt A, Stachmann A, Beropoulis E, Bisdas T. Efficacy and safety of transbrachial access for iliac endovascular interventions. *J Endovasc Ther*. 2016;23(3):454–60

[7]   Millon A, Della Schiava N, Brizzi V, Arsicot M, Boudjelit T, Herail J, Feugier P, Lermusiaux P. The antegrade approach using transbrachial access improves technical success rate of endovascular recanalization of TASC C-D aortoiliac occlusion in case of failed femoral access. *Ann Vasc Surg*. 2015;29(7):1346–52

[8]   Grenon SM1, Reilly LM, Ramaiah VG. Technical endovascular highlights for crossing the difficult aortic bifurcation. *J Vasc Surg*. 2011;54(3):893–6.

[9]   Jongkind V1, Akkersdijk GJ, Yeung KK, Wisselink W. A systematic review of endovascular treatment of extensive aortoiliac occlusive disease. *J Vasc Surg*. 2010;52(5):1376–83.

[10] Leville CD1, Kashyap VS, Clair DG, Bena JF, Lyden SP, Greenberg RK, O'Hara PJ, Sarac TP, Ouriel K. Endovascular management of iliac artery occlusions: extending treatment to TransAtlantic Inter-Society Consensus class C and D patients. *J Vasc Surg*. 2006;43(1):32–9.

[11] Sixt S1, Krankenberg H, Möhrle C, Kaspar M, Tübler T, Rastan A, Brechtel K, Macharzina R, Neumann FJ, Zeller T. Endovascular treatment for extensive aortoiliac artery reconstruction: a single-center experience based on 1712 interventions. *J Endovasc Ther*. 2013;20(1):64–73

[12] Haulon S, Mounier-Véhier C, Gaxotte V, Koussa M, Lions C, Haouari BA, Beregi JP. Percutaneous reconstruction of the aortoiliac bifurcation with the "kissing stents" technique: long-term follow-up in 106 patients. *J Endovasc Ther*. 2002;9(3):363–8.

[13] Simons PC, Nawijn AA, Bruijninckx CM, Knippenberg B, de Vries EH, van Overhagen H. Long-term results of primary stent placement to treat infrarenal aortic stenosis. *Eur J Vasc Endovasc Surg*. 2006;(6):627–33.

[14] Klonaris C, Katsargyris A, Tsekouras N, Alexandrou A, Giannopoulos A, Bastounis E. Primary stenting for aortic lesions: from single stenoses to total aortoiliac occlusions. *J Vasc Surg*. 2008;47(2):310–7.

[15] lvarez-Tostado JA, Clair DG, Greenberg RK, Lyden SP, Srivastava SD, Eagleton M, Sarac TS, Kashyap VS, Moise MA. Endovascular management of chronic infrarenal aortic occlusion. *J Endovasc Ther*. 2009;16(1):84–928.

[16] Kim TH, Ko YG, Kim U, Kim JS, Choi D, Hong MK, Jang Y, Shim WH. Outcomes of endovascular treatment of chronic total occlusion of the infrarenal aorta. *J Vasc Surg*. 2011;53(6):1542–9.

[17] Lun Y, Zhang J, Wu X, Gang Q, Shen S, Jiang H, Duan Z, Xin S. Comparison of midterm outcomes between surgical treatment and endovascular reconstruction for chronic infrarenal aortoiliac occlusion. *J Vasc Interv Radiol*. 2015;26(2):196–204.

[18] Setacci C, Galzerano G, Setacci F, De Donato G, Sirignano P, Kamargianni V, Cannizzaro A, Cappelli A. Endovascular approach to Leriche syndrome. *J Cardiovasc Surg* (Torino). 2012;53(3):301–6.

[19] Aihara H, Soga Y, Iida O, Suzuki K, Tazaki J, Shintani Y, Miyashita Y; REAL-AI Registry Investigators. Long-term outcomes of endovascular therapy for aortoiliac bifurcation lesions in the real-AI registry. *J Endovasc Ther*. 2014;21(1):25–33.

[20] Kasemi H, Marino M, Dionisi CP, Di Angelo CL, Fadda GF. Seven-year approach evolution of the aortoiliac occlusive disease endovascular treatment. *Ann Vasc Surg*. 2016;30:277–85.

[21] Rossi M, Iezzi R. Cardiovascular and Interventional Radiological Society of Europe guidelines on endovascular treatment in aortoiliac arterial disease. *Cardiovasc Intervent Radiol*. 2014;37(1):13–25.

[22] Udoff EJ, Barth KH, Harrington DP, Kaufman SL, White RI. Hemodynamic significance of iliac artery stenosis: pressure measurements during angiography. *Radiology*. 1979;132(2):289–93.

[23] Ye W, Liu CW, Ricco JB, Mani K, Zeng R, Jiang J. Early and late outcomes of percutaneous treatment of TransAtlantic Inter-Society Consensus class C and D aorto-iliac lesions. *J Vasc Surg*. 2011;53(6):1728–37.

[24] Wressnegger A, Kinstner C, Funovics M. Treatment of the aorto-iliac segment in complex lower extremity arterial occlusive disease. *J Cardiovasc Surg* (Torino). 2015;56(1):73–9.

[25] Klein AJ, Feldman DN, Aronow HD, Gray BH, Gupta K, Gigliotti OS, Jaff MR, Bersin RM, White CJ; Peripheral vascular disease committee for the society for cardiovascular angiography and interventions. SCAI expert consensus statement for aorto-iliac arterial intervention appropriate use. *Catheter Cardiovasc Interv*. 2014;84(4):520–8.

[26] Kufner S, Cassese S, Groha P, Byrne RA, Schunkert H, Kastrati A, Ott I, Fusaro M. Covered stents for endovascular repair of iatrogenic injuries of iliac and femoral arteries. *Cardiovasc Revasc Med*. 2015;16(3):156–62.

[27] Toggweiler S, Leipsic J, Binder RK, Freeman M, Barbanti M, Heijmen RH, Wood DA, Webb JG. Management of vascular access in transcatheter aortic valve replacement: part 2: vascular complications. *JACC Cardiovasc Interv*. 2013;6(8):767–76.

Permissions

All chapters in this book were first published in PAD&AETPAD, by InTech Open; hereby published with permission under the Creative Commons Attribution License or equivalent. Every chapter published in this book has been scrutinized by our experts. Their significance has been extensively debated. The topics covered herein carry significant findings which will fuel the growth of the discipline. They may even be implemented as practical applications or may be referred to as a beginning point for another development.

The contributors of this book come from diverse backgrounds, making this book a truly international effort. This book will bring forth new frontiers with its revolutionizing research information and detailed analysis of the nascent developments around the world.

We would like to thank all the contributing authors for lending their expertise to make the book truly unique. They have played a crucial role in the development of this book. Without their invaluable contributions this book wouldn't have been possible. They have made vital efforts to compile up to date information on the varied aspects of this subject to make this book a valuable addition to the collection of many professionals and students.

This book was conceptualized with the vision of imparting up-to-date information and advanced data in this field. To ensure the same, a matchless editorial board was set up. Every individual on the board went through rigorous rounds of assessment to prove their worth. After which they invested a large part of their time researching and compiling the most relevant data for our readers.

The editorial board has been involved in producing this book since its inception. They have spent rigorous hours researching and exploring the diverse topics which have resulted in the successful publishing of this book. They have passed on their knowledge of decades through this book. To expedite this challenging task, the publisher supported the team at every step. A small team of assistant editors was also appointed to further simplify the editing procedure and attain best results for the readers.

Apart from the editorial board, the designing team has also invested a significant amount of their time in understanding the subject and creating the most relevant covers. They scrutinized every image to scout for the most suitable representation of the subject and create an appropriate cover for the book.

The publishing team has been an ardent support to the editorial, designing and production team. Their endless efforts to recruit the best for this project, has resulted in the accomplishment of this book. They are a veteran in the field of academics and their pool of knowledge is as vast as their experience in printing. Their expertise and guidance has proved useful at every step. Their uncompromising quality standards have made this book an exceptional effort. Their encouragement from time to time has been an inspiration for everyone.

The publisher and the editorial board hope that this book will prove to be a valuable piece of knowledge for researchers, students, practitioners and scholars across the globe.

List of Contributors

Mei-Ling Sharon Tai, Julia Sien Yuin Liew, Sheun Yu Mo and Mohamed Abdusalam Elwaifa
Division of Neurology, Department of Medicine, Faculty of Medicine, University of Malaya, Malaysia

Yoshiaki Yokoi
Kishiwada Tokushukai Hospital, Osaka, Japan

Amir-Houshang Shemirani and Katalin Szilvia Zsóri
Faculty of Medicine, Clinical Laboratory Research Division, Laboratory Medicine, University of Debrecen, Debrecen, Hungary

András Jávor
Debrecen University, Debrecen, Hungary

Zoltán Csiki
Faculty of Medicine, Institute of Internal Medicine, University of Debrecen, Debrecen, Hungary

Osami Kawarada
Department of Cardiovascular Medicine, National Cerebral and Cardiovascular Center, Osaka, Japan

Omer Tanyeli
Department of Cardiovascular Surgery, Meram Medicine Faculty, Necmettin Erbakan University, Konya, Turkey

Akihiro Higashimori
Kishiwada Tokushukai Hospital, Osaka, Japan

Mirela-Anca Stoia, Mihaela Mocan, Cerasela Mihaela Goidescu, Diana Larisa Hognogi Mocan and Roxana Chiorescu
Department of Cardiology, County Clinical Emergency Hospital, University of Medicine and Pharmacy "Iuliu Hatieganu", Cluj-Napoca, Romania

Masahiko Fujihara
Kishiwada Tokushukai Hospital, Osaka, Japan

Keisuke Fukuda
Kishiwada Tokushukai Hospital, Osaka, Japan

Index

www.ingramcontent.com/pod-product-compliance
Lightning Source LLC
Chambersburg PA
CBHW061952190326
41458CB00009B/2853